T0323687

Advance Praise for *Atlas of EEG, Seizure Semiology, and Management*

"The *Atlas of EEG, Seizure Semiology, and Management* is a tour de force, integrating the essential features of normal and abnormal EEGs and how these relate to understanding seizures and diagnosing and treating the diverse epilepsy syndromes that neurologists and epileptologists are confronted with. This Atlas will help both the novice and the expert to better integrate neurophysiology, clinical observations, and patient care."

—Orrin Devinsky, MD, Professor of Neurology and Neuroscience,
NYU Grossman School of Medicine

"This is an excellent and detailed book that includes basic principles of electronics and electrophysiology, as well as the origins of EEG activity with a description of the role in EEG and diagnosis and management. The book includes definitions and classifications of epilepsies and has over 500 images, particularly of basics of electrophysiology as well as EEG patterns and excellent examples of EEG tracings. The book also includes a nice, concise overview of the various anti-epileptic drugs, their mechanism of action, indications, and side effects, and has excellent tables. This book is very well written, detailed, and provides a very good source of information as well as a review for those interested in clinical neurophysiology and epilepsy."

—Tulio E. Bertorini, MD, Professor of Neurology,
Director of Clinical Neurophysiology Fellowship,
University of Tennessee Health Science Center

THIRD EDITION

ATLAS OF EEG, SEIZURE SEMIOLOGY, AND MANAGEMENT

KARL E. MISULIS, MD, PHD, FAAN
Professor of Clinical Neurology
Professor of Clinical Biomedical Informatics
Division Chief, Inpatient General Neurology
Director, Neurology Hospitalist Service
Vanderbilt University Medical Center
Nashville, Tennessee, USA

HASAN H. SONMEZTURK, MD
Associate Professor of Neurology
Program Director Epilepsy Fellowship
Program Director Clinical Neurophysiology Fellowship
Medical Director Neurological ICU CEEG Monitoring Service
Medical Director Intraoperative Neuromonitoring Service
Vanderbilt University Medical Center
Nashville, Tennessee, USA

KEVIN C. ESS, MD, PHD, FAAN, FANA
Gerald M. Fenichel Chair in Neurology
Division Chief, Pediatric Neurology
Divisions of Pediatric Neurology and Epilepsy
Departments of Pediatrics, Neurology, Cell & Developmental Biology
Vanderbilt University Medical Center
Nashville, Tennessee, USA

BASSEL ABOU-KHALIL, MD
Professor of Neurology
Vanderbilt University School of Medicine & Division Chief, Epilepsy
Vanderbilt University Medical Center
Nashville, Tennessee, USA

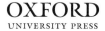

OXFORD
UNIVERSITY PRESS

OXFORD
UNIVERSITY PRESS

Oxford University Press is a department of the University of Oxford. It furthers
the University's objective of excellence in research, scholarship, and education
by publishing worldwide. Oxford is a registered trade mark of Oxford University
Press in the UK and certain other countries.

Published in the United States of America by Oxford University Press
198 Madison Avenue, New York, NY 10016, United States of America.

Library of Congress Cataloging-in-Publication Data
Names: Misulis, Karl E., author. | Sonmezturk, Hasan H., author. | Ess, Kevin C., author. |
Abou-Khalil, Bassel, author.
Title: Atlas of EEG, seizure semiology, and management / Karl E. Misulis, Hasan H. Sonmezturk,
Kevin C. Ess, Bassel Abou-Khalil.
Description: Third edition. | New York, NY : Oxford University Press, [2022] |
Includes bibliographical references and index.
Identifiers: LCCN 2021047423 (print) | LCCN 2021047424 (ebook) |
ISBN 9780197543023 (hardback) | ISBN 9780197543047 (epub) |
ISBN 9780197543054 (online) Subjects: MESH: Electroencephalography—methods |
Seizures—diagnosis | Seizures—therapy | Atlas
Classification: LCC RC386.6.E43 (print) |
LCC RC386.6.E43 (ebook) | NLM WL 17 |
DDC 616.8/047547—dc23
LC record available at https://lccn.loc.gov/2021047423
LC ebook record available at https://lccn.loc.gov/2021047424

DOI: 10.1093/med/9780197543023.001.0001

9 8 7 6 5 4 3 2 1

Printed by Integrated Books International, United States of America

CONTENTS

PART 1

Introduction to EEG

1.1

Overview of Seizures and Epilepsy

KARL E. MISULIS

Electroencephalography (EEG) is an invaluable tool for evaluating patients with suspected seizures or encephalopathy, yet EEG is only one source of data so information from this technology must be integrated with knowledge of basic science and clinical neurology.

This work has a principal focus on EEG, but interleaves that discussion with information on seizures, epilepsy, encephalopathy, and other neurologic conditions for which EEG can be a useful diagnostic tool.

SEIZURES AND EPILEPSY

Here we discuss some of the important terms used in the definition and classification of seizures and epilepsies. Extensive detail is presented in Part 3, "Seizure Semiology and Classification" and Part 4, "Epilepsy Classification and Epileptic Syndromes."

A foundational distinction is between the terms "seizure" and "epilepsy." A *seizure* is defined by Robert Fisher as "a transient occurrence of signs and/or symptoms due to abnormal excessive or synchronous neuronal activity in the brain,"[1] whereas *epilepsy* is a disorder in which the patient has recurrent unprovoked seizures. This definition is the reason that we do not use the term *psychogenic nonepileptic seizure*; since events of this type were not seizures, there is no specific neuronal activity, hence it is a *psychogenic nonepileptic event* (PNE).

In 2014, the definition of epilepsy was revised by Fisher and the International League Against Epilepsy (ILAE) as follows[2]:

Epilepsy is a disease of the brain defined by any of the following conditions:
- At least two unprovoked (or reflex) seizures occurring >24 h apart;
- One unprovoked (or reflex) seizure and a probability of further seizures similar to the general recurrence risk (at least 60%) after

two unprovoked seizures, occurring over the next 10 years;
- Diagnosis of an epilepsy syndrome.

The traditional definition of epilepsy has been that it takes at least two unprovoked seizures to fulfill the definition. The new definition states that one unprovoked seizure is sufficient to diagnose epilepsy if there is also evidence of enduring seizure tendency, such as epileptiform activity on the EEG.[3]

All patients with epilepsy have seizures, whereas not all patients who have had a seizure have epilepsy. For example, seizures due to severe hyponatremia do not quality as epilepsy even if multiple.

CLASSIFICATIONS

Before discussing the types of seizures, an introduction to seizure symptoms and signs is appropriate.

Symptoms and Signs

- *Prodrome* is an abnormal sensation preceding the seizure in some patients, not associated with epileptiform discharge.
- *Aura* is a subjective sensation that can immediately precede a seizure. This represents the initial portion of the epileptiform discharge.
- *Clonic activity* is episodic muscle contraction associated with a seizure.
- *Tonic activity* is increased muscle tone during a seizure.
- *Automatism* is a stereotyped movement that occurs as part of a seizure, such as lip smacking.
- *Post-ictal period* is an episode of disordered neurologic functioning following a seizure until return to baseline status.

Classification of Seizures and Epilepsies

The 1981 International Classification[4] was a major advance, but there have since been revisions in classifications of seizures[5] and epilepsies[6] which are described in detail in this book in Part 3 for seizures and Part 4 for epilepsies. There are two broad categories: *focal-onset* seizures and *generalized* seizures. The terms *partial* including *simple partial* and *complex partial* are no longer used.

Focal-onset seizures refer to seizures occurring in one hemisphere, whether from a defined focus or diffusely involving the one hemisphere. *Generalized* seizures refer to seizures of generalized onset.

Awareness is used as an important part of the new classification scheme, referring to whether the patient retains awareness during the event; this does not refer to whether the patient is aware that they have had a seizure.

Table 1.1.1 presents a summary of the new classification of seizures.

Focal-onset seizures are subdivided into *aware* or *impaired awareness seizures*. These are then divided into motor onset or nonmotor onset seizures. Some seizures with focal onset will progress to bilateral involvement, so these are termed focal to bilateral tonic-clonic seizures.

Generalized-onset seizures are divided into *motor* and *nonmotor*. Motor is either *tonic-clonic* or *other motor*. *Nonmotor* generalized-onset seizures are *absence* seizures.

Unknown-onset seizures are classified into *motor*, *nonmotor*, or *unclassified*.

TABLE 1.1.1 CLASSIFICATION OF SEIZURES

Onset type	Attribute	Value
Focal onset	Awareness	Aware
		Impaired awareness
	Onset	Motor onset
		Nonmotor onset
	Focal to bilateral tonic clonic seizures	
Generalized	Motor onset	
	Nonmotor onset – Absence	
Unknown onset	Motor onset	Tonic-clonic
		Epileptic spasms
	Nonmotor onset – Behavioral arrest	
	Unclassified	

TABLE 1.1.2 CLASSIFICATION OF EPILEPSIES

Parameter	Value	
Epilepsy types	Focal	
	Generalized	
	Combined generalized and focal	
	Unknown	
Etiologies	Structural	
	Genetic	
	Infectious	
	Metabolic	
	Immune	
	Unknown	
Epilepsy syndromes	Idiopathic generalized epilepsies	Childhood absence Juvenile absence Juvenile myoclonic Generalized tonic-clonic
	Self-limited focal epilepsies	With centro-temporal spikes Self-limited occipital epilepsies Other self-limited frontal, temporal, and parietal epilepsies

The new 2017 Classification of Epilepsies[7] was designed in conjunction with the classification of seizures. Changes were made in terminology and an emphasis placed on etiologic diagnosis. The new classification scheme for epilepsies presumes that the patient has a definite diagnosis of an epileptic seizure.

Table 1.1.2 presents a summary of the new classification of epilepsies.

Details of the classification scheme are presented in Part 4, but a synopsis follows here.

Epilepsy types were classified into *focal, generalized, combined generalized and focal*, and *unknown*. We can see how this correlates with the seizure types presented earlier.

Etiologies are divided into *structural, genetic, infectious, metabolic, immune*, and *unknown*.

The classification progresses to *epilepsy syndromes*, which are defined on the basis of seizure types, EEG, and imaging, along with other clinical data such as onset age, comorbidities, and associated clinical details such as intellectual and developmental disturbances.

1.2

Role of EEG in Diagnosis and Management

KARL E. MISULIS AND HASAN SONMEZTURK

ROUTINE EEG

Routine electroencephalogram (EEG) is commonly performed in patients with episodic disorders or encephalopathies in whom the differential diagnosis includes seizures.

Valid indications for EEG include:

- Seizure or possible seizure;
- Well-controlled epilepsy, to evaluate risk of recurrence upon withdrawal of treatment;
- Syncope without definite cardiac or vascular cause;
- Unexplained loss of consciousness, especially if presentation could be a seizure;
- Dementia when prion, virus, or autoimmune condition is considered as an etiology;
- Determination of whether myoclonic movements are epileptic;
- Stupor, coma, or altered mental status of unclear etiology;
- Psychosis of unclear etiology especially without prior psychiatric history;
- Other spells of unknown nature (e.g., intermittent motor event).

Not valid indications for EEG include those which are highly unlikely to be epileptic:

- Headache;
- Chronic behavioral disorder unless presentation suggests neurologic cause such as psychosis and epilepsy;
- Dizziness or vertigo;
- Chronic deficits, such as dementia or one-sided weakness;
- Movement disorders such as tremor or dyskinesia.

Some epileptic syndromes are likely underdiagnosed. Nonconvulsive seizures, including nonconvulsive status epilepticus, may be incorrectly assumed to be metabolic encephalopathy, drug intoxication, or critical illness encephalopathy. Similarly, episodic focal deficits may be assumed to be transient ischemic attacks (TIA) yet are ultimately diagnosed as partial seizures. In these patients a positive motor component may be subtle or the history merely incomplete.

Table 1.2.1 presents some of the common EEG modalities used in routine neurology practice.

TABLE 1.2.1 ELECTROENCEPHALOGRAM (EEG) MODALITIES

Modality	Use
Routine 20-min EEG	Screening study to look for predisposition to seizures or to characterize EEG background associated with disordered brain function.
Routine 2- to 12-hour video-EEG	Screening study for capture of frequent episodes or for determination of seizure predisposition.
12- to 26-hour video-EEG	Extended EEG with video recording to determine whether relatively frequent episodes are seizures and to look for nonconvulsive seizures in unexplained altered mental status.
Epilepsy monitoring unit	Used to capture video-EEG correlates to suspected seizures in a controlled inpatient environment.
Ambulatory EEG	Capture EEG correlates in patients with suspected seizures in their home environment.
Home video EEG	Similar to EMU except that an expert is not available to examine patients during seizure and medications cannot be discontinued for study.

Note that while the routine 20-min EEG is listed and is commonly ordered, a 2-hour video-EEG is preferable, with better diagnostic yield. Epilepsy monitoring unit (EMU) admission should only be conducted by neurologists with advanced training in epilepsy diagnosis and management.

The diagnostic yield of EEG for detecting epilepsy is difficult to determine, but this question has been studied in several ways. McGinty and colleagues found that routine 20-min EEGs in patients with known epilepsy were positive on the first EEG in 22% patients, rising to 34% yield by the fourth EEG.[1]

Mahuwala and colleagues studied whether a second study after a negative 30-min EEG should be 30 min or 2 hours. The diagnostic yield when the second EEG was 30 min was 3.3% whereas when the second EEG was 2 hours, the yield was 4.2%.[2]

The take-home message from these and related data is that repeated and/or long-term video-EEG monitoring should be performed for patients with suspected seizures if the initial studies are unrevealing. The data also highlight the low yield of a single routine EEG regardless of length.

VIDEO-EEG MONITORING

Video-EEG monitoring refers to prolonged EEG with simultaneous video recording, intended to capture clinical events. It allows the correlation of brain electrical activity with clinical manifestations.

Video-EEG monitoring is performed most commonly for the following indications[3]:

- Evaluate for subclinical or nonconvulsive status epilepticus in patients with unexplained cognitive impairment;
- Spell-capture, to characterize events as either epileptic or nonepileptic;
- Classification of seizure type to assist especially in medication selection;
- Quantification of seizures, especially when they are frequent or not consistently recognized by the patient;
- Evaluation for interictal epileptiform discharges to classify seizure and epilepsy types;
- Localization of the epileptogenic zone in the presurgical evaluation of patients with seizures; performed in the EMU by epileptologists.

Less common indications for video-EEG include

- Quantification of response to treatment;
- Studying seizure precipitants, particularly in reflex epilepsy;

- Evaluating the clinical correlate of EEG discharges that are unclear as to whether they are ictal or interictal;
- Remote history of seizure-like events.

INTRACRANIAL TECHNIQUES

Intracranial techniques are discussed in more detail in Chapter 5.7, but some of the key techniques will be introduced here.

Stereotactic electroencephalography (SEEG): This is the technique predominantly (80–90%) used for invasive seizure focus localization in United States and around the world. It has replaced other techniques such as subdural grids or strips or depth electrodes because it can be done without craniotomy and is minimally invasive. The SEEG electrodes are placed through small burr holes (2.4 mm in diameter) using stereotactic navigation. This technique could not be co-applied with subdural grids or strips because they require craniotomy, and precise stereotactic navigation is not possible once a craniotomy is performed.

Subdural grids aid in the identification of seizure focus, especially in eloquent regions of the cortex, since they are not inserted into the brain. This technique was often used with depth electrodes; however, within the past decade, both grids and depths have been nearly completely replaced by SEEG.

Subdural strip recordings have been performed for years and are still used for presurgical evaluation.[4,5]

Epidural strip electrodes are easier to place than subdural electrodes by virtue of their extradural location, but they are of less localizing value.

Depth electrodes have been used for both diagnosis and management. For diagnosis, depth electrodes can reveal discharges which are invisible from scalp or subdural electrodes. This has especially been found to be helpful for recordings from deep temporal structures, including the amygdala.[6,7]

Epidural peg electrodes are placed through the skull but not into the substance of the brain. They can visualize discharges which might be contaminated by muscle artifact and can also show where discharges are not present, although they are not able to precisely map a focus.

Foramen ovale electrodes have been used especially for the evaluation of seizures with medial temporal lobe focus. They are seldom used now because of improvements in other technologies.

Neurostimulation is a treatment for refractory epilepsy using depth electrodes. While the data are not robust, there is evidence of effectiveness in patients who have not responded adequately to other therapies.[8]

PART 2

Basic Science of EEG

2.1

Physiology

KARL E. MISULIS

This chapter is a brief review of brain physiology as it pertains to the electroencephalogram (EEG). A detailed discussion of basic neurophysiology can be found in the excellent text by Purves et al.[1]

MEMBRANE PHYSIOLOGY

The earliest membranes in evolutionary history were likely composed of protein, but membranes in all tissues now are composed of lipid bilayers (Figure 2.1.1). The lipid bilayer is composed of long sheets of phospholipids.

Neuronal membranes are replete with transmembrane proteins. Some of these form channels with differing ionic permeabilities. In general, ions flow down their electrochemical gradient through these channels when they are open. The *sodium-potassium pump* uses energy to maintain these ionic gradients.

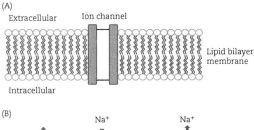

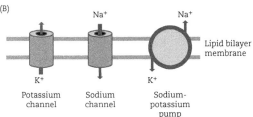

FIGURE 2.1.1 Membrane structure. A: Lipid bilayer membrane is impermeable to ions, but the ion channels allow for and control ion flow. B: Simplified diagram showing differential permeabilities of the sodium and potassium channels and the sodium-potassium pump, which maintains the chemical gradient required for resting and action potentials.

RESTING MEMBRANE POTENTIAL

The resting membrane potential is generated by the properties of all ions on the inside and outside of the cell, but the relative contribution of each is determined by its individual *conductance*. The term "conductance" refers to the ability of a specific ion to move charge, whereas the term "permeability" refers to the ability of a specific atom to pass through a medium, so these terms are related but have distinct implications.

At rest, there is a greater permeability of the membrane to potassium than to other ions. Since the potassium concentration is greater inside the cell than outside, positively charged potassium ions exit the cell through potassium channels, and a membrane potential is built up, with the inside being negative.

The magnitude of the membrane potential can be measured, but it can also be calculated if the concentrations of the ions inside and outside the cell are known and the permeability to the ions is known.

The *equilibrium potential* is the potential at which the electrical gradient is sufficient to exactly counterbalance the chemical gradient. In other words, this is the potential which the membrane would have if the membrane was only permeable to one ion.

The equilibrium potentials for the three most important ions are:

- Potassium = −88 mV
- Sodium = +60 mV
- Chloride = −61 mV

The *resting membrane potential* is a summation of the equilibrium potentials for all of the ions weighted by the conductance of each ion.

If there was no method of maintaining the concentration gradient of potassium as well as other ions, then the ion flow would reduce the chemical gradient, thereby altering the equilibrium potential, and, eventually, there would be little potential difference across the membrane. This happens with cell death. The sodium-potassium pump moves sodium out of the cell while it moves potassium into the cell, using energy from adenosine triphosphate (ATP). For every three sodium ions expelled from the cell, two potassium ions are brought into the cell, so the pump does create a small charge differential (responsible for only about −12 mV of the membrane potential), but it is not the main direct generator of the membrane potential.

POSTSYNAPTIC POTENTIALS

Excitatory transmitters such as acetylcholine and glutamate produce depolarization by opening sodium and/or calcium channels. The depolarization can be recorded intracellularly as an *excitatory postsynaptic potential* (EPSP).

Inhibitory transmitters such as gamma-aminobutyric acid (GABA) produce opening of potassium and/or chloride channels, which results in loss of excitability not so much by hyperpolarization of the membrane but rather by clamping of the membrane potential near the equilibrium potential for these ions, far from the action potential threshold. The potential produced is the *inhibitory postsynaptic potential* (IPSP).

An action potential is generated when EPSPs produce sufficient depolarization to activate additional voltage-gated channels that can then enhance the depolarization.

Postsynaptic potentials terminate because of closure of the channels. This is due to a limited open time of channels as well as cessation of the effect of the transmitter on the receptor. Cessation of transmitter action is due first to release of the transmitter by the receptor. Generally, transmitter is only bound to the receptor for about 1 ms. In many cases, the same transmitter can then bind to that or another receptor. Ultimately, the transmitter is removed from receptor locus in one of three ways:

- Diffusion
- Reuptake
- Degradation

Diffusion occurs because there is a chemical gradient for free transmitter molecules to diffuse away from the synapse.

Reuptake occurs when the presynaptic terminal which just released the transmitter internalizes free transmitter molecules for repackaging and reuse. This occurs especially with GABA, glutamate, dopamine, and other catecholamines.

Degradation occurs when the transmitter is metabolized to inactive constituents. The most common example is acetylcholine, which is metabolized by acetylcholinesterase to acetate and choline. Degradation also consumes some of the neuropeptide transmitters.

EPSPs and IPSPs are key neuronal activities generating scalp-recorded EEG signals.

ACTION POTENTIAL GENERATION AND TERMINATION

An *action potential* occurs when there is marked increase in conductance to sodium ions, depolarizing the cell until it overshoots zero potential to become interior-positive. An action potential developing in a specific portion of a neuron membrane is usually due to propagation of the action potential from another part of the same neuron or from EPSPs produced by synaptic transmission, but it can also be from direct mechanical effects on the neuron.

As sodium conductance increases, the membrane potential approaches the equilibrium potential for sodium, which is interior-positive (+60 mV). During the course of the action potential, the sodium channels eventually close, producing a reduction in sodium conductance; hence the membrane becomes inside-negative again as the membrane potential returns closer to the equilibrium potential for potassium (Figure 2.1.2).

This basic physiology is key to generation of EEG activity.

Summation of potentials is essential for central neural transmission. Often the depolarization associated with a single synaptic event does not cause the release of sufficient transmitter to activate the subsequent neuron. Therefore, the potential changes produced by multiple incoming synaptic events are summed so that depolarization of the next-order neuron can reach threshold.

Spatial summation occurs when potentials developing on different parts of the neuron sum to produce a larger depolarization.

Temporal summation occurs when repetitive activation of a single input results in additive depolarization sufficient to activate the next-order neuron.

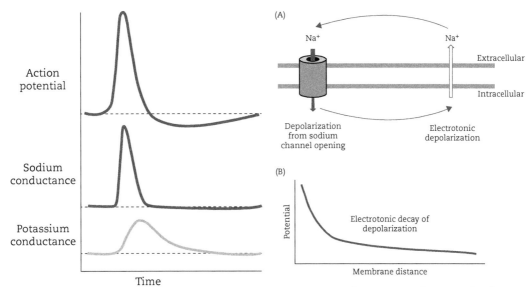

FIGURE 2.1.2 Action potential. Sequence of changes in membrane conductance associated with an action potential. Potassium conductance predominates during rest. Sodium conduction predominates during the action potential.

FIGURE 2.1.3 Electrotonic conduction. A: Lipid bilayer membrane with a sodium channel that is opened, resulting in depolarization not only at that site but downstream by electrotonic conduction. B: Graph of exponential decay in depolarization as a function of distance.

ACTION POTENTIAL PROPAGATION

Depolarization of one segment of membrane results in depolarization of adjacent membrane by electrotonic conduction (Figure 2.1.3). The depolarization spreads but decays along the length of the membrane. If the electrotonic depolarization of the membrane is sufficient, an action potential can develop at a locus distant from the region of primary depolarization.

2.2

Electronics

KARL E. MISULIS

The conceptual parallel between electrical circuits and biologic circuits is of more than passing interest to neurophysiologists. The general physical properties of current flow in biologic tissues are comparable to those in electrical devices, although the systems are far different.

CIRCUIT ELEMENTS

Circuit elements are connected with conductors to form complex circuits. Traditional circuitry used boards to hold the elements and wires to connect them. The next development was the printed circuit board, where strips of conductor were painted onto a board to connect elements. Modern design involves some individual circuit elements plus layers of conducting, semi-conducting, and nonconducting materials that are etched to form transistors, capacitors, resistors, and conductors (Table 2.2.1).

Conductors and Nonconductors

Conductors are able to allow electrons to move because they have unpaired electrons in their outer electron orbitals. Some of these atoms can accept an "extra" electron, resulting in a net negative charge, but with atomic stability. The spot for this extra electron is a *hole*. Other atoms can more easily donate an unpaired electron, which results in a net positive charge but is also atomically stable since every orbital is then full (Figure 2.2.1). During the process of conduction, electrons move from hole to hole, driven by a potential gradient that is established by either the power supply or biologic tissue (Figure 2.2.2).

Nonconductors do not have unpaired electrons that can be donated, nor do they have holes to accept electrons. Therefore, electrons cannot pass through nonconductors unless there is such a large potential gradient across the material that electrons spark through the material.

Resistors

Resistors are composed of material that conducts less well than conductors, dissipating some of the energy associated with the moving electrons as heat (Figure 2.2.3).

TABLE 2.2.1 CIRCUIT ELEMENTS

Element	Features
Conductor	Material that easily conducts current by allowing the flow of electrons. This requires an atomic structure conducive to mobilization of electrons.
Non-conductor	Material that does not conduct current.
Semiconductor	Material that conducts better than a nonconductor but less well than a conductor. Used to make diodes and transistors.
Power supply	Source for power that imparts energy to electrons, thereby causing them to move.
Resistor	Element that opposes the flow of electrons, dissipating energy as heat.
Capacitor	Element that stores energy in the form of separation of charge.
Inductor	Element that stores energy in the form of magnetic field.
Diode	Device made by layering two pieces of semiconductor. Conducts current in only one direction.
Transistor	Device for controlling current flow, made by layering semiconductor materials. Integral for amplifiers.
Amplifier	Device to amplify signals.

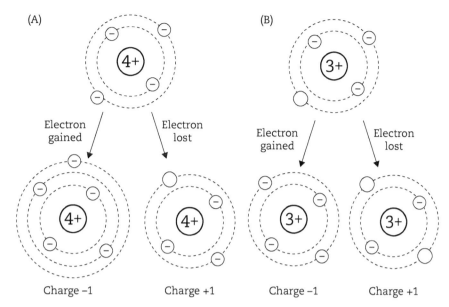

FIGURE 2.2.1 Conductors and nonconductors. Atomic structure of the outer orbitals of some important elements. A is a nonconductor, B is a conductor. A: The atom is electrically neutral and all orbitals are filled so it is unable to easily donate or receive an electron. An electron donated to this atom would not be welcome, and formation of a new orbital does not occur. Losing an electron would require a large amount of energy and would not occur in an electronic circuit. B: Electrically neutral but has one empty orbital spot. Can easily receive an electron. Gaining an electron is favored since it fills the outer orbital even though there is electrical negative charge. Likewise, the single outer orbital electron can be donated easily.

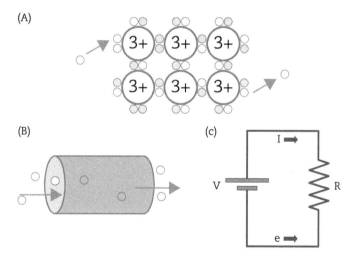

FIGURE 2.2.2 Anatomy of a conductor. A: Atomic structure of a conductor. Adjacent atoms share electrons, shown as small gray circles. The small white circles are "holes," which are unfilled portions of orbitals. Electrons move from hole to hole through the conductor. B: Less enlarged view of a conductor, showing electron flow through the conductor. By convention, current flow is defined as the flow of positive charge—therefore, in the opposite direction to the flow of electrons. C: Simple circuit diagram of a conductor. The symbol for a battery "V" has the positive terminal upward. Electrons flow from the negative terminal (bottom) through the conductor to the positive terminal. Current flow is opposite to the flow of electrons.

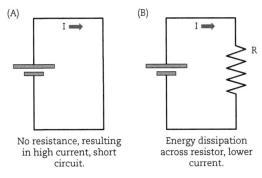

No resistance, resulting in high current, short circuit.

Energy dissipation across resistor, lower current.

FIGURE 2.2.3 Resistor. A: A conductor connects the terminals of a battery. Current will flow from the positive terminal to the negative terminal through the conductor. Electrons are flowing in the opposite direction. The magnitude of current will quickly destroy the battery. B: A resistor is inserted into the conductor circuit. This reduces the current flow by an amount proportional to the resistance of the resistor.

Resistors are integral components of circuits since they regulate current flow. Insertion of resistors into a circuit reduces the rate of charge movement, or *current*. When current flows through resistors, energy is dissipated, referred to as *voltage drop*. Some resistors are purely designed for current regulation, whereas other circuit elements incorporate resistance as a mechanism to produce heat or light.

Capacitors

Capacitors are composed of plates of conducting material separated by nonconducting material (Figure 2.2.4). Therefore, current cannot flow directly through a capacitor, although *capacitive current* can flow. Capacitive current is virtual current; the electrons arriving on one plate of the capacitor are not the same electrons leaving the opposite plate. The capacity or *capacitance* is a measure of the ability of the capacitor to store energy by separation of charge producing an electric field.

When the power supply is turned on, electrons flow and build up on one plate of the capacitor. Because of a repulsive effect on electrons on the opposite plate, electrons stream off this plate, leaving a positive charge. Eventually, the potential developed across the capacitor is sufficient to oppose the flow of current, and net electron flow stops. At this point, the charge across the capacitor is equal and opposite to that of the power supply.

When the power supply is switched off, the only potential difference in the circuit is across the capacitor. Electrons flow from the negatively charged plate through the circuit and onto the positively charged plate.

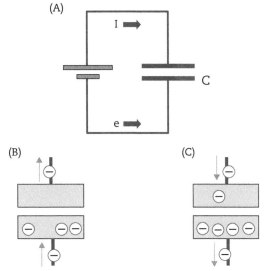

FIGURE 2.2.4 Capacitor. A: Simple circuit of a battery charging a capacitor. When the battery is switched on, electrons flow from the negative terminal and onto the lower plate of the capacitor. Electrons leave the upper plate and travel through the conductor to the positive terminal of the battery. B: Close-up of the capacitor during the charging phase. Electrons accumulate on the lower plate and depart from the upper plate. C: When the battery is switched off, electrons flow off the lower plate and onto the upper plate. The motivation for electron movement is the charge separation across the plates of the capacitor.

Capacitors alter the frequency response of electronic circuits and additionally are used for a variety of electronic applications requiring pulsed current, such as strobe lights.

Inductors

Inductors are a coil of conducting wire (Figure 2.2.5). They capitalize on the general property of conductors to build up a magnetic field when current flows. As electrons flow through a straight conductor, a weak magnetic field is created. This field is large enough to be detected by sensitive equipment but not typically enough to significantly influence the flow of current. However, when the conducting wire is coiled, the magnetic fields from multiple turns of the coil are summed, so the magnetic field can be substantial.

One use of an inductor is as an *electromagnet*, where a constant current through the coil creates a stable magnetic field with north and south poles, just like a permanent magnet. Consider a power supply connected to an inductor (Figure 2.2.6). When the power supply is switched on and

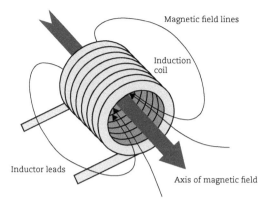

Magnetic field lines

Induction coil

Inductor leads

Axis of magnetic field

FIGURE 2.2.5 Inductor. Diagram of an inductor coil. The coil of wire results in the magnetic fields being in effectively the same direction, producing a summation of the fields. This makes for a powerful field that is dependent on the amount of current flowing through the coiled wire and the number of turns of the coil.

the magnetic field builds up, there is a lag in current until the field is maximally developed. At that point, the impedance abates and current freely flows. This is because the energy is taken from the system in creating the magnetic field.

The energy stored in the magnetic field is reclaimed when the power supply is switched off. In this case, the current ceases to flow from the power supply, and the magnetic field begins to collapse, but this collapse in magnetic field causes current to flow through the system in the same direction as it initially did during the charging phase. The production of electric current by a changing magnetic field is *induction*.

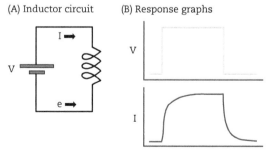

(A) Inductor circuit   (B) Response graphs

I

V

V

e

V

I

FIGURE 2.2.6 Inductor theory. A: Circuit diagram of a power supply (V), inductor, and current (I) flowing through the circuit. Electrons flowing through the inductor coil produce a magnetic field. B: Graph of the response to a step in voltage (V). The current builds up but more slowly than expected because some of the energy of the current flow is used to generate the magnetic field.

Inductors are important for radios and a variety of equipment in which flow of current through a circuit needs to be controlled. But the biggest implication of inductors for neurophysiology purposes is *stray inductance*. This is unintentional inductance due to the presence of wires all around us. While they may not have all of the turns and tight structure of a commercial inductor, they can produce sufficient inductance to cause stray current flow and thereby noise in sensitive neurophysiologic equipment. Since line power is alternating current (AC), these wires can produce a constantly changing magnetic field which in turn induces fluctuating current in leads and equipment.

Semiconductors

Semiconductors are so called because they semiconduct: they conduct better than nonconductors but less well than conductors. They are composed of a nonconducting material that has a few atoms of conducting material intermixed.

The base material is usually silicon or germanium, and the atoms inserted within the base material are elements that can be electron donors or electron acceptors. For our example, we can use arsenic as donor and gallium as acceptor, although other elements are often used. This is *doping*, and the type of the intermixed material determines the type of semiconductor. Silicon and germanium have four outer electrons, making them essentially nonconductors (Figure 2.2.7). Arsenic has five outer electrons, so, in a lattice with silicon, there is tight binding of four of these electrons and one is a "spare" in that it is not tightly bound and therefore can dissociate from its nucleus and move through the material. This is an *N-type semiconductor* since it has spare electrons from an orbital point of view although they are not spare in terms of electrical neutrality. Doping a semiconductor with gallium, which has three outer electrons and therefore an unfilled electron orbital, creates a *P-type semiconductor*. The P-type indicates that the semiconductor has properties of a positive material in that it can easily accept an electron.

Diodes

Diodes are composed of two wafers of semiconductor, which are then joined. When the two are placed together, electrons migrate from the N side to the adjacent P side (Figure 2.2.8). This creates a junction potential, which develops to the point at which the charge differential opposes the further flow of electrons.

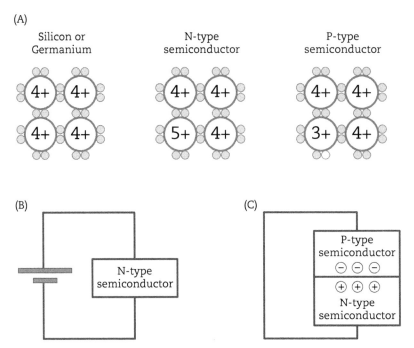

FIGURE 2.2.7 Semiconductor. A: Atomic structure of semiconductor material. Pure silicon (*left*) is a nonconductor. Doping of this material with a conducting element results in either available electrons for flow (*center*, N-type) or available empty electron orbitals, which can temporarily host a flowing electron ("hole" or P-type, *right*). B: A piece of semiconductor material as part of a circuit can conduct electric current although not as well as a conductor. C: Two semiconductor pieces are placed together without a battery. Some of the spare electrons of the N-type semiconductor move to occupy partially filled orbitals of the P-type semiconductor. This is analogous to the diffusion potential of biological membranes.

Therefore, at rest, the junction between these materials is polarized with a positive charge on the N-type side and a negative charge on the P-type side.[1]

When a power supply is applied to deliver potential difference across the diode, current can easily flow in only one direction. If the negative side of the power supply is applied to the N side, then the junction potential is negated so current can flow. On the other hand, if the polarity is reversed, electrons delivered to the P side serve to augment the junction potential. There are no unpaired electrons or holes available to facilitate further current flow.

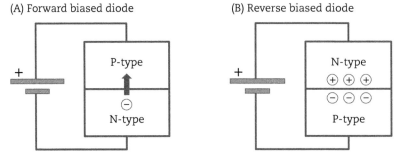

FIGURE 2.2.8 Diode. A: A battery is connected to the N-P semiconductor complex. In this diagram, current can flow, since the junction potential between the two materials is negated by the applied voltage. B: The position of the semiconductor materials is reversed so that the applied voltage serves to augment the junction potential. Current cannot flow. Since the N-P semiconductor junction allows for current flow in only one direction, this is a diode.

There are diodes in electrophysiological equipment, such as for rectifying AC voltage. However, the main purpose of semiconductors in EEG equipment is for the manufacture of transistors.

Transistors

Transistors are typically composed of three layers of semiconductor. One of the most common types is the *junction bipolar transistor*, shown in Figure 2.2.9. With no applied voltage, junction potentials develop at the NP junctions. The left side of the circuit is the *controlling* side and the right side is the *controlled* side. The left side power source could be the biological voltage of the patient, and the right side would then be the rest of the amplifier circuitry.

The upper NP junction is reverse biased, and normally electrons would not flow. The lower PN junction is forward biased. When voltage is applied to the controlled side, this alters the potential developed at the upper PN junction, resulting

(A)

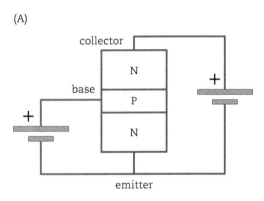

(B)

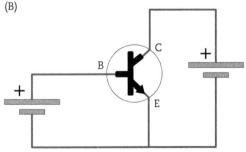

FIGURE 2.2.9 Transistor. A: A transistor is constructed from three layers of semiconductor material. Voltage supplied on the left side of the circuit controls the conductance across the entire transistor. Therefore, a small amount of voltage on the controlling side governs current flowing on the controlled side. B: Circuit diagram of the transistor.

in allowance of current flow. The voltage applied by the EEG machine's power supply to the controlled side is much larger than the voltage of the controlling side, so a small amount of current flow in the controlling side alters the current flowing on the controlled side to a much greater extent. For most transistors of this type, the amplification is linear over a defined range of input voltages.

AMPLIFIERS

Overview

Biological potentials are of such small magnitude that amplification is required in order to analyze and display the signals. The first stage of amplification is commonly at the head stage of the device. This simple amplifier raises the magnitude of the signal so that it exceeds the magnitude of electrical noise. Noise already in the electrode system will be amplified, however. Shielded cables then conduct current to the EEG machine.

The EEG machine further amplifies the raw signal and converts it to digital in preparation for data manipulation and display.

Amplification needed for computer input is many orders of magnitude greater than most biologic signals, so multiple stages are required for amplification. For example, if each amplifier stage provides approximately 10× amplification, a gain of 1,000× requires three stages, producing 10^3 amplification. This would amplify a 50-microvolt signal to 50 millivolts. Further amplification is needed since most computers need signals in the range of 1 or more volts to convert analog signal into digital data.

Single-Ended Versus Differential Amplifiers

Single-ended amplifiers amplify signal delivered to the active input in reference to a ground (Figure 2.2.10A). The output of a single-ended amplifier is a magnified representation of the input to the amplifier.

Differential amplifiers (Figure 2.2.10B) are composed of two elementary single-ended amplifiers plus a subtracting circuit. Two signal inputs are used. Both are amplified by single-ended amplifiers. Then the amplified output from one is subtracted from the amplified output of the other. This difference is displayed and represents the differential output. The output of a differential amplifier is the amplified difference between the signal at two inputs.

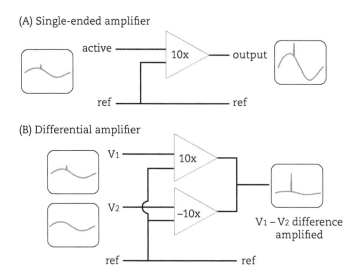

(A) Single-ended amplifier

(B) Differential amplifier

FIGURE 2.2.10 Single-ended versus differential amplifier. A: Single-ended amplifier in which the input and output are in reference to a common level so the amplified output is similar to the input, just larger. B: Differential amplifier in which there is amplification, inversion, then summation so that the output is the amplified difference between the two inputs.

CIRCUIT LAWS

Overview

The basic laws that govern electric circuits are many, but the most important are these:

- Ohm's law,
- Kirchhoff's current law,
- Kirchhoff's voltage law.

In addition, two basic additional concepts are instructive to remember.

- Summation of resistors in series,
- Summation of resistors in parallel.

Table 2.2.2 presents a summary of these laws.

Ohm's Law

Ohm's law states that, for any resistive circuit, the voltage is equal to the current times the resistance or

$$V = 1 \times R$$

As the voltage increases across a fixed resistance, the current flow increases. On the other hand, as the resistance increases with a fixed voltage, the current drops (see Figure 2.2.11).

TABLE 2.2.2 SUMMARY OF IMPORTANT CIRCUIT LAWS

Law	Features
Ohm's law	For a resistive circuit, the current flowing is equal to the applied voltage divided by the resistance. Or, $I = V/R$. Rearranged, this is $V = I \times R$, where V is applied voltage, I is current, and R is resistance.
Kirchhoff's current law	For a node, or junction point of conductors, all of the current flowing into the node must equal to the current flowing out of the node. Since outward flow can be considered reverse of incoming, then: $\Sigma I_i = 0$, where I_i represents the individual currents.
Kirchhoff's voltage law	For a circuit loop, the sum of the voltage sources is equal to the voltage drops, where voltage drop is dissipation across a resistance. Or, $\Sigma V_S = \Sigma V_R$.
Summation of resistors in series	For two or more resistors in series, the equivalent resistance is equal to the sum of the individual resistances. Or, $R_T = \Sigma R_i$, where R_T is total resistance and R_i is resistance of the individual resistors.
Summation of resistors in parallel	For two or more resistors in parallel, the reciprocal of the equivalent resistance is equal to the sum of the reciprocals of the individual resistances. Or, $1/R_T = \Sigma (1/R_i)$.

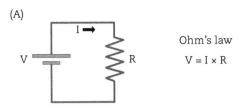

Ohm's law

$$V = I \times R$$

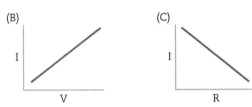

FIGURE 2.2.11 Ohm's law. A: Circuit diagram of a resistor-capacitor (RC) circuit. The power supply provides a voltage (V), which drives electrons around the circuit in the opposite direction to positive current (I) through the resistor (R). B: Linear positive relationship between applied voltage and current. C: Linear inverse relationship between resistance of the resistor and current flow. Higher resistance means less current.

Permutations of Ohm's law apply and are useful in circuit theory.

Current of a resistive circuit is equal to the voltage divided by the resistance or

$$I = \frac{V}{R}$$

Similarly, resistance in a resistive circuit is equal to the voltage divided by the current or

$$R = \frac{V}{I}$$

Kirchhoff's Current Law

Kirchhoff's current law is easy to conceptualize (Figure 2.2.12).

The sum of the currents flowing into a node, or connector, in a circuit is zero. In other words, the sum of the current flowing into a node is equal to the sum of the current flowing out. This is evident since a connector point has no ability to store or modify energy. Kirchhoff's current law is presented as

$$\sum I_i = \sum I_o$$

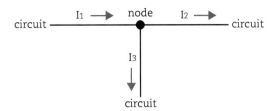

FIGURE 2.2.12 Kirchhoff's current law. The sum of the currents flowing into and out of a node is zero. The node cannot store or modify energy.

where I_i represents the incoming currents to the node and I_o represents the outgoing currents from the node.

This indicates that the sum of the incoming currents is equal to the sum of the outgoing currents. However, since outgoing currents are in the opposite direction from incoming currents (from the viewpoint of the node), they can be considered negative currents (although this means = negative from a mathematical point of view, not a charge point of view).

Therefore,

$$\sum I = 0$$

where I in this formula represents all of the individual currents into and out of the node.

Kirchhoff's Voltage Law

Kirchhoff's voltage law states that, for any circuit loop, the sum of the voltage sources is equal to the sum of the voltage drops (Figure 2.2.13). *Voltage drop* means dissipation of voltage across a circuit element. Since voltage drops are of opposite direction to voltage sources, the law really says that the sum of the voltages around a circuit loop is zero.

A *circuit loop* is any closed loop of connectors and their circuit elements. Figure 2.2.13 shows both a simple single loop circuit and a more complex circuit with three loops: top loop, bottom loop, and the large loop encompassing both power supplies and resistors, without the central horizontal connector. So, for each of the loops in these diagrams,

$$\sum V_S = \sum V_R$$

where V_S represents the individual voltage sources such as batteries or biologic signals and V_R is the voltage drop across each resistor.

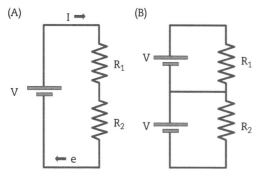

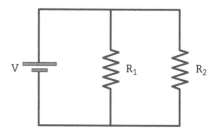

FIGURE 2.2.15 Resistors in parallel. The reciprocal of the total resistance of two resistors in parallel is equal to the sum of the reciprocals of the individual resistances.

FIGURE 2.2.13 Kirchhoff's voltage law. A: The sum of the voltage sources and drops in a circuit loop is zero. B: Kirchhoff's voltage law applies to all circuit loops, including each of the smaller loops in this diagram and the large loop encompassing both batteries and both resistors.

Summation of Resistors in Series

Two or more resistors in series can be replaced conceptually with a single resistor with a total equivalent resistance (Figure 2.2.14). The intuitive assumption is that the total equivalent resistance is the sum of the individual resistances, and this is correct.

Expressed mathematically,

$$R_T = \Sigma R_i$$

where R_T is the total equivalent resistance of the system and R_i is the resistance of the individual resistors.

Summation of Resistors in Parallel

Two or more resistors in parallel (Figure 2.2.15) can also be replaced conceptually by a single resistor with an equivalent resistance.

The total resistance is less than the resistance of any of the resistors, which may not be intuitively obvious. This discrepancy occurs because each resistor is a conduit for electron flow, so, the more conduits in parallel, the lower overall resistance.

For electron flow, conductance is the reciprocal of resistance.

$$G = \frac{1}{R}$$

where G is conductance and R is resistance.

The greater the resistance, the less the conductance. If there are two or more routes of conductance, then each route increases the overall conductance. The total conductance is equal to the sum of the individual conductances. Or,

$$G_T = \Sigma G_i$$

where G_T is the total conductance and G_i is the conductance of the individual resistors.

If we then substitute 1/R for the conductances, we have the following formula:

$$\frac{1}{R_T} = \Sigma \frac{1}{R_i}$$

where R_T is the total equivalent resistance of the resistors in parallel and R_i is the resistance of the individual resistors.

COMPUTERS AND DIGITAL DATA

Computers are considered "black boxes" in our era. It is not crucial to know how they work, and certainly an in-depth understanding of computer architecture is not essential to the performance

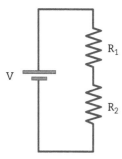

FIGURE 2.2.14 Resistors in series. The total resistance of two resistors in series is equal to the sum of the individual resistances.

and interpretation of EEGs, but we should have some idea of what computers do.

Computers do math. At the core of a computer is the central processing unit (CPU) and attached to that are memory modules, devices, inputs, and outputs. The CPU is composed of a control unit and a logic unit, the latter of which is often called the *arithmetic logic unit* (ALU). It is called this because it has two main basic functions. One is to do arithmetic, such as adding numbers. The other function is logic, such as determining whether one number is larger than another number. But these are both really arithmetic functions. Math is foundational whether the CPU is tasked with calculating the product of two numbers, performing spell-checking on a document, or displaying an EEG signal.

Analog-to-Digital Conversion

The calculations for EEG data presume that the data have been converted into digital format, and, for this, an *analog-to-digital converter* (ADC) is used and is an integral part of all neurophysiological equipment.

The analog signal recorded from the brain is amplified so that the signal is substantially larger than noise encountered during the acquisition process. Subsequently, the analog signal is converted to digital format by the ADC. The ADC samples the signal at specified times and makes measurements. Figure 2.2.16 illustrates the concept.

The rate of sampling is dependent on the hardware, but generally most electrophysiological equipment samples fast enough to have a good representation of time-dependent changes in the biological signal. The sample is taken in a small fraction of a second, then the converter waits until it is time to sample again. The interval between samples is the *intersample interval*. The number of samples per second is the *sampling rate*.

In practice, the time resolution (sampling rate) and voltage resolution (amplitude of smallest voltage resolution levels) is so good that the reconstructed waveform would be virtually indistinguishable from the native waveform and not a rough approximation, as in Figure 2.2.16.

SIGNAL PROCESSING

Signal processing begins on the analog signal prior to the ADC, but most of what concerns us as neurophysiologists are the calculations performed on the digitized data.

Calculations can accomplish various tasks, including

- Removing high frequencies;
- Removing low frequencies;
- Removing specific frequencies, such as 60-Hz line power artifact;
- Determining amounts of specific frequency bands (power spectral analysis);
- Identifying potentials that might be epileptiform activity (spike detection);
- Identifying sleep stages.

These calculations are not perfect. Frequency and timing distortion can occur, including phase shifts. Also, some functions, such as spike detection and sleep stage analysis, are particularly difficult for computers, so these functions are used for screening, and human review is needed for final determinations.

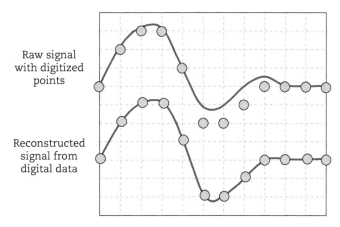

Raw signal with digitized points

Reconstructed signal from digital data

FIGURE 2.2.16 Analog-to-digital conversion. An analog (continuously variable) signal is essentially placed on an X/Y grid where the X axis is time and samples are taken at specific times. The Y axis is voltage with specific voltage levels and the measurement is of the voltage level exceeded or met by the analog signal at each of the sample times. Connecting the dots produces a digital representation of the analog signal.

FILTERS

Overview

Filters alter the frequency composition of the EEG signal so that we can more easily see those frequencies of interest. Raw EEG signal is composed of a broad range of frequencies, only some of which are relevant to routine interpretation. Frequencies slower than 0.5 Hz and faster than 70 Hz are of lesser value and can obscure other frequencies.

Frequency composition of the signal can be altered by three basic filter types:

- High-frequency filter (HFF)
- Low-frequency filter (LFF)
- 60-Hertz (or notch) filter

The HFF attenuates the higher frequencies, whereas the LFF attenuates the lower frequencies. The 60-Hz filter attenuates frequencies around 60 Hz. The mechanism of filters, however, is complicated. There is not a precise cut-off, but rather a decay in the amplitude of these frequencies near the selected set frequency. This decay is called a *transfer function*, and the steepness is termed the *roll-off*. Sometimes the term "cut-off frequency" is used but this implies an absolute barrier to frequencies, which is not the case. The signal drops off by a certain amount per octave of frequency. Therefore, the filter effect is described by the filter type (high vs. low vs. notch), the cut-off frequency, and the roll-off.

Filters are often used to remove artifacts from EEG signals. Some artifacts have frequencies different from most EEG frequencies of interest. Common artifacts are

- Electrical artifact,
- Cardiac (EKG),
- Muscle (EMG),
- Tongue movement (glossokinetic),
- Eye movement,
- Sweat,
- Head movement,
- Respiratory movement.

The first three are high-frequency and can be attenuated by an HFF, but use of the HFF may also attenuate important fast activity, such as spikes and sharp waves. Therefore, it is best if we can remove some of these electrical artifacts without more filtering. Careful attention to the technical details of EEG performance often removes most of these artifacts.

Slow artifacts can be attenuated by an LFF, but this also can attenuate some of the slower physiological signals, such as frontal intermittent rhythmic delta activity (FIRDA) or polymorphic delta activity (PDA) and can actually change the morphology of some slow activity to appear as faster transients.

A note about terminology: we use the terms "high-frequency filter," "low-frequency filter," and "60-Hz filter" to indicate what they are intended to filter from the desired signal potentials. Literature sometimes uses the terms "high-pass filter" and "low-pass filter" to indicate what they allow to pass, meaning that a high-pass filter allows frequencies over a certain set frequency and a low-pass filter allows frequencies below a certain set frequency. But, for technical and convention reasons, we do not use these terms.[2]

Physics of Filters

There are three basic types of filters:

- Passive filters
- Active filters
- Digital filters

Passive filters are described because they illustrate the mechanism of filters. However, most filters in modern EEG equipment are *active* and *digital*. Passive filters are so called because they modify the signal without use of an exogenous power source, typically using only resistors and capacitors and sometimes inductors. *Active filters* use transistors and a power supply in addition to resistors and capacitors to filter the signal. *Digital filters* are calculations performed on the digital data. These are discussed in more detail later.

The basic construction of the simplest passive filter is the RC circuit (resistor-capacitor circuit; Figure 2.2.17). The RC circuit is a resistor and a capacitor in series with a power supply. Current flows through the conductor from the positive side of the power supply to the negative side. We are speaking of "positive current," which is an electrical convention. In reality, current is electrons flowing from the negative end of the power supply to the positive end. The effect of the RC circuit can be best seen if meters are placed across the resistor and capacitor and a measurement of current is made (Figure 2.2.17).

Meters will show a potential difference, which in the case of a resistor is the voltage drop. For the capacitor, the measured voltage difference is the charge built up across the plates.

Recordings that would be obtained are shown in Figure 2.2.18. For this illustration, a square-wave pulse is delivered by the power supply. A meter placed across the terminals of the power supply would show the square-wave. The voltage

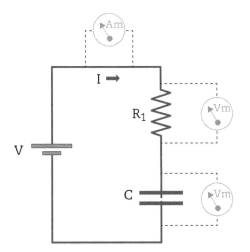

FIGURE 2.2.17 RC circuit. RC where meters are placed to measure the voltage differences across the resistor and capacitor and to measure the current.

(*V*) causes current (*I*) to move through the circuit. Current charges the capacitor (*C*). The voltage measured across the capacitor has a gradual increase because it takes time for the capacitor to charge. The voltage plateaus because the maximum voltage that can develop across the capacitor is the voltage of the power supply. When the power source is turned off, the voltage across the capacitor gradually decays because it takes time for the electrons displaced on either side of the capacitor plates to return to their base state—equal electrons on both sides.

The current flowing through the device (*I*) as measured by the ammeter has a complex waveform because of the capacitor. When the voltage is first turned on, there is a lot of current flowing through the circuit, giving the high spike of current. With current flow, there is buildup of charge across the capacitor, and this potential difference opposes the further flow of current. Therefore, the current is dependent on the difference in voltages of the power supply and capacitor, giving the gradual decline. When the voltage across the plates of the capacitor is equal and opposite to the voltage of the power supply, current ceases.

When the power supply voltage is switched off, the charged capacitor is now the only source of electromotive force (EMF) in the circuit, so current flows in the reverse direction to the initial current, hence the negative current spike.

The voltage measured across the resistor looks exactly like the current measurements because the voltage drop across a resistor is equal to current multiplied by resistance—from Ohm's Law.

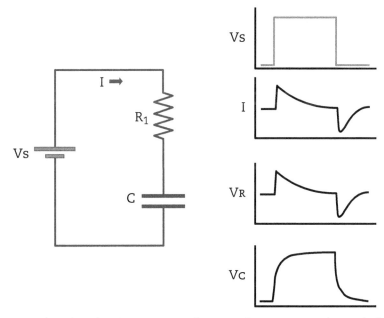

FIGURE 2.2.18 Recordings from the RC circuit. A step change in voltage, positive 1 volt, is applied; the graphs show the changes in voltage difference and current with onset and offset of the step voltage. Current is initially large, but as the capacitor is charged, that voltage opposes the supply voltage, and, as the capacitor becomes fully charged, current stops. When the applied voltage is zeroed, the capacitor discharges with current moving in the opposite direction. Voltage across the resistor varies directly with current, from Ohm's law.

What does this have to do with filters? The RC circuit is the simplest filter. Looking at the single-step voltage just presented, the voltage measured across the capacitor looks like the signal voltage but with the high-frequency component filtered out—you can see what the signal voltage was, but not how fast it got there. In contrast, the voltage measured across the resistor looks like a differential (dV/dt) of the signal voltage. We can see the positive change in potential as the pulse starts and the negative change as the pulse stops, but we cannot see the plateau in voltage; essentially, the low-frequency component has been filtered out.

For the RC circuit, the voltage across the capacitor looks like a high-frequency filtered signal and the voltage across the resistor looks like a low-frequency filtered signal.

This is a demonstration of passive filters and their simplest version: the RC circuit.

Filters in Practice

Passive filters, such as the RC circuit, have greater importance in the generation of noise and distortion of signal than in equipment design. The electrode leads have inherent resistance, and the proximity of leads and other wires provides capacitance. Therefore, unintentional RC circuits can distort the signal voltage arising from the brain in unpredictable and changing ways.

Active filters are circuits using semiconductors that amplify and attenuate the signal in a frequency-dependent fashion. Though the exact mechanism is not presented here, suffice it to say that frequency-dependent amplification involves feedback circuits that attenuate certain frequencies, and the active filters are not constrained by the high- versus low-frequency filtering function: specific frequency bands can be accentuated or attenuated.

Digital filters are calculations performed on the digital data. The calculations can be of many types, including smoothing across multiple data points, often with weighting, and attenuation of specific frequencies.

Signal distortion occurs when the filtering process alters the appearance of signals within the frequency band of interest. For example, if the low-frequency filter setting is high, then slow delta activity will not only be reduced in amplitude, but also mathematically differentiated, making a faster component that was not in the original signal. Similarly, if a high-frequency filter is set too low, spike activity will be blunted, perhaps giving the appearance of a normal physiological potential of lower frequency—again, not part of the original biological signal. A 60-Hz filter can also attenuate spikes, although with modern equipment this is not as problematic as it once was.

Phase shift occurs when a rhythm is passed through a filter. The most common manifestation of this is a *phase lead*; this is when the rhythm appears to move ahead in time due to a differentiating effect of the filter system. Consider a sine wave as shown in Figure 2.2.19.

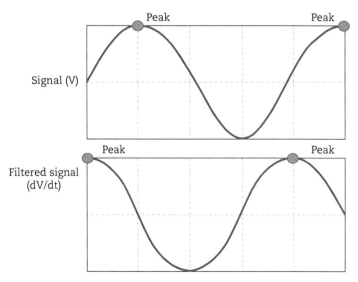

FIGURE 2.2.19 Sine wave with phase shift. Filters not only alter the frequency response of the signal but can also produce a phase shift, where the peaks of the waves are not simultaneous with those of the input signal. In this example, a filter has caused a phase-lead, where the filtered signal is quarter-cycle or 90 degrees ahead of the native signal.

The original signal wave is shown on top, with peak positivity a quarter cycle from the beginning (i.e., 90 degrees). In this example the wave is differentiated, which can help to remove some slow frequencies. Every point of the lower wave is *dV/dt*, or the change in voltage over time: *dV/dt* is most positive during the rising phase of the native wave, most negative during the falling phase of the native wave, and zero at the flat points—peak positivity and negativity. When the points of peak positivity are highlighted by dots to show a marker of the cycle of the wave, you can see that the filtered wave is a quarter cycle or 90 degrees ahead of the native wave.

Phase shift is not important for most EEG applications. Spikes may appear slightly earlier because of this phase-shifting effect, though this small effect is not clinically important. Note that phase shift can occur with digital filters as well as with analog filters.

Filter Settings

Filters are set to default values when the EEG machine is started. The most commonly used default values are

- Low-frequency filter = 1 Hz;
- High-frequency filter = 70 Hz;
- 60-Hz filter = off.

The LFF may be decreased to better see some slow activity, though most physiologic and pathologic slow activity is seen well with default settings. The LFF is increased if there is slow activity that at least partially obscures the recording, including, specifically, sweat artifact. Unfortunately, increasing the LFF may also attenuate and thereby obscure some slow activity of clinical interest, such as focal or generalized slowing.

The HFF is almost never increased. Reduction of the HFF is usually done to attenuate fast activity such as electrical artifact or muscle activity (EMG). The former is best dealt with by the 60-Hz filter as well as by improving the recording technique and environment. Unfortunately, lowering the HFF may attenuate and blunt physiologic fast activity such as epileptiform discharges.

The 60-Hz filter is often needed when performing EEGs in the ICU or in other portable situations.

ELECTRODES

Overview

Electrodes are often given an afterthought in the performance of EEG; however, electrode properties are a critical part of the EEG system, and even minor deviations in the quality or placement of electrodes can greatly alter the recording.

Electrode Basics

Electrodes are connected to the scalp with a conducting gel, which serves as a malleable extension of the electrode. Without this extension, any minor movement of the head would result in mechanical disturbance of the electrode–scalp interface, producing electrical artifact.

Some important technical requirements of electrodes and electrode placement are as follows:

- Electrodes of the same type and manufacturer,
- Equal lead length,
- Equal electrode impedances,
- Leads are not in proximity to other devices,
- Leads are not coiled.

ELECTRODE THEORY

The electrode–amplifier interface is crucial to the understanding of electrode theory. Referring to Figure 2.2.20, the signal voltage (V_s) is generated by the brain and conducted to the scalp. The electrode resistance (R_e) is really impedance, which indicates frequency-dependent resistance. The

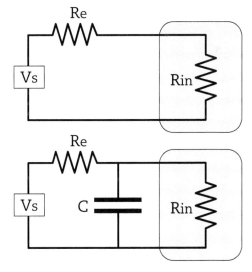

FIGURE 2.2.20 Electrode theory. *Top*: Diagram of the electrode-amplifier interface. V_s is the signal voltage from the body. R_e is the electrode resistance. R_{in} is the input resistance of the amplifier. The signal voltage is equal to the sum of voltages across the electrode (R_e) and the input resistance of the amplifier (R_{in}). *Bottom*: Same diagram as in A, but a small capacitance (C) is inserted into the circuit. This capacitance is created by proximity of the electrode leads.

current flows from these electrodes through the leads and to the input of the amplifier. The input of the amplifier is high resistance, which results in little charge movement being required to detect a voltage. Therefore, the input resistance (R_{in}) should be much larger than R_e and the resistance of the body from which the recording is made. Again, although we are speaking of "resistance" for the purpose of calculation, "impedance" is a more accurate term.

In the second diagram, there is a small capacitor between the electrode leads. This is not a structural capacitor but rather is due to proximity of the leads. This capacitance, along with the resistance of the electrode–patient interface, creates an RC circuit that can modify the recorded signal. The effect of this capacitance is to distort the incoming signal, essentially acting as a filter.

The signal seen by the amplifier is the most faithful representation of the input from the brain when all of the technical requirements for electrodes noted earlier are met and when the effects of noise-causing errors have been minimized.

Electrode Composition

Electrodes are composed of a variety of metals. While silver and gold have been traditionally used, a variety of other metals are in use. Electrodes are *reversible* or *nonreversible*. Reversible electrodes include the typical silver chloride electrodes. Reversible electrodes permit easy bidirectional chemical reactions that account for the movement of charge. Nonreversible electrodes have difficulty with electron flow in one direction, essentially conducting electric charge mainly in one direction well and in the opposite direction less well. A junction potential can be developed across interfaces, which can create electrode pops and distort the frequency response of the recording system.

DIGITAL DISPLAYS

Computer displays are almost universally used. Paper records are obsolete and as such are not discussed.

The mechanisms to show data on the screen are part of the computer's operating system, and the programming consists of calculations that tell the computer what you want the picture on the screen to look like. Few modern programs are written from scratch using low-level instructions. More commonly, they are written in high-level languages that rely on sub-applications or runtime routines to perform the elementary processes of input, analysis, and display,

The displays required for the interpretation of EEG are generally of higher resolution than most budget displays.

2.3

Generators of EEG Activity

KARL E. MISULIS

Electroencephalographic (EEG) activity is due to charge movement in neuronal membranes. It is attractive to think of EEG activity as originating in defined nuclei, but, in general, the electrical potentials represent the summed electrical activity from millions of neurons. Rather than representing the electrical activity of specific tracts and nuclei, scalp EEG is a complex representation of fluctuating and shifting dipoles.

EEG signals recorded from the scalp are generated mainly by the cerebral cortex, with the portion of the cortex adjacent to the skull being the greatest contributor. However, subcortical activity and pathology influences and drives cortical activity.

GENERATORS OF NORMAL EEG ACTIVITY

Cortical Potentials: Most cortical efferents are oriented perpendicular to the cortical surface. The gyration of the cortex results in only a fraction of the cortical efferents being oriented perpendicular to the scalp. Therefore, those neurons would be expected to have a disparate contribution to the surface-recorded EEG. Electrical activity at the large cortical neurons produces dipoles that are summed to generate the scalp EEG. It is thought that summated excitatory postsynaptic potentials (EPSPs) and inhibitory postsynaptic potentials (IPSPs) are responsible for most of the EEG activity recorded at the scalp. Action potentials probably have a minor contribution to the scalp-recorded EEG.

Scalp Potentials: Synchronous activity of numerous neurons is required if there is to be a recordable wave from the scalp leads. One estimate is that approximately 6 cm² of cortical surface must be synchronously activated in order for there to be a potential recorded at the scalp. Scalp potentials are volume conducted through the skull and scalp, which results in considerable attenuation of the activity.

Generators of Specific Potentials

Posterior Dominant Rhythm: The posterior dominant rhythm (PDR) is the idling rhythm seen over the occipital regions with eyes closed. In adults the most visible rhythms are in the 8–13 Hz (alpha frequency) range, whereas they are much slower in young children. The PDR is attenuated by eye opening and mental effort.

The exact generator is not completely understood, but it is believed that thalamic pacemakers guide occipital generation of the rhythm, although recent data suggest that the reverse may be true—an occipitally generated alpha rhythm.[1]

Sleep spindles are seen in light sleep and disappear in the awake state, as well in deeper stages of sleep. There is evidence that neurons in the thalamic reticular nucleus change firing pattern, generating approximately 20 Hz activity in approximately the same circadian relationship.[2] These drive thalamocortical neurons, which then help to generate the scalp-recorded potentials that we see as sleep spindles. While the exact purpose is not known, they may play a role in memory consolidation, which is the integration of short-term working memory into long memory.[3]

Vertex waves accompany the sleep spindles, sometimes fusing with one to produce a K complex. Vertex waves are present in light sleep and drowsiness, disappearing with deeper stages of sleep. As with many potentials, the generator is not completely identified but seems to involve thalamocortical connections with particular involvement of sensorimotor cortex related to vision, hearing, and touch.[4] From this localization, it has been hypothesized that vertex waves are involved in sensory experiences during sleep.

Mu rhythm is an arch-shaped potential with negative polarity which is present in the waking state, chiefly around C3 and/or C4 electrodes. It is suppressed by moving the contralateral arm or even thinking about moving the arm. The origin seems to be in the motor cortex but is likely modulated by prefrontal projections which may be related to movement initiation.[5]

GENERATION OF ABNORMAL EEG ACTIVITY

Abnormal EEG activity can be *epileptiform* or *nonepileptiform*. The most important nonepileptiform activities are slowing and suppression. *Slowing* and *suppression* indicate a disordered function of the neurons, whereas epileptiform activity indicates abnormal synchronous activity.

Attenuation and Suppression

Attenuation and suppression are terms sometimes used interchangeably, but they have different causes and implications. *Attenuation* refers to reduction in the amplitude of the EEG. *Suppression* is a lower amplitude but, in addition, it is often associated with a loss of faster frequencies.[6] Attenuation can be normal, as when the PDR is attenuated by eye opening. Suppression is always pathologic.

Focal attenuation can indicate a cortical lesion or reversible cortical dysfunction. Focal attenuation could also result from an increase in tissue between the cortex and the recording electrode (e.g., subdural hematoma). Focal attenuation can also occur when there is smear of electrode gel between electrodes.

Generalized attenuation may suggest a generalized cortical injury or transient dysfunction. However, an attenuated EEG in adults could be normal as long as the frequency composition is normal; a tense individual may have a low-voltage fast background, not showing the normal appearance of relaxed wakefulness.

Slow Activity

Focal irregular slow activity is usually due to a localized subcortical structural lesion (or dysfunction). Focal slow activity seems to be a result of deafferentation of the cortex from subcortical structures.

Generalized bisynchronous slow activity can be intermittent or continuous. It may be due to disordered circuit loops between the cortex and thalamus. This type of abnormality is reported in conditions affecting both cortical and subcortical structures, as well as in a number of toxic/metabolic encephalopathies and in deep midline lesions.

Generalized asynchronous slow activity has a broad differential diagnosis, though it usually indicates encephalopathy of some sort. This pattern is likely due to poor synchrony and rhythmicity of regions of the cortex.

Epileptiform Activity

Epileptiform activity involves abnormal synchronous activation of many neurons. Corresponding to focal epileptiform activity at the cellular level is a wave of depolarization called the paroxysmal depolarization shift (PDS).

Paroxysmal Depolarization Shift (PDS): The PDS is the fundamental electrophysiological substrate of focal epileptiform activity. The PDS cannot be recorded with scalp electrodes but requires cortical microelectrodes for detection. The PDS is an extracellular field potential in which there is a wave of depolarization followed by a wave of repolarization. High-amplitude afferent input to the cortex produces depolarization of cortical neurons sufficient to trigger repetitive action potentials, which in turn contribute to the potentials recorded at the surface. Repolarization due to inactivation of interneurons is followed by a brief period of hyperpolarization.

Cyclic depolarization and repolarization is believed to be the cortical counterpart to rhythmic spike-wave discharges. The rhythmicity may be at least in part due to the inability of cortical neurons to sustain prolonged high-frequency discharges but, in addition, is likely due to built-in circuitry to inhibit repetitive discharges. The repetitive discharge is not terminated by neuronal exhaustion but rather by this mechanism of inactivation. There may be membrane effects independent of active inhibition to terminate seizures, yet the exact mechanisms of seizure termination are not completely understood.

Seizures: There is a gray zone between interictal activity and ictal activity. Repetitive discharge on the crest of the PDS may be prolonged to produce a seizure. In addition, a prolonged discharge of one neuron may then entrain a group of adjacent neurons to depolarize and repetitively discharge, thereby producing expansion of the region of epileptogenic activity and prolongation of the discharge to a duration which is clearly ictal.

Spikes and Sharp Waves: Sustained depolarization of a neuron can result in multiple action potentials on the crest of the depolarization. If one neuron is activated by this burst, there will likely be no neurologic symptoms, and the discharge will not be recorded from scalp electrodes. However, if there is synchronous activation of multiple neurons, this can be recorded on scalp electrodes as a spike or sharp wave.

Traditional teaching has been that at least 6 cm² of cortex has to have synchronized activity for a spike to be seen by scalp electrodes. However, more recent data indicate that more than 90% of spikes with a cortical area of at least 10 cm² were detected extracranially, whereas only 10% of spikes of cortical area less than 10 cm² were detected, and none of spikes of less than 6 cm² synchronous cortical activity was detected.[7] These are lower limits: most scalp-recorded spikes are associated with synchronous cortical activity of 20–30 cm².

PART 3

Seizure Semiology and Classification

3.1

Definitions

KARL E. MISULIS AND BASSEL ABOU-KHALIL

In this chapter, we discuss some of the important terms used in the definition and classification of seizures.

Semiology is the study of signs and *seizure semiology* is the study of the signs and symptoms that are due to the electrocerebral activity which produces seizures. The semiologic findings of a seizure are as important as electrographic findings in determining the seizure type and, when focal, the localization of its focus.

A *seizure* is defined by the International League Against Epilepsy (ILAE) as "a transient occurrence of signs and/or symptoms due to abnormal excessive or synchronous neuronal activity in the brain."[1] Thus seizures are events, whereas *epilepsy* is a disorder, one important manifestation of which is recurrent unprovoked seizures. In 2005, the ILAE defined epilepsy as "a disorder of the brain characterized by an enduring predisposition to generate epileptic seizures and by the neurobiological, cognitive, psychological, and social consequences of this condition." In 2014, the ILAE revised the definition of epilepsy as "a disease of the brain defined by any of the following conditions[2]:

- At least two unprovoked (or reflex) seizures occurring >24 hours apart;
- One unprovoked (or reflex) seizure and a probability of further seizures similar to the general recurrence risk (at least 60%) after two unprovoked seizures, occurring over the next 10 years;
- Diagnosis of an epilepsy syndrome."

The traditional definition of epilepsy required at least two unprovoked seizures. The new definition states that one unprovoked seizure is sufficient to diagnose epilepsy if there is also evidence of enduring seizure tendency such that the risk of another unprovoked seizure is similar to that expected after two unprovoked seizures. Examples of this may include a single seizure occurring more than a month after a stroke or a single seizure with epileptiform activity on electroencephalogram (EEG). In these situations the neurologist is likely to prescribe an anti-seizure medication (ASM) due to the high risk of recurrence.

All patients with epilepsy have seizures, whereas not all patients who have had a seizure have epilepsy. For example, seizures due to severe hyponatremia do not qualify as epilepsy even if multiple since severe hyponatremia is known to provoke seizures, and the seizure tendency is resolved after the hyponatremia is corrected.

As a note on terminology, we use the convention of *anti-seizure medication* rather than the former *anti-epileptic drug* (AED). The reason for this is based on the argument that the medications do not directly solve the disorder of epilepsy but rather address the seizures as manifestations of the epilepsy.

3.2

Overview of Seizure Semiology

BASSEL ABOU-KHALIL

Ictal semiology refers to the signs and symptoms associated with seizures.[1] Many of the definitions are derived from the glossary of descriptive terminology for ictal semiology, reported by the International League Against Epilepsy (ILAE) task force on classification and terminology.[2]

MOTOR MANIFESTATIONS

Motor manifestations are most often positive, with a muscle contraction that produces a movement. Negative motor manifestations, with a decrease in muscle contraction, are less common.

Elementary motor manifestations include

- *Tonic activity*: Sustained muscle contraction:
  - May result in a posture (usually involving contraction of several muscles)
  - *Versive*: Sustained deviation of the eyes or the head to one side
  - *Dystonic*: Abnormal posture with a rotatory motion
- *Epileptic spasms*: Proximal and truncal tonic activity more sustained than a myoclonic jerk but yet very short in duration
- *Myoclonic activity*: Very brief contraction usually lasting less than 100 msec
- *Negative myoclonic activity*: Interruption of muscle tone for a fraction of a second
- *Clonic activity*: Sustained rhythmic jerking
  - *Without a march*: Remains in the same body part
  - *With Jacksonian march*: Spreads unilaterally to adjacent body parts as a result of the spread of seizure activity along the motor strip
- *Tonic-clonic activity*: Initial tonic posturing that evolves to clonic activity
- *Atonic activity*: Decreased muscle tone usually lasting more than 1 sec

Automatisms are repetitive coordinated motor activity that is not purposeful, though it may look voluntary. Automatisms are usually associated with altered sensorium and amnesia.

- *Perseverative automatisms* involve continuation of pre-ictal activity
- De novo *automatisms* start after seizure onset. Automatisms can be classified by the body part involved.
  - *Oro-alimentary automatisms*: Lip smacking, chewing, swallowing, lip licking
  - *Manual automatisms*: Involving the hand
  - *Pedal automatisms*: Involving the feet
- *Reactive or manipulative automatisms* imply interaction with nearby objects, for example picking on bedsheets or fumbling with an object.
- *Nonmanipulative automatisms* are rhythmic movements that are independent of environment. If involving the hand they are referred to by the acronym RINCH—*rhythmic ictal nonclonic hand movements*.
- *Gestural automatisms* are movements commonly used to enhance speech.
- *Hyperkinetic automatisms* imply a rapid sequence of movements with frenetic character. Examples are thrashing, kicking, pelvic thrusting, body rocking, or bicycling motions.
- *Gelastic automatisms* produce involuntary laughter.
- *Dacrystic automatisms* produce involuntary crying.

SENSORY PHENOMENA

There are a broad range of sensory manifestations of seizures. Sensory phenomena may involve any sensory modality.

- *Elementary sensory manifestation*: Unformed sensations involving a single primary sensory modality, including
  - *Somatosensory*: Tingling, numbness, pain, or a sense of movement; may have a Jacksonian march with sensation moving to adjacent body parts, reflecting

spread of electrical activity over the sensory strip.

- *Visual*: Flickering or flashing lights, simple patterns, spots, sensation of the eyes moving, visual loss.
- *Auditory*: Single tones or buzzing, humming, or ringing sounds; loss of hearing.
- *Vertigo*: Dizziness.
- *Olfactory hallucinations*: Most often unpleasant.
- *Gustatory hallucinations*: Most commonly metallic taste.
- *Cephalic sensation*, and nonspecific sensation with variable descriptions including tingling, fullness, pressure, or lightheadedness.
- *Complex sensory manifestations*: Seeing people or hearing music.
- *Sensory illusions*: Alteration/distortion of perception.

AUTONOMIC MANIFESTATIONS
Autonomic manifestations include

- *Subjective autonomic experiences*, such as an epigastric sensation, nausea, feeling hot, a sense of palpitation, or a sense of flushing;

- *Objective clinical manifestations*, such as pupillary dilation, pallor or flushing, tachycardia or bradycardia, piloerection, vomiting, borborygmus, or flatulence.

EXPERIENTIAL PHENOMENA
Experiential phenomena include:

- *Affective experiences*, such as fear, euphoria, sadness;
- *Dysmnesic phenomena*: *Déjà vu* (inappropriate feeling of familiarity); *jamais vu* (inappropriate feeling of unfamiliarity), or *déjà vecu* (sensation that present events have been experienced before);
- *Dyscognitive phenomena*: Altered cognition, such as altered awareness, perception, attention, memory, or executive function.

In the new classification these were reclassified into two groups: *Emotional/Affective* (including agitation, anger, anxiety, crying, fear, laughing, paranoia, pleasure) and *Cognitive* (including acalculia, aphasia, attention impairment, *déjà vu* or *jamais vu*, dissociation, dysphasia, hallucinations, illusions, memory impairment, neglect, forced thinking, responsiveness impairment).

3.3

Seizure Classification

BASSEL ABOU-KHALIL

Seizure classifications schemes have evolved over time. The International League Against Epilepsy (ILAE) 1981 classification scheme was the most widely used until 2017.[1] This divided seizures into *partial*, *generalized*, and *unclassified* based on their onset. A newly revised classification scheme was released in 2017.[2] This citation should be in every neurologist's core reference list. The drives to revise the classification were multiple; among the enumerated reasons were

- Some seizure types, such as tonic seizures, can have either focal or generalized onset.
- Seizures that have an unobserved onset cannot be further classified in the 1981 classification scheme.
- The 1981 classification required a specification of level of consciousness, which is often not available in seizure description.
- Some terms in the 1981 classification, such as "simple partial" or "complex partial" are not easily understood by the public.
- The classification of partial seizures does not allow visualization of the ictal clinical activity.
- Some seizure types are not included in the 1981 scheme.

The new classification offers the following changes:

- Updates terminology for greater clarity and accessibility to the lay public;
- Identifies awareness as the aspect of consciousness to be used as one optional level for classification of focal seizures;
- Expands the classification categories for focal seizures based on the initial clinical manifestation; optional additional descriptors can be added in parentheses to describe manifestations during seizure progression;
- Allows some seizure types to have either a focal or generalized onset;

- Allows subclassification of seizures that have unknown onset;
- Includes previously unclassified seizure types.

As seen in Figures 3.3.1 and 3.3.2, there are a number of specific changes and among these are

- The term *focal* is used rather than *partial*.
- *Awareness* is the specific aspect of consciousness used to classify focal seizures.
- Multiple terms are no longer used, including "simple partial" (replaced by *focal aware*), "complex partial" (replaced by *focal impaired awareness*), "secondarily generalized" (replaced by *focal to bilateral tonic-clonic*), "psychic," and "dyscognitive."
- Certain seizure types can be of focal or generalized onset, including atonic, clonic, epileptic spasms, myoclonic, and tonic seizures.
- New focal seizure types include *automatisms*, *behavior arrest*, *hyperkinetic*, *autonomic*, *cognitive*, and *emotional*.
- New generalized seizure types include *absence with eyelid myoclonia*, *myoclonic absence*, *myoclonic-atonic*, and *myoclonic-tonic-clonic*.
- Seizures with unknown onset still have features that can be classified as *tonic-clonic*, *other motor*, or *nonmotor*.

Some specific characteristics of the revised classification deserve attention.

Focal refers to onset in one hemisphere, whether discrete in one restricted locus or more diffusely located throughout the hemisphere.

Generalized is still used to indicate seizures of generalized onset, but not for seizures which began focal and then became bilateral. The term *generalized* is reserved for seizures with generalized onset. The term *bilateral* is applied for tonic-clonic activity involving the whole body when the onset is focal.

ILAE 2017 Classification of Seizure Types Basic Version

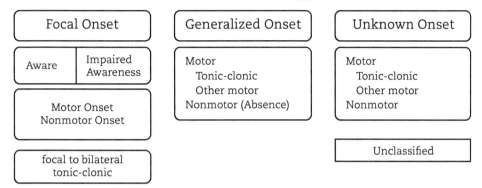

FIGURE 3.3.1 New 2017 seizure classification (basic) from the International League Against Epilepsy (ILAE).

Seizures of unknown onset can now be classified. The most common scenario is that of tonic-clonic seizures, where the beginning was unobserved or otherwise obscured. Another scenario is that of an episode of staring and unresponsiveness that can be either a focal impaired awareness seizure or a generalized absence seizure.

The term "*unclassified seizure*" should be used to designate an event which is likely to be a seizure but that occurs without sufficient information to otherwise classify it. The term should not be used for events that are probably not seizures.

Awareness specifies preserved awareness during a seizure, rather than awareness of whether a seizure has occurred. Awareness can be on a continuum so that any change in awareness results in classification with impaired awareness, even if not totally unaware. Also, impaired awareness is used to describe a seizure that has impairment during

ILAE 2017 Classification of Seizure Types Expanded Version

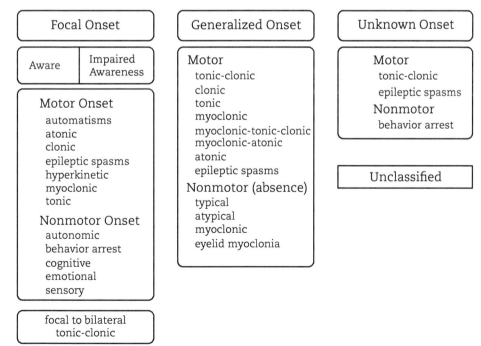

FIGURE 3.3.2 New 2017 seizure classification (expanded) from the International League Against Epilepsy (ILAE).

any phase of the seizure, not necessarily during the entirety of the episode.

Listed here are some examples of how focal seizures would be classified based on their early manifestations.

A seizure where a patient was unable to understand language and then had impaired awareness and then clonic left arm jerks would be termed *focal, impaired awareness, cognitive seizure (progressing to clonic left arm activity)*.

A seizure that starts with altered awareness, then oro-alimentary automatisms, then dystonic posturing of the right arm would be termed *focal, impaired awareness, automatisms seizure (progressing to right arm dystonic posturing)*.

A seizure that starts with a rising epigastric sensation followed by a feeling of fear, where it is not known if awareness was impaired, would be classified as *focal, autonomic seizure (progressing to emotional manifestation or progressing to fear)*. This illustrates that classification of awareness is optional and can be bypassed if not known.

A seizure that starts with fear then right arm tonic posturing without altered awareness would be classified as *focal aware emotional seizures (progressing to right arm tonic posturing)*.

3.4

Seizure Semiology by Seizure Type and Seizure Localization

BASSEL ABOU-KHALIL

FOCAL ONSET SEIZURES BY TYPE

Focal Aware Seizures

Focal aware seizures are associated with preserved consciousness throughout the seizure.

Focal aware seizures may have:

- Motor signs,
- Somatosensory or special sensory symptoms,
- Autonomic symptoms or signs,
- Emotional or cognitive manifestations (previously referred to as psychic or experiential),
- Combinations of the above.

The new proposal by the International League Against Epilepsy (ILAE) suggested dividing these seizures into *motor* or *nonmotor* (including autonomic, behavior arrest, cognitive, emotional, or sensory dysfunction). When focal aware seizures are purely subjective they may be called *auras* or *isolated auras*.

The clinical manifestations of focal aware seizures depend on the brain region involved in the ictal discharge. This brain region may or may not be the epileptogenic zone; at times, the clinical manifestations reflect seizure spread to adjacent or even distant regions. Despite that, seizure manifestations may have important lateralizing and localizing value. Focal clonic or tonic motor activity, somatosensory experiences, visual auras, and auditory auras have value in the localization and lateralization of the epileptogenic zone. However, some auras, such as an odd feeling in the head or generalized body tingling, are nonspecific with respect to localization.

Focal Impaired Awareness

Focal impaired awareness seizures involve altered awareness during the seizure, ranging from subtle confusion to complete loss of contact. There may be some recollection of events or total amnesia. They may start with loss of awareness or may have a focal aware onset.

It is not always possible to tell if a seizure is focal aware or focal impaired awareness since decreased ability to respond verbally may be due to aphasia or motor inhibition as well as to altered awareness. Focal impaired awareness seizures may manifest only with altered awareness or may include motor activity, most commonly automatisms. Focal impaired awareness seizures may arise from any brain region, but they most often originate in the temporal lobe, followed by the frontal lobe.[1] The manifestations of focal impaired awareness seizures can vary with lobe of origin, as will be discussed later.

As noted earlier, the classification of awareness can be bypassed if information is not available. The motor-onset and nonmotor-onset categories applied to focal aware seizures also apply to focal impaired awareness seizures. The motor-onset category includes seizure types that were previously only listed under generalized onset. This includes tonic, atonic, myoclonic, and clonic seizures, and epileptic spasms. These focal seizure types most often originate in the frontal lobe. The motor activity can affect one side or one part of the body, or it can be bilateral as a result of rapid propagation of the ictal discharge. The remaining focal motor seizure categories "automatisms" and "hyperkinetic" are not shared with generalized-onset seizures. The nonmotor-onset category includes autonomic, behavioral arrest, cognitive, emotional, and sensory seizures.

Focal Seizure Evolving to Bilateral Tonic-Clonic Seizure

Focal to bilateral tonic clonic seizures may evolve directly from focal aware onset, directly from focal impaired awareness onset, or may evolve from focal aware to focal impaired awareness to bilateral tonic-clonic seizure. The transition usually involves some lateralizing features, the most important of which is versive head turning opposite the side of seizure onset. There may also be contralateral tonic or clonic motor activity.

During generalized tonic contraction, there may be an asymmetry, with arm extension contralateral and arm flexion ipsilateral to the seizure focus.[2] This is designated *figure-of-four* posturing. The clonic activity may be symmetrical and synchronous, or it may have some asymmetry and asynchrony. The clonic activity may be more pronounced on the side of seizure onset, but may also become more prominent on the ipsilateral side late in the seizure. The clonic activity may even stop earlier on one side of the body. Late ipsilateral head deviation may be seen in some individuals. Asynchrony may produce some relatively low-amplitude side-to-side head or trunk motions.

Clonic activity usually decreases in frequency progressively, such that longer pauses develop between jerks over time. The generalized tonic-clonic phase rarely lasts more than 2 min. Following the end of the clonic activity, it is common to observe stertorous respiration (deep, loud, snoring respiration).

The speed of recovery from a focal to bilateral seizure depends to a large extent on seizure duration and severity. Tongue biting is common, most often involving the side of the tongue. Incontinence of urine, and less often of stool, may also occur. After awakening, patients commonly report headache and generalized muscle soreness.

Focal Seizure Semiology by Localization

Symptoms and signs of focal-onset seizures can, to a certain extent, help to localize the site of origin of the discharge to one of the following localizations:

- Frontal,
- Temporal,
- Parietal,
- Occipital,
- Insular.

Of the focal seizures, temporal origin is the most common, with frontal origin next in frequency, followed by parietal, occipital, and insular origin.[3]

Temporal

Temporal lobe epilepsy (TLE) is the most common symptomatic/cryptogenic focal epilepsy. While some characteristic manifestations of temporal lobe seizures have long been recognized, the advent of video electroencephalogram (EEG) monitoring and its use in presurgical evaluation have had a great impact on the full understanding of temporal lobe seizure semiology. TLE is often refractory to medical therapy and is often amenable to surgical treatment. The surgical outcome depends on accurate localization of the epileptogenic zone. The analysis of clinical semiology in patients who were seizure-free after temporal lobectomy versus those still experiencing seizures has helped to identify manifestations characteristic of temporal lobe origin and those that suggest extratemporal localization. In addition, specific seizure manifestations were analyzed for their lateralizing and localizing value within the temporal lobe.

Aura

Most patients with TLE report a seizure aura. This is particularly true in mesial TLE, by far the largest TLE group. In a selected patient group with proven mesial temporal lobe origin, more than 90% of patients reported an aura. An aura is most common with right TLE and least common with bitemporal epilepsy. Most common was an epigastric aura. Although no aura is totally specific for temporal lobe seizures, some are very strongly associated with a temporal lobe origin, particularly viscerosensory (such as epigastric sensation) and experiential or psychic auras (such as *déjà-vu*). Both of these types of aura are more likely with right temporal foci, but this is only a trend. Whereas viscerosensory auras are generally more common in mesial TLE associated with hippocampal sclerosis, experiential auras and especially *déjà-vu* are more common in the benign familial TLE syndrome.[4]

Multiple sequential auras in the same seizure suggest a nondominant localization, most often temporal. Chills and goosebumps are more common with left temporal foci, and if they are unilateral, they are usually ipsilateral to the seizure focus. Olfactory and gustatory auras are uncommon mesial TLE auras. They are associated with mesial temporal tumors. An auditory aura is very suggestive of lateral temporal origin. This can be a positive (buzzing or ringing sound) or negative symptom (loss of hearing). The auditory aura is a hallmark of an autosomal dominant form of TLE. Cephalic auras (nonspecific sensation in the head) are more likely extratemporal. The same is true of somatosensory and visual auras. Absence of an aura is more likely with bitemporal epilepsy.

Motor

The focal impaired awareness phase of mesial temporal lobe seizures usually starts with motor arrest or motionless staring, oro-alimentary automatisms, or nonspecific extremity automatisms.

Oro-alimentary automatisms, mainly lip smacking, chewing, and swallowing movements, are suggestive of temporal lobe involvement. However, they are not specific for TLE. They may reflect the spread of seizure activity to the temporal lobe from other locations and can also be seen in a more subtle form in absence seizures or postictally in a variety of seizure types.

Spitting and drinking automatisms suggest right temporal localization.[5] Automatisms with preserved responsiveness also favor right temporal localization.[6,7]

Extremity automatisms are less specific and can be seen in temporal as well as extratemporal epilepsy. However, the progression of these automatisms is more gradual in TLE. In extratemporal epilepsy, they tend to have an abrupt bilateral onset and a frenzied character. The most common upper extremity automatisms are manipulative, involving interaction with the environment, for example, picking on clothing or bedsheets or fumbling with objects. Manipulative automatisms in isolation have no lateralizing value. However, the extremity contralateral to the side of the focus is often involved in dystonic posturing or immobility and may therefore not demonstrate automatisms.[8] In this instance, manipulative automatisms will predominate in the extremity ipsilateral to the seizure focus. This may lead to confusion for the inexperienced observer who may interpret repetitive automatisms as clonic activity. The less common nonmanipulative upper extremity automatisms involve rhythmic repetitive motions that are either distal (milking, pill rolling, grasping, fist clenching, or opening–closing motions) or proximal (often with a circular motion like waving or stirring). These automatisms tend to be contralateral and often precede dystonic posturing.[9,10,11,12]

Seizures originating in the temporal pole often manifest with hyperkinetic automatisms, similar to what is seen in orbitofrontal focal impaired awareness seizures. This is related to seizure spread to the orbitofrontal region.[13,14]

Defined in the strictest manner, dystonic posturing is an unnatural position that includes a rotatory component. Dystonic posturing has been associated with ictal activation in the contralateral putamen. There is evidence of a spectrum of posturing, with classical dystonic posturing at one extreme and simple immobility of an extremity at the other, including subtle posturing without a clearly demonstrated rotatory component in between. Dystonic posturing has a strong lateralizing value in TLE. However, as with any other manifestations, late occurrence could represent activation of the contralateral side and may therefore have a lesser value.

Head turning in TLE has been the subject of great controversy. Current evidence suggests that early head turning, particularly that associated with dystonic posturing, tends to be ipsilateral to the epileptogenic temporal lobe.[15] Its mechanism is not well-defined. Some have suggested it could represent neglect of the contralateral hemisphere. However, in many instances, the early head turning is of a tonic nature, which raises the possibility of a motor drive, possibly from the basal ganglia. In one study, head turning within 30 sec of seizure onset, in association with dystonic posturing and not leading to bilateral tonic-clonic activity, was strictly ipsilateral to the temporal lobe of seizure origin. Late head turning, on the other hand, is more likely to be contralateral.[16] Head turning that leads to bilateral tonic-clonic activity can have a tonic or clonic character and has been termed *versive* or *adversive*. Versive head turning is almost always contralateral to the hemisphere of seizure origin. However, an ipsilateral versive head turn has been noted toward the end of a focal to bilateral tonic-clonic seizure in some patients.

Language

Language manifestations are potentially very valuable in lateralizing temporal lobe seizure origin. Ictal speech arrest does not seem to have lateralizing value. It may be due to disruption of language mechanisms, loss of awareness/responsiveness, or a positive or negative motor effect. There is a suggestion, however, that in temporal focal aware seizures, speech arrest could represent aphasia and may thus be lateralizing to the dominant temporal lobe. Global aphasia may occur in association with localized focal aware seizures restricted in the temporal lobe, including the basal temporal language area. Chronic temporal lobe lesions do not produce global aphasia. However, acute electrical stimulation of Wernicke's area and basal temporal language area does produce global aphasia, perhaps because compensatory mechanisms have not had the chance to be activated. Global aphasia in focal aware seizures therefore could be consistent with a temporal localization.

Well-formed ictal language strongly suggests a nondominant (usually right) temporal lobe involvement. The well-formed ictal language in some patients with right temporal lobe seizures has a tinge of fear. For example, it is not uncommon for patients to utter "I'm sick, I'm sick," or "I'm going to die, don't let me die." In most instances, however, the patient does not remember these utterances, and fear may not be a known component of the semiology. This has been referred to as "ictal verbal help-seeking."[17]

Single words or nonverbal vocalizations have no lateralizing value.

Ictal jargon is rare but has been associated with dominant temporal lobe foci. It may reflect a partial disruption of language mechanisms, as seen in Wernicke's aphasia.

Post-ictal aphasia is strongly associated with a left dominant temporal localization. In one study, all patients with right temporal seizures were able to correctly read a test sentence within 1 min of seizure termination, while patients with dominant left temporal foci had disruption of reading for more than 1 min. In patients with atypical language representation, the lateralizing significance of language dysfunction has to be reinterpreted.[18,19]

Other Manifestations
A variety of other ictal manifestations may have lateralizing value.

- Ictal vomiting has been associated with right-sided temporal foci. However, this is not uniform, and vomiting may also be a manifestation of extratemporal foci.
- Ictal spitting, ictal flatulence, and ictal drinking are more common with right temporal foci.
- Unilateral eye blinking tends to be ipsilateral to seizure origin.
- Focal facial motor activity early in the seizure favors a lateral neocortical origin.[20]

Transition from Focal to Bilateral
The motor manifestations during transition to bilateral tonic-clonic activity can be very valuable in lateralization. Versive head turning, focal tonic posturing, and focal clonic activity are most often contralateral to seizure origin.[21] Occasionally, however, they can be falsely lateralizing if there is contralateral seizure spread prior to bilateral tonic-clonic activity.

Post-ictal Manifestations

- Post-ictal cough has been found predominantly following right temporal seizures.

- Post-ictal nose wiping tends to be performed with the hand ipsilateral to the seizure focus.
- Post-ictal urinary urgency suggests a right temporal localization.

None of the above signs is sufficient in isolation. However, the combination of several signs and symptoms can be a powerful tool in localizing and lateralizing TLE. The addition of semiological information unquestionably enhances the localizing ability of the presurgical evaluation.

Frontal
The frontal lobe is the second most common source of seizures after the temporal lobe. A great variety of seizure manifestations can be related to frontal lobe origin.[22]

Aura
An aura is less common with frontal lobe origin than with temporal lobe origin. There is only a limited specificity in auras. Autonomic auras with abdominal sensation are more likely to be of temporal lobe origin. However, frontal lobe limbic seizures may have autonomic auras including epigastric sensation. These autonomic auras have been ascribed to the orbitofrontal and cingulate regions.

Somatosensory auras are generally ascribed to activation of the primary sensory cortex. However, frontal lobe seizures originating in the supplementary sensorimotor area are frequently associated with a sensory aura due to activation of the supplementary sensory area. The sensory auras related to supplementary motor seizures generally do not have a march, are more often proximal, and may be bilateral in distribution, although a contralateral occurrence is most likely. Forced thinking may be seen with dorsolateral frontal lobe origin.

Perhaps the most common aura in frontal lobe seizures is the nonspecific cephalic sensation, which has no localizing value. It has been suggested that isolated auras are a common feature of temporal lobe but not frontal lobe epilepsy.

Motor
Activation of the primary motor cortex is well-known to be associated with clonic activity. Focal clonic or tonic-clonic seizures therefore are most likely originating in the primary motor cortex. Focal cortical myoclonus is another ictal manifestation originating in the primary motor cortex. If motor activity involves the lower extremity, this

suggests mesial localization, while facial involvement suggests inferior frontal localization. The localizing value of clonic activity is greatest when awareness is totally preserved. If awareness is impaired, it is likely that the motor seizure manifestations reflect seizure spread to the motor cortex from elsewhere.

Seizures originating in the supplementary sensorimotor area tend to be asymmetrical tonic or postural seizures. They are characterized by posturing that can affect one limb, two limbs, or all four extremities. If the seizure origin is in the supplementary motor area, they will usually be focal aware seizures, with no alteration of consciousness. Supplementary motor seizures are a notable exception to the rule that bilateral seizure activity should be accompanied by loss of consciousness. These seizures tend to be brief in duration, tend to cluster, and tend to be predominantly nocturnal, arising out of sleep. The posturing of the extremities is predominantly proximal, while the hands and fingers or feet and toes seem to be free. Patients will frequently wiggle the distal extremities. There is often a vocalization of moaning or groaning, and the patient reports being unable to breathe. Supplementary sensorimotor seizures are occasionally precipitated by startle, most commonly by unexpected auditory stimuli, less often by unexpected somatosensory stimuli.

Seizures originating in the supplementary sensorimotor area may occasionally manifest with inhibition of movement. There may be ictal paralysis or just inhibition of motion without paralysis, with loss of ability to move or speak. These seizures are usually focal aware or may start as focal aware seizures with later impaired awareness. The ictal paralysis may be followed by positive motor (tonic or clonic) activity in the same affected extremity or may be accompanied by positive motor activity in a different body part on the same side. The ictal inhibition is presumed secondary to seizure activity in a negative motor area, often seen adjacent to the supplementary sensorimotor area. Since the seizure origin is in the mesial frontal cortex, there is often no recorded interictal or ictal EEG activity due to unfavorable dipole orientation. These seizures are frequently misdiagnosed as psychogenic. The correct diagnosis is often reached on observation of evolution to bilateral tonic-clonic seizure activity after the withdrawal of anti-seizure medications in the epilepsy monitoring unit.

Bizarre focal impaired awareness seizures have been ascribed to seizure origin in the cingulate gyrus or orbitofrontal region, but they may also arise in other regions of the frontal lobe and even outside the frontal lobe, usually manifesting after spread to the cingulate gyrus or orbitofrontal region. A longer latency between electrical seizure onset and hypermotor behaviors suggests an extrafrontal origin.

Hypermotor seizures are characterized by frenetic gestural automatisms (also referred to as hypermotor behavior) that are often bilateral, unless there is associated contralateral posturing. These automatisms can be bizarre and can be associated with bizarre vocalizations and verbalizations, including expletives. These seizures tend to be short and associated with only brief post-ictal manifestations unless there is spread to the temporal lobe.

The presence of *unilateral posturing and rotation along the body axis*, such as with turning prone, favor a mesial frontal origin, while severe agitation favors an orbitofrontal localization.[23] Again, the clinical features and the frequent absence of interictal epileptiform activity, as well as absence of rhythmic ictal EEG activity or its masking by artifact, have frequently resulted in the misdiagnosis of psychogenic seizure events.

Ictal pouting (also referred to as "*chapeau de gendarme*"), defined as a symmetrical and sustained lowering of labial commissures with contraction of chin, is suggestive of anterior cingulate involvement. This sign is usually associated with hypermotor behavior.[24]

Gelastic seizures are short seizures characterized by sudden unprovoked laughter and are best known as a seizure type originating from hypothalamic hamartomas.[25] However, they may also be seen with frontal cingulate as well as mesial-basal temporal seizure origin. Frontal and hypothalamic gelastic seizures are usually not associated with emotion, while temporal gelastic seizures seem to be. The gelastic seizures of frontal cingulate and hypothalamic origin may have preserved awareness, while those of temporal origin are associated with altered awareness after the initial sense of mirth. Frontal gelastic seizures may be accompanied by hypermotor manifestations or tonic posturing.

Seizures originating in the anterior-mesial frontal region at times imitate absence seizures through rapid secondary bilateral synchrony. These seizures are frequently referred to as *frontal absences*. They can clinically be characterized by altered responsiveness and arrest of activity for a few seconds with rapid return to baseline and minimal post-ictal manifestations. Such seizures can be totally indistinguishable from generalized absence seizures, except for the presence of a frontal lesion and at times the presence of consistent asymmetry on EEG. Frontal lobe origin seizures can imitate a variety of other generalized seizure types, including generalized tonic, generalized atonic, and generalized tonic-clonic seizures. Frontal lobe seizures are recognized to have a more rapid spread to the contralateral hemisphere. This is partly why falling (drop attacks) and incontinence seem more likely with frontal lobe seizures.

Seizures originating in the frontal operculum are characterized by hypersalivation, oral-facial apraxia, and, at times, facial clonic activity.

Seizures originating in the dorsolateral frontal lobe may manifest with tonic posturing of the extremities and versive eye and head deviation. The head deviation preceding evolution to tonic-clonic activity is contralateral, but early head turning can be in either direction.

The lateralizing value of signs in frontal lobe seizures may be less than with temporal lobe seizures due to the propensity for rapid contralateral spread and contralateral hemisphere activation.

It is important to recognize that seizures originating in the frontal lobe, particularly in the orbitofrontal region, may manifest after propagating to the temporal lobe, with a semiology typical of mesial temporal lobe seizures.

Parietal

The parietal lobe is the next most likely source of seizures after the temporal and frontal lobes.

Aura

The best recognized manifestation of parietal lobe origin is a sensory aura, particularly if there is an associated march. The sensation can be described as numbness, tingling, pins and needles, burning, or pain. It can also be nondescript. Less common auras that suggest parietal lobe origin include vertigo, difficulty localizing body position in space, or sensation that a body part is moving or an extremity is absent.

Sensory

Sensory march is strongly suggestive of a post-central, primary sensory cortex involvement, contralateral to the ictal discharge. Sensory aura without march can originate in the second sensory area, which is located over the parietal operculum. The sensory manifestations from the second sensory area are most often contralateral, but they are occasionally ipsilateral or bilateral.

Motor

Focal weakness has also been described with parietal foci. Seizures with focal weakness have been referred to as *focal inhibitory motor seizures* or *focal atonic seizures*.[26] They frequently have a preceding sensory aura.

Most patients with parietal lobe epilepsy have no parietal lobe symptoms but instead manifestations resulting from spread to the occipital, temporal, or frontal lobe.

Common manifestations with frontal lobe propagation include

- Contralateral tonic posturing;
- Focal clonic activity;
- Generalized asymmetrical tonic posturing;
- Head and eye deviation, described in almost 50% of patients.

When there is propagation to the temporal lobe, focal impaired awareness seizures can be characterized by

- Staring,
- Relative immobility with minimal automatisms,
- Oro-alimentary automatisms.

Occipital

Aura

Sensory auras suggesting occipital origin are

- *Visual aura*, and this is the key manifestation that suggests occipital lobe origin.
- *Elementary visual hallucinations* strongly suggest involvement of primary visual cortex. These hallucinations may be black or white or colored. They can be flashing or steady. They can be stationary or moving. There may be distortion of vision, and there may also be a loss of vision. Ictal blindness can be a blackout or a whiteout. If this is in one field, it strongly suggests seizure activity contralateral to that field. More complex visual hallucinations, such as ones involving scenes, suggest involvement of the occipitotemporal junction.
- *Auditory hallucinations, vertigo, and focal sensory experiences* may also be seen but

suggest seizure spread to the lateral temporal or parietal regions.

Motor

Motor symptoms suggesting occipital origin include

- Bilateral blinking,
- Nystagmoid eye movements,
- Eye deviation, usually contralateral.

One distinctive feature of occipital lobe seizures that develop and propagate posteriorly is the slow progression of ictal manifestations. For example, the eye deviation that is seen with occipital lobe origin tends to be much slower than that noted with frontal lobe origin. However, clinical assurance of occipital localization is less than perfect.[27]

Some studies suggest that manifestations of seizures originating in the occipital lobe are most commonly related to seizure spread to the temporal or frontal lobe. Seizure spread to the temporal lobe commonly manifests with oro-alimentary automatisms, while seizure spread to the frontal lobe may produce asymmetrical tonic posturing. Evolution to bilateral tonic-clonic activity is common with frontal lobe propagation. When different seizures in the same patient alternate between temporal and frontal semiology, an occipital origin should be suspected, with variable routes of seizure propagation.

Insular

Insular epilepsy cannot be analyzed with scalp video-EEG studies since it is not possible to record from the insula with scalp electrodes. The semiology of insular epilepsy was elucidated only with analysis of seizures recorded with depth electrodes implanted in the insula.[28] Insular epilepsy may imitate temporal, parietal, or frontal epilepsy.

Aura

The most common subjective aura of seizure activity in the insula is laryngeal discomfort/constriction, shortness of breath, and paresthesias around the mouth. Sensory manifestations may also involve other body parts, usually contralaterally. With sensory manifestations, insular origin is suspected when paresthesias have large cutaneous territories, bilateral, painful, or accompanied by early olfactory, gustatory, viscerosensory, or auditory symptoms. Autonomic manifestations are common, with visceral sensations in the chest or abdomen.

Motor

Dysarthria or dysphonia may occur, at times extreme, with resultant muteness. Hypersalivation is very common. Seizure propagation to the frontal lobe may manifest with tonic spasm of the contralateral face and upper extremity and contralateral head and eye deviation. There may be hypermotor manifestations mimicking frontal lobe focal impaired awareness seizures. There may also be typical temporal semiology with spread to the temporal lobe.

Other Regions

Seizures very rarely start in subcortical regions. The best recognized are hypothalamic seizures from hypothalamic hamartomas.[29] The most typical seizure type is gelastic seizures (seizures with laughter), and some of these patients may also have dacrystic seizures (seizures with crying).

However, patients with hypothalamic hamartomas may also have other seizure types that seem to develop over time, including focal impaired awareness seizures, nongelastic focal aware seizures, focal to bilateral tonic-clonic seizures, and some other seizure types that appear generalized, such as atonic and tonic seizures and epileptic spasms.

There are also rare reports of seizures starting in cerebellar gangliogliomas, usually in infants.[30] These seizures are characterized by hemifacial twitching ipsilateral to the lesion and at times contralateral head and eye deviation or contralateral nystagmus.

GENERALIZED-ONSET SEIZURES

Generalized-onset seizures start simultaneously in both hemispheres. They vary considerably in severity of clinical manifestations. At one extreme are generalized tonic-clonic seizures and at the other are generalized absence seizures. The reason that generalized absence seizures are generalized yet so mild in clinical manifestations is that they involve a restricted bilateral frontoreticular network.

Generalized Absence Seizures

In the new classification scheme, these are classified as *generalized onset—nonmotor seizures*.

These seizures can occur in a variety of epileptic syndromes, particularly *childhood absence epilepsy* and *juvenile absence epilepsy*.[31] These seizures are characterized by a sudden onset without an aura, brief duration (usually less than 15 sec), and sudden termination without any post-ictal state. Typical generalized absence seizures are associated with generalized 2.5–4 Hz spike-and-wave activity.

Typically, there is suspension of awareness and arrest of activity during the episodes, but some motor manifestations are quite common. Absence seizures with only altered awareness or responsiveness are sometimes called *simple absence seizures*.

When absence seizures are associated with motor activity or autonomic manifestations, they were previously sometimes referred to as *complex absence seizures*. This term is not part of the official classification. Simple automatisms are the most common associated motor activity, particularly perseverative automatisms. Automatisms may include fumbling with an object that the patient was holding, rubbing a body part, or mouth movements such as licking lips. Automatisms are more likely with longer duration of absence seizure activity. Myoclonus is the next most common motor manifestation. This includes blinking and subtle twitching of fingers. Less commonly, there may be tonic features such as up-rolling of the eyes and slight stiffening of the neck with neck extension, or atonic components such as slight decrease of tone and slumping. Autonomic manifestations may occur, including pupillary dilation, piloerection, and, infrequently, incontinence.

At times, consciousness is partially preserved. This is more likely to occur in adults who have had persistent absence seizures from childhood. When there is some preservation of awareness but loss of responsiveness, patients may describe some subjective experiences that could erroneously suggest an aura. For example, lightheadedness or spaciness may be reported. In addition, some patients report confusion after the seizure. This usually reflects the effects of missing parts of a conversation rather than true confusion.

Atypical Absence Seizures

This variant of generalized absence seizures tends to occur in symptomatic generalized epilepsy, such as Lennox-Gastaut syndrome. The main distinction between typical and atypical absence seizures is electrographic, as the latter have a slower frequency of less than 2.5 Hz. Clinical distinctive features reported are a slower loss of awareness and a more gradual recovery, as well as perhaps more prominent motor manifestations.

Myoclonic Absences

These seizures differ from absence seizures by the presence of a very prominent clonic activity at the same frequency as the spike-and-wave discharges. They are associated with the typical 2.5–3.5 Hz spike-and-wave activity seen with typical absence seizures. The seizures in this syndrome tend to be harder to control.

Eyelid Myoclonia

These seizures consist of brief repetitive jerks of the eyelids with eyes rolling back and frequent associated neck extension. They occur predominantly in women, as part of an epileptic syndrome called *epilepsy with eyelid myoclonia* or *Jeavons syndrome*. Eyelid myoclonia may occur with or without associated absence and spike-and-wave activity.[32] Women with this condition are usually photosensitive and also have eye closure sensitivity.

Generalized Myoclonic Seizures

Generalized myoclonic seizures last a fraction of a second. They vary in severity from mild with a barely visible twitch to severe with massive myoclonus associated with falling. The myoclonic jerk may involve the whole body or the upper extremities or the head alone. Although they are usually bilateral, they could be unilateral with shifting lateralization. Myoclonic seizures are not associated with appreciable loss of consciousness because of their very brief duration. However, they often occur in clusters, and patients occasionally report some disruption of consciousness with a cluster of closely spaced generalized myoclonic seizures.

Generalized myoclonic seizures need to be distinguished from nonepileptic myoclonus, which can originate at any level of the central nervous system.

Generalized myoclonic seizures can be negative, with very brief loss of tone that may not be appreciated unless the affected extremities are elevated or engaged in other activity.

Generalized Clonic Seizures

These seizures, characterized by rhythmic clonic jerking, start with loss of consciousness. They are infrequent. They are seen in children with severe myoclonic epilepsy of infancy (Dravet syndrome) and in patients with progressive myoclonic epilepsies.

Generalized-Onset Tonic-Clonic Seizures

Generalized-onset tonic-clonic seizures do not have an aura, although they may be preceded by a prodrome, sometimes as a prolonged feeling of being seizure-prone. The onset is abrupt, with loss of consciousness, then generalized tonic contraction. In patients with juvenile myoclonic epilepsy, it is common for generalized tonic-clonic seizures to start with repetitive myoclonic jerks, then called myoclonic-tonic-clonic seizures.

Generalized tonic-clonic seizures may also evolve from generalized absence seizures. The tonic phase may be symmetrical, but asymmetries may be seen. In particular, versive head turning is common and may change direction from one seizure to the other. Versive head turning alone does not mean that the seizure onset was focal.[33] The tonic phase may show evolution from flexion to extension. The eyes are usually half open and the mouth is open. A loud vocalization may result from contraction of the diaphragm and contracted glottis. Cyanosis is most likely to occur during the tonic phase of the seizure. Clonic activity evolves from the tonic phase, initially with high frequency, but progressing to lower frequency and larger amplitude. After the jerking stops, the individual is limp and unresponsive, with stertorous respiration. Post-ictal confusion and sleep are common. The post-ictal manifestations are similar to that noted with focal to bilateral tonic-clonic seizures.[34] The duration of the post-ictal period can be from minutes to hours.

Generalized Tonic Seizures

These seizures occur most often in neurologically impaired individuals. They are more likely to occur out of sleep. They are characterized by sudden loss of consciousness with associated increased tone. The posturing/stiffening can be generalized and massive or minimal, manifesting only with eye opening or with slight neck extension. The tonic contraction may end with one or more pauses that result in a few clonic jerks. The posturing may be asymmetric. The pattern of muscle involvement may evolve, producing a change in body and limb position over the course of the seizure.

Tonic seizures can be abrupt or can manifest with slow posturing. The most common pattern of generalized tonic seizure posturing involves flexion of the trunk and extension of the extremities with abduction at the shoulders. There may be associated vocalization, particularly with massive and abrupt generalized tonic seizures.

Generalized tonic seizures are typically quite brief but may have a post-ictal state with a duration and severity that are disproportionate to the clinical seizure duration. This may be because tonic seizures may be followed by atypical absence, referred to as tonic-absence seizure.[35]

These seizures can be difficult to distinguish from focal-onset tonic seizures of frontal origin.

Epileptic Spasms

Epileptic spasms is the term now recommended to replace *infantile spasms*, because these seizures may occur after infancy.[36,37] Epileptic spasms are shorter than generalized tonic seizures but longer than generalized myoclonic seizures. The intensity of contraction is greater in the middle of the spasm than at onset or termination, while the contraction seen with tonic seizures is more likely to be sustained. The classic epileptic spasm involves flexion of the neck and trunk with arm abduction. These seizures typically occur in clusters, with a seizure every few seconds to a minute, and demonstrate increasing then decreasing intensity over the course of the cluster.

Generalized Atonic Seizures

These seizures can vary in manifestation from subtle drooping of the head to a massive loss of tone with falling. They are more common in children. They are associated with drop attacks. Drop attacks can be due to tonic seizures as well, and the distinction between the two can be difficult without direct observation.

Generalized atonic seizures are associated with brief loss of consciousness. The duration is usually not more than a few seconds. More prolonged atonic seizures are seen in association with Lennox-Gastaut syndrome and related epilepsies.

Myoclonic-Atonic Seizures

These seizures are commonly part of the syndrome of myoclonic astatic epilepsy, also referred to as *Doose syndrome*. In these seizures, a myoclonic jerk precedes the loss of tone. The seizures are very brief, with rapid recovery. However, injuries are not uncommon from a fall due to loss of tone.

Generalized-Onset Seizures with Focal Evolution

This seizure type is not officially recognized by the ILAE. Just as focal-onset seizures may secondarily generalize, generalized-onset seizures rarely evolve to become focal.[38,39] This focal evolution can occur with generalized myoclonic or generalized absence seizures. Such seizures most often manifest with prolonged staring and arrest of activity, at times with subtle automatisms. Focal clonic activity may also occur. Post-ictal confusion is common and results in misdiagnosis as focal impaired awareness seizures.

UNKNOWN-ONSET SEIZURES

When the seizure onset is missed, it may be difficult to classify a seizure as focal-onset or generalized-onset. However, it is usually still possible to classify the seizure as motor or nonmotor. The most common seizure type of unknown onset in adults is tonic clonic. A number of clinical features have been evaluated in an attempt to determine if tonic clonic seizures are focal or generalized in onset. However, none of these is definitive on an individual basis. Features more commonly encountered with focal to bilateral tonic-clonic seizures include versive head turning, asymmetrical tonic posturing including figure-of-four posturing, asymmetrical clonic activity, asynchronous clonic activity resulting in side-to-side head or body motions, and asymmetric seizure termination. However, all of these features may also be seen less frequently in primary generalized tonic-clonic seizures. Hence, there is no reliable clinical features during the bilateral tonic or clonic phase to help classify seizure onset if it was not captured.

PART 4

Epilepsy Classification and Epileptic Syndromes

4.1

Epilepsy Classification

BASSEL ABOU-KHALIL

Since seizures are *events* while epilepsy is a *disease* with unprovoked recurrent seizures as its main clinical manifestation, there are separate classifications. The International League Against Epilepsy (ILAE) scheme of classification of epilepsy and epileptic syndromes from 1989 (Box 4.1.1) was used for many years until the most recent reclassification of 2017 (Figure 4.1.1). The 1989 classification will be described first, followed by the new 2017 classification.

OLD CLASSIFICATION
The 1989 classification divided epilepsies into those that are "localization-related" (synonymous with partial, focal, or local) and those that are "generalized," based on the fact that most patients will have either focal-onset seizures only or generalized-onset seizures only. Each of these major categories was further subclassified as *idiopathic*, *symptomatic*, or *cryptogenic*.

Idiopathic meant that the epilepsy had no known etiology and that it was pure, with no associated neurological manifestations such as ataxia or dementia. Idiopathic epilepsies were presumed to be genetic.

Symptomatic epilepsies were due to a known insult or lesion.

Cryptogenic epilepsies were presumed to be the result of an insult or lesion that is not known, that is hidden.

Most of the localization-related epilepsies were symptomatic or cryptogenic, whereas most of the generalized epilepsies were idiopathic.

Examples of idiopathic localization-related epilepsy include benign epilepsy with centrotemporal spikes and idiopathic childhood occipital epilepsy. Examples of symptomatic/cryptogenic localization-related epilepsy include temporal lobe epilepsy with hippocampal sclerosis and epilepsy secondary to cavernous malformation or tumor.

Examples of idiopathic generalized epilepsy include childhood absence epilepsy, juvenile absence epilepsy, and juvenile myoclonic epilepsy. Examples of symptomatic/cryptogenic generalized epilepsy include West syndrome and Lennox-Gastaut syndrome.

The classification also included two smaller categories: "epilepsies and syndromes undetermined as to whether there are focal or generalized," either because they had both focal-onset and generalized-onset seizures or because the seizure onset was not known, and a category of "special syndromes."

NEW CLASSIFICATION
The new classification adopted by the ILAE in 2017 proposed three levels of diagnosis: *seizure type*, *epilepsy type*, and *epilepsy syndrome* (Figure 4.1.1). While satisfying all three levels of diagnosis is ideal, it is not always possible. The classification may at times be limited to the first level of seizure type either because there is too little information (e.g., when only one seizure occurred) or because of limited resources (e.g., when the testing needed to achieve additional levels is not available).

Seizure Type
The first level of *seizure type* is based on the seizure classification discussed in Chapter 3.3. Seizures are classified based on onset as either *focal*, *generalized*, or *unknown*.

Epilepsy Type
The second level of *epilepsy type* includes four categories: *focal*, *generalized*, *combined generalized and focal*, and *unknown*. The first two categories correspond to the first two categories of the 1989 classification. The diagnosis of *generalized epilepsy* typically requires demonstration of generalized spike-and-wave discharges on electroencephalogram (EEG). An exception may be situations

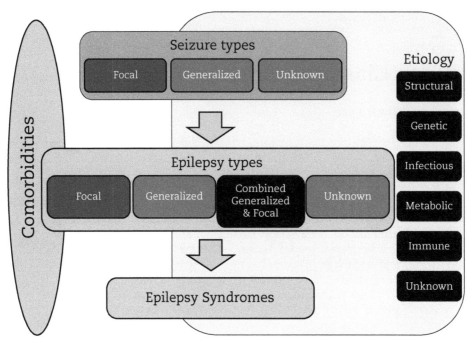

FIGURE 4.1.1 International League Against Epilepsy (ILAE): Three levels of diagnosis.

BOX 4.1.1   INTERNATIONAL CLASSIFICATION OF EPILEPSIES AND EPILEPTIC SYNDROMES

1. Localization-related (partial, focal, local) epilepsies and syndromes
    1.1 Idiopathic (with age-related onset)
    1.2 Symptomatic
    1.3 Cryptogenic (probably symptomatic)
2. Generalized epilepsies and syndromes
    2.1 Idiopathic
    2.2 Cryptogenic or symptomatic
    2.3 Symptomatic (probably symptomatic)
3. Epilepsies and syndromes undetermined as to whether they are focal or generalized
4. Special syndromes

From Commission on Classification and Terminology of the International League Against Epilepsy. Proposal for revised classification of epilepsies and epileptic syndromes. *Epilepsia*. 1989 Jul–Aug;30(4):389–399. doi:10.1111/j.1528-1157.1989.tb05316.x. PMID: 2502382.

---

where there is a combination of generalized myoclonic seizures and generalized tonic-clonic seizures suggesting the diagnosis of juvenile myoclonic epilepsy. In such cases, focal epilepsy may be more likely. On the other hand, the diagnosis of focal epilepsy can be made on clinical grounds and does not require demonstration of focal epileptiform discharges on EEG, even though such finding would support and strengthen the diagnosis. The category of *combined generalized and focal* is new and includes epilepsies that include both focal-onset and generalized-onset seizures. Dravet syndrome, Lennox-Gastaut syndrome, and genetic epilepsy with febrile seizures plus are examples of conditions that include both focal- and generalized-onset seizures. While the diagnosis can be made on clinical grounds, EEG demonstration of both generalized spike-and-wave discharges and focal epileptiform discharges is very helpful to support the diagnosis. The "unknown" category is reserved for instances where available information is insufficient to determine if seizures are focal or generalized.

Epilepsy Syndrome

The third level of level of diagnosis is *epilepsy syndrome*. An epilepsy syndrome is defined by a group of characteristics such as typical age at onset, seizure types (including seizure types that are required to diagnose the syndrome and seizure types that exclude the syndrome), EEG features (including features that are required and features that are exclusionary), natural course and expected response to therapy, associated clinical signs and symptoms, imaging features, and pathophysiological mechanisms. In some cases, there may be specific seizure triggers and a diurnal seizure pattern. There may be specific associated cognitive, psychiatric, or medical comorbidities. This chapter discusses some of the epilepsy syndromes encountered in adults.

Epilepsy Etiology

The classification requires consideration of *epilepsy etiology* from the first level and at every step of diagnosis. Etiological categories recognized include *structural, genetic, infectious, metabolic, immune*, and *unknown* cause. More than one etiology may be applicable for some patients. For example, tuberous sclerosis is both genetic and structural. Epilepsy as a long-term consequence of limbic encephalitis that resulted in unilateral hippocampal sclerosis is both immune and structural.

Comorbidities

The classification also requires consideration of *comorbidities* from the very first level and at every step of diagnosis. Comorbidities can be cognitive, psychiatric, behavioral, or, in some cases, may be other neurological or medical disorders. These comorbidities should be identified early in the process of diagnosis and managed appropriately.

New Terminology

The new classification also changed some other terminology. For example, the term "benign" was replaced by *self-limited* or *pharmacoresponsive*, depending on the intended meaning of "benign." For example, "benign epilepsy with centrotemporal spikes" became *self-limited epilepsy with centrotemporal spikes*, since it is known that the condition tends to remit at puberty. The terms "malignant epilepsy" and "catastrophic epilepsy" were dropped and replaced by *developmental encephalopathy, epileptic encephalopathy*, or both. The term *epileptic encephalopathy* suggests that the epilepsy is responsible for neurological decline, while *developmental encephalopathy* suggests that neurological decline is not a result of the epilepsy. It is, of course, possible that neurological decline could be a result of both the epilepsy and underlying pathology.

4.2

Select Epilepsy Syndromes Seen in Adulthood

BASSEL ABOU-KHALIL

GENERALIZED EPILEPSY SYNDROMES: IDIOPATHIC GENERALIZED EPILEPSIES

Childhood Absence Epilepsy

Childhood absence epilepsy typically starts with generalized absence seizures between 4 and 10 years of age in children with normal development and normal neurological status. Generalized typical absence seizures recur multiple times daily. Seizure duration is usually less than 15 sec. When the syndrome is strictly defined, other generalized seizure types such as generalized tonic-clonic seizures are absent during the active stage of absence seizures, although they may be seen later in the natural course and in a minority of patients. Complete seizure remission commonly occurs before age 20, but a small percentage of patients have persistent seizures. In some instances, childhood absence epilepsy evolves into juvenile myoclonic epilepsy (JME) in the second decade, with appearance of myoclonic seizures. Childhood absence epilepsy is thought to be genetically determined, although the exact mode of inheritance is unknown in most patients. Ethosuximide is the treatment of choice when absence seizures occur in isolation.

Juvenile Absence Epilepsy

Juvenile absence epilepsy is very similar to childhood absence epilepsy, except that the age at onset is in the second decade, with a peak between ages 10 and 12. The absence seizures are not as frequent as in childhood absence epilepsy. In addition, most patients also have generalized tonic-clonic seizures. This condition has a greater tendency for persistence of seizures into adulthood than does childhood absence epilepsy.

Juvenile Myoclonic Epilepsy

JME is common, accounting for up to 10% of all cases of epilepsy. The age at onset is typically between 12 and 18. However, a subgroup of patients are diagnosed with childhood absence epilepsy in the first decade of life. Generalized myoclonic seizures are required for the diagnosis. These typically occur after awakening, particularly following sleep deprivation. They are often not recognized as seizures and not brought to medical attention.

About 90% of patients develop generalized tonic-clonic seizures, typically after sleep deprivation or alcohol binge. This is when they usually seek medical attention. The diagnosis of juvenile myoclonic epilepsy may not be apparent unless the physician specifically inquires about myoclonic jerks. Approximately one-third of patients also have generalized absence seizures.

The diagnosis of JME is based on the clinical history and electroencephalogram (EEG), which shows bursts of generalized irregular 4–6 Hz spike-and-wave activity. The EEG is most likely to be positive when obtained in the morning, after awakening.

JME is predominantly a lifelong condition, with fewer than 25% of patients achieving a medication-free remission in long-term follow-up. However, the majority of patients respond to medication therapy. Classical JME is usually the most treatment responsive, while patients who start out with childhood absence epilepsy tend to be more treatment-resistant.

Valproate appears to be the most effective medication for all three seizure types seen in JME. However, valproate's teratogenicity limits its use in women of childbearing age. Generalized myoclonic and generalized absence seizures may be aggravated by several narrow-spectrum anti-seizure medications that are specific for focal epilepsy (such as carbamazepine).

Epilepsy with Generalized Tonic-Clonic Seizures Alone

Epilepsy with generalized tonic-clonic seizures alone includes so-called *epilepsy with grand mal on awakening* as well as epilepsy with generalized tonic-clonic seizures that are random in timing. The onset of seizures is most often in the second decade of life, but there is a very wide range. Sleep deprivation is a frequent seizure precipitant and seen with other idiopathic generalized epilepsies. Seizures generally respond well to treatment, as noted with JME.

FOCAL EPILEPSY SYNDROMES

Familial Mesial Temporal Lobe Epilepsy

Familial mesial temporal lobe epilepsy is a heterogeneous condition, including a pharmacoresponsive variety and a more drug-resistant variety. In the pharmacoresponsive syndrome, there are no prior febrile seizures. The most prominent aura is *déjà vu* with frequent focal aware seizures, infrequent focal impaired awareness seizures, and rare focal to bilateral tonic-clonic seizures.

Magnetic resonance imaging (MRI) is normal with no hippocampal sclerosis. The epilepsy is frequently not recognized when the only seizure type is subjective focal aware seizures, but when recognized is very responsive to medical therapy.

Other forms of familial mesial temporal lobe epilepsy may be associated with prior febrile convulsions, hippocampal sclerosis on MRI, and less responsiveness to medical therapy. Surgical treatment is often required for seizure control.

Mesial Temporal Lobe Epilepsy with Hippocampal Sclerosis

Mesial temporal lobe epilepsy with hippocampal sclerosis is one of the most common epilepsies, particularly in epilepsy referral centers. Patients frequently have a history of antecedent febrile seizures, in up to 80% of individuals. The febrile seizures are often prolonged, even satisfying criteria for status epilepticus. They may also be focal. The age at onset of afebrile seizures is variable but most commonly is in late childhood or adolescence. The clinical features of mesial temporal lobe seizures were described previously (Chapter 3.4).

Clinical seizure characteristics cannot reliably distinguish mesial temporal lobe epilepsy due to hippocampal sclerosis from that due to tumors or vascular malformations. Hippocampal sclerosis is usually identified on MRI by decreased hippocampal volume and increased hippocampal T2 signal. Patients commonly have material-specific memory dysfunction, with impaired verbal memory when the left hippocampus is involved or visual-spatial memory when the right hippocampus is involved.

This epilepsy is often drug-resistant. However, the natural course may include periods of remission alternating with relapses. Eventually the epilepsy may become consistently drug-resistant. Response to surgical therapy is excellent, with 60–80% of patients seizure-free after temporal lobectomy or selective amygdalohippocampectomy.

Autosomal Dominant Nocturnal Frontal Lobe Epilepsy

Autosomal dominant nocturnal frontal lobe epilepsy most often manifests in patients younger than 20 years, with a mean between 8 and 11 years. The seizures are usually stereotyped and arise out of sleep. They are often hypermotor, with vigorous frenetic movements, including thrashing, kicking, or bicycling. The seizures may also be asymmetrical tonic or may have a mixture of hypermotor and tonic manifestations. Occasionally, they simply manifest with paroxysmal arousal. They are typically short in duration, lasting less than 30 sec. The condition is often misdiagnosed as a sleep disorder or psychogenic seizures. The seizures respond very well to carbamazepine or oxcarbazepine.

Autosomal Dominant Epilepsy with Auditory Features

Autosomal dominant epilepsy with auditory features usually first manifests in adolescence or early adulthood. There is typically an elementary auditory aura such as buzzing, ringing, humming, or even loss of hearing. Reflex auditory precipitation is common. Aphasia may be noted when seizure onset is in the dominant lateral temporal lobe.

Rasmussen Syndrome

Rasmussen syndrome is a chronic progressive disorder of unknown etiology and probably heterogeneous. Focal motor seizures most commonly start between 1 and 14 years of age. The seizures pattern may evolve to focal impaired awareness or focal to bilateral tonic-clonic seizures. Seizures become progressively more frequent but typically localize in the same hemisphere. Episodes of status epilepticus are common.

Progressive hemiparesis occurs together with general intellectual decline and other manifestations depending on the affected hemisphere. Imaging shows progressive hemiatrophy. This condition is suspected to be autoimmune in nature, but there is limited benefit from immunotherapy, and hemispherectomy is usually required to achieve complete seizure control. Rasmussen syndrome is discussed in more detail in Chapter 6.3.

EPILEPSY SYNDROMES WITH BOTH FOCAL AND GENERALIZED SEIZURES

Lennox-Gastaut Syndrome

Lennox-Gastaut syndrome is defined by a triad of (1) a combination of seizure types, (2) a characteristic interictal EEG abnormality of generalized slow spike-and-wave discharges in waking and paroxysmal fast activity in sleep, and (3) cognitive dysfunction. The age of onset is between 3 and 10 years with a peak between 3 and 5 years.

The most commonly encountered seizure types are generalized tonic, generalized atonic, and atypical absence seizures, but focal seizures also commonly occur. Drop attacks due to either generalized atonic or generalized tonic seizures, tend to be debilitating because of associated injuries.

Seizures tend to be drug-resistant. Lennox-Gastaut syndrome tends to be a chronic disorder even though epilepsy may become less active over time. Almost half of patients may appear normal before the onset of seizures, but intellectual deterioration occurs over time.

Genetic Epilepsy with Febrile Seizures Plus

Genetic epilepsy with febrile seizures plus (GEFS+) appears to be autosomal dominant in inheritance. The condition has a heterogeneous phenotype in affected individuals, even within the same family. Some individuals have only typical febrile seizures remitting at 6 years. Other individuals have febrile seizures plus, which refers to febrile seizures persisting beyond 6 years of age or febrile seizures intermixed with afebrile generalized tonic-clonic seizures. Other individuals even have other seizure types, such as generalized absence or myoclonic seizures. Less common seizure types are myoclonic-atonic and focal seizures typical of temporal lobe origin.

PART 5

Clinical EEG

5.1

Terminology and Definitions

KARL E. MISULIS AND BASSEL ABOU-KHALIL

Interpretation of a clinical electroencephalogram (EEG) begins with identification of the clinical state and events, and then identifying the EEG correlates to them. For most patients, diagnosis can be accomplished by a routine EEG, but for some with uncommon events which need to be captured, a prolonged recording is needed.

TABLE 5.1.1 CLINICAL EVENTS

Term	Definition
Epileptic seizure	Episodes of change in neurologic behavior due to abnormal neuronal activity in the brain
Epilepsy	Brain disorder in which there are epileptic seizures
Psychogenic nonepileptic events	Episodic neurologic events that can resemble epileptic seizures but that are due to psychological issues rather than due to a change in neuronal activity in the brain
Physiologic nonepileptic events	Episodic neurologic events that can resemble seizures but that are due to physiological issues rather than abnormal neuronal activity or psychological events (e.g., convulsive syncope, movement disorder)
Behavioral events	Cognitive and motor deficits that result in movements that are behavioral and not epileptic

TABLE 5.1.2 ELECTROENCEPHALOGRAM (EEG) EVENTS

Term	Definition
Spike	Epileptiform transient with a duration of 25–70 msec
Sharp wave	Epileptiform transient with a duration of 70–200 msec
Slow wave	Individual waves in the theta (4–7.9 Hz) or delta (<4 Hz) range
Sharply contoured slow wave	Sharp transient with a duration >200 msec
Epileptiform discharge	Episodic waves or complexes that stand out from the background and suggests a predisposition to epilepsy
Spike-and-wave complex	Spike followed by a slow wave
Suppression	Reduction in voltage not due to technical or non-electrocerebral factors; related to reduction in cortical synaptic activity

Table 5.1.1 describes some common clinical events, and Table 5.1.2 describes some common EEG events. These and additional entities are subsequently discussed in the text.

5.2

EEG Basics

KARL E. MISULIS AND BASSEL ABOU-KHALIL

PERFORMANCE

Electroencephalogram (EEG) has migrated from paper to digital and from EEG-only to EEG with physiologic and video monitoring. We recommend that EEG labs transition to modern video-EEG technology for office and hospital studies.

Electrode Placement
10–20 Electrode Placement System

The 10–20 electrode placement system is a standard for placement of scalp electrodes. The 10–20 system uses a systematic measurement process to create reproducible electrode positions based on landmarks. Figure 5.2.1 shows a diagram of the electrode positions, and a variation of this diagram appears as a display option on some EEG software packages.

Terminology for most electrodes is one or two letters that indicate region and a number that reflects laterality and position with respect to the midline. The regions are

- Frontopolar (Fp)
- Frontal (F)
- Central (C)
- Temporal (T)
- Parietal (P)
- Occipital (O)
- Auricular (A)

The second character of most electrode position designations follows these rules:

- Odd numbers are left-sided.
- Even numbers are right-sided.
- Lower-case "z" is midline.
- Lower numbers are more medial (in the case of F7 vs. F3) or anterior (in the case of T3 vs. T5) than higher numbers.

Additional electrode positions are sometimes used, as discussed later.

Therefore, the left central electrode is C3, and the corresponding position on the right is C4. Cz is in the midline. F7 is lateral to F3, and T4 is anterior to T6.

Notice that F7 and F8 have several names, reflecting that they can record both anterior temporal or inferior frontal activity (see Figure 5.2.2). Examining the field of discharges can be essential to determining the source of recorded activity (see Figure 5.2.3). F7 and F8 are physically over inferior frontal cortex, but they can record both anterior temporal (most often) or inferior frontal activity. Deciding the source of discharges depends on the field of these discharges. For example, if the field is F8 and T4, then F8 activity is anterior temporal, while if the field is F4 and F8, then F8 is likely recording inferior frontal activity. If F8 alone is involved, or if the field involves F8 and Fp2 (Fp2 records

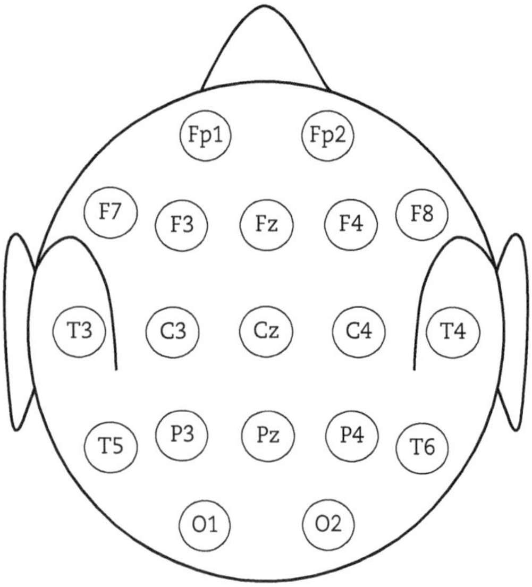

FIGURE 5.2.1 10–20 Electrode placement system. Final electrode placement positions are shown.

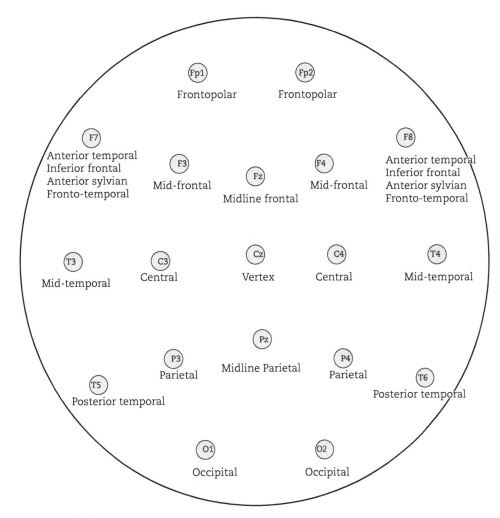

FIGURE 5.2.2 Additional electrode names.

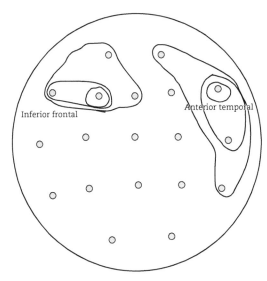

FIGURE 5.2.3 Potential fields.

frontopolar activity but could also detect dipoles originating at the temporal tip), then it is not clear if F8 is anterior temporal or inferior frontal. This uncertain status of F7/F8 has resulted in the exploration of "true" anterior temporal electrodes (discussed later).

Other leads of interest include

- Ear (auricular) with left being A1 and right being A2,
- Ground (G) electrode.

Electrode placement is based on precise measurement, which can usually be completed in less than 10 minutes by an experienced technologist. The measurements start with marking the inion, nasion, and preauricular points. The inion is the occipital protuberance. The nasion is the indentation between the forehead and the nose. The preauricular points are immediately posterior to the indentation of the zygoma, anterior to the tragus. The first measurement is for the distance between the nasion and inion along the sagittal line, passing over the top of the head. The frontopolar plane is marked at 10% of the distance from the nasion. Another 20% from that will mark the frontal plane, then another 20% from that will mark the central plane, then another 20% will mark the parietal plane, then another 20% will mark the occipital plane. Next, the distance between the preauricular points is measured, marking Cz where it intersects the central plane. The circumferential plane is at 10% of the distance from the left preauricular point, then the parasagittal plane is at 20% from that. Similar measurements are then made on the right side (Figures 5.2.4 and 5.2.5 are steps 1 and 2).

Next, the midline electrode positions are marked based on the position of Cz (Figure 5.2.5).

Next, measurements are made in the circumferential plane to mark the positions of the coronal planes at that level (Figure 5.2.6). The positions of T3 and T4 are then finalized, followed by the positions of other electrodes at that level (Figure 5.2.7).

Next, the positions of C3 and C4 as well as the frontal plane (midpoint between Fp1 and C3 and between Fp2 and C4) and parietal planes (midpoint between C3 and O1 and between C4 and O2) are marked (Figure 5.2.8).

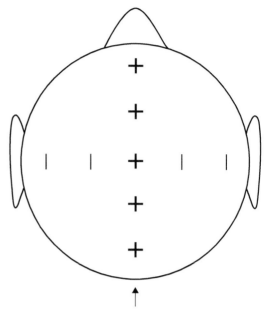

Step 3 - Sagittal plane + marks

FIGURE 5.2.5 Marking midline positions.

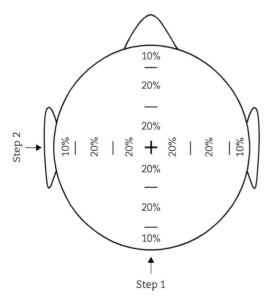

Step 1

FIGURE 5.2.4 Measurement of the head in 10% and 20% intervals, anterior-posterior and left-right.

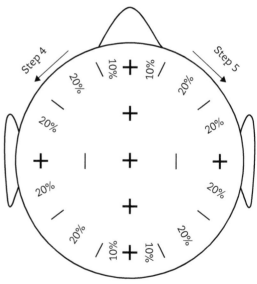

FIGURE 5.2.6 Measurement in circumferential plane.

Next, electrode locations are finalized in the coronal frontal and parietal planes (Figure 5.2.9).

The importance of accurate electrode placement cannot be overemphasized. Electrode placement based on "guesstimates" results in inaccurate cortical localization.

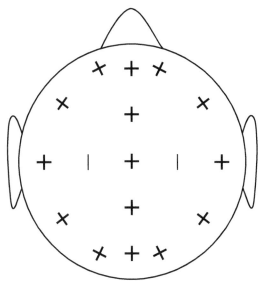

Step 6 - circumferential plane + marks

FIGURE 5.2.7 Marking positions on the circumferential planes.

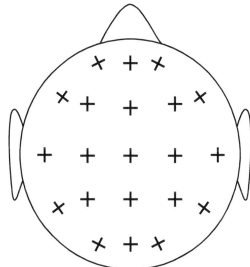

Step 9 and 10 - Frontal and parietal planes + marks

FIGURE 5.2.9 Final positions of the electrodes.

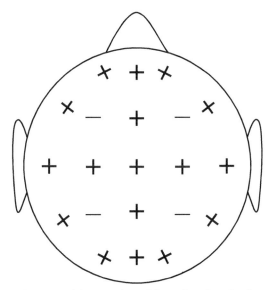

Step 7 and 8 - Location of frontal and parietal planes and + marks for C3 and C4

FIGURE 5.2.8 Marking C3 and C4, and Fp1 and Fp2.

Additional Electrodes Outside the 10–20 System

Additional leads are occasionally placed, although not as part of routine EEG performance (see Figure 5.2.10). These include

- Silverman "true" anterior temporal (T1 and T2) electrodes to monitor anterior temporal activity,
- Zygomatic electrodes and cheek electrodes for monitoring of lateral-basal temporal lobe activity,
- Supraorbital electrodes for monitoring anterior orbitofrontal activity,
- Infraorbital electrodes for differentiation of cerebral frontal slow-wave activity from vertical eye movements or tongue movements.

T1 electrode placement: The distance from the auditory canal to the outer canthus of the eye is measured and divided into thirds. T1 will be 1 cm superior to the mark closest to the ear canal.

The reason for the T1/T2 electrodes is that F7/ F8, which are the anterior temporal electrodes, are physically located over the lateral inferior-posterior frontal region. They do record anterior temporal lobe activity, but may also record frontal activity. To monitor mesial-basal temporal activity, the most commonly used electrodes are *sphenoidal electrodes*. *Nasopharyngeal electrodes* were frequently used in the past but are rarely used now because they are unstable, easily dislodged, and become more uncomfortable over time. Deep sphenoidal electrodes are inserted just below the zygomatic arch, 2 cm anterior to the line between the tragus and the condyle of the mandible. The needle is directed horizontally and approximately 10 degrees posteriorly. The tip should rest close to

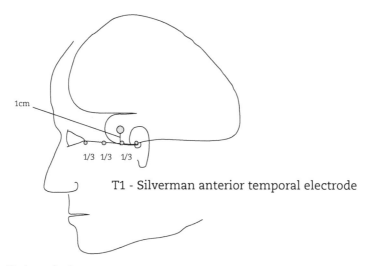

FIGURE 5.2.10 T1 electrode placement.

the foramen ovale (at a depth of 4–5 cm). Although their insertion is painful, sphenoidal electrodes are well-tolerated and stable, making them ideal for recording seizures with long-term monitoring. Mini-sphenoidal electrodes are inserted in the same location to a depth of only 1 cm. This makes them possible to insert by EEG technologists. Although they are not as good as sphenoidal electrodes for detecting mesial-basal activity, their ease of insertion makes them useful for short-term recordings.

10–10 Electrode Placement System

The 10-10 electrode placement system is based on the same landmarks as the 10–20 system, but involves the addition of electrodes between 10–20 electrode positions (see Figure 5.2.11). The purpose is to enhance localization of potentials using scalp

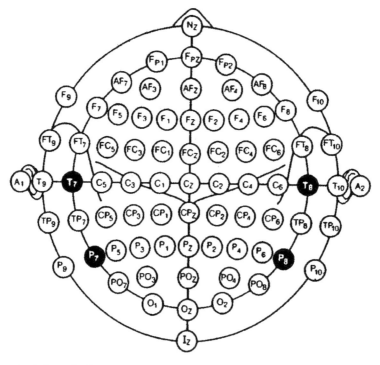

FIGURE 5.2.11 10–10 electrode placement system.

electrodes. Higher density arrays using the 10–10 system can be useful for dipole source analysis.

Although there have been several nomenclatures for this system, the one recommended by the American Clinical Neurophysiology Society[1] is the modified combinatorial nomenclature. In this nomenclature system, the letters identify the coronal plane location, and the number (or z) refers to the position relative to the midline. The odd numbers (1 to 9) belong on the left, the even numbers (2 to 10) belong on the right, and z still stands for the midline. The smaller numbers refer to positions close to the midline and the larger numbers to positions farther away from the midline. In this new nomenclature, the 10–20 electrode names could be preserved, with the exception of T3/T4 and T5/T6. These electrodes lie in the same sagittal planes as F7 and F8 and needed to have the same numbers. T3 and T4 were therefore changed to T7 and T8. T5 and T6, the posterior temporal electrodes, are close to the temporo-parieto-occipital junction, and, because they are in the same coronal plane as P3 and P4, were named P7 and P8. In this Atlas, both new and old names for these electrodes are used. It is important to keep in mind that for P7/P8 and P9/P10, the letter P stands for posterior temporal, while P stands for parietal when the number following P is smaller than 7.

The following are the new and old names for the revised 10–20 system:

- T7 = T3
- T8 = T4
- P7 = T5
- P8 = T6

The additional coronal electrode planes created in the 10–10 system are AF for anterior frontal, FC and FT for frontocentral/ frontotemporal plane, CP for centroparietal plane, TP for temporoparietal plane, and PO for parieto-occipital plane.

Additional electrodes in the 10–10 system are rarely used in routine EEG recording. Even in epilepsy monitoring, it would be very impractical to use all the 10–10 electrodes. However, when the field of certain activity has to be clarified, selected additional electrodes can be used in a region of interest. For example, in suspected mesial frontocentral foci, FC1, FCz, FC2, C1, C2, CP1, CPz, and CP2 could be added for best delineation of the field. In left temporal lobe epilepsy, FT7, FT9, and T9 could be added and may obviate the need for T1 and T2 electrodes.

IFCN Extended Array

The International Federation of Clinical Neurophysiology (IFCN) recommended routine use of an extended 25 electrode array with 3 inferior temporal electrodes on each side added to the 10–20 electrode system (Figure 5.2.12). This would improve coverage of the inferior temporal region.[2] The additional electrodes are F9, T9, and P9 on the left and F10, T10, and P10 on the right. These additional electrodes can also allow source analysis for focal epilepsy, although higher density arrays are better for dipole source analysis.[3]

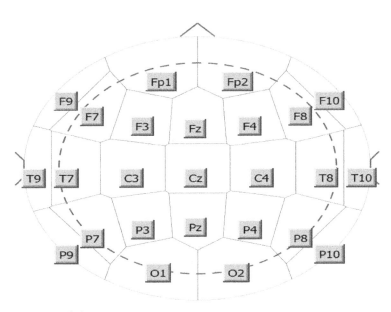

FIGURE 5.2.12 FCN extended array.

Applying Electrodes

Which to Use: Paste or Collodion

Electrodes are attached by either paste or collodion. Paste is commonly used for routine short-duration EEG recordings. Collodion is also sometimes used for routine recording but is more commonly used for long-term recordings such as extended inpatient and ambulatory studies. Collodion takes longer to apply and remove so that paste is preferentially used for routine recording. Before application of electrodes by either method, the skin must be prepared.

The electrodes and scalp are bridged using conductive gel, which is a malleable extension of the electrode. The gel serves to maximize skin contact and allow for fixation on the skin, which minimizes the effect of small amounts of movement. The gel lowers the impedance of the electrode–skin interface.

Physiologic Monitoring

It is often important to monitor physiological parameters in conjunction with the EEG (see Table 5.2.1). Electrocardiogram (EKG) is the most important and needs to be monitored in all patients. One reason is that EKG artifact often appears on EEGs and could result in confusion regarding the origin of some sharp potentials.

Additional electrodes for physiological monitoring need to be used predominantly in neonatal EEGs, in brain death recordings, and in select situations, particularly for intensive care unit (ICU)

recordings. They include, but are not restricted to the following:

- Eye movement electrodes:
  - Infraorbital electrodes (these are placed immediately below each eye, for distinguishing vertical eye movements from frontal EEG activity)
  - Electro-oculogram leads (both electrodes are lateral to the eyes, one above the right eye and another electrode below the left eye). These leads record eye movements. They are used mainly for neonatal EEG and for sleep recordings.
- Electromyogram (EMG) electrodes (submental or over a muscle selected based on clinical picture)
- Respiration monitor (to monitor respiratory effort):
  - Air flow monitor

EEG technologists should be encouraged to be proactive and creative, adding electrodes as needed. For example, if the patient has right arm jerks and EEG potentials that may possibly be linked to these, the tech could add an electrode over the right arm, which would help the electroencephalographer in identifying a consistent relationship between the two.

EKG electrodes are almost always placed for routine EEG, but especially are useful during long-term EEG monitoring and sleep studies. EKG monitoring is particularly helpful for patients having routine EEG when there are sharp

TABLE 5.2.1 PHYSIOLOGIC MONITORING

Parameter	Recording method	Clinical use
EKG	Electrodes below the right clavicle and left fifth intercostal space on the mid-clavicular line.	EKG artifact commonly contaminates EEG recordings, and EKG monitoring is essential to differentiate this from cortical sharp waves and spikes.
Eye movements	Electrodes placed above and to the side or below the eyes in an array to map eye movements.	Eye movements are seen on scalp EEG and can be misinterpreted as frontal EEG. Also used during some sleep studies.
EMG	Disc electrode is placed usually on chin and/or arm or leg, or on muscle that is being monitored.	Recording muscle activity especially in neonates during sleep. Of limited value in adults, unless the EEG correlate of twitches is being evaluated.
Respiratory	Chest transducer or airflow transducer.	Especially for polysomnography. May be helpful in epilepsy monitoring if there is concern over ictal or post-ictal apnea.
	Oximeter	Especially for polysomnography. May be helpful in epilepsy monitoring if there is concern over ictal or post-ictal apnea.

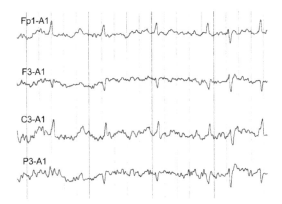

FIGURE 5.2.13 Electrocardiogram (EKG) artifact. LB montage, left parasagittal region.

transients that might be EKG or slow transients that may be pulse artifact (see Figure 5.2.13). Because of the common cardiac and vascular contamination of the recordings, routine EKG lead placement is recommended.

Eye movement electrodes are used to evaluate eye movement artifact due to the polarization of the globe. The globe can be considered to be a dipole, with the corneal region positive compared to the posterior retinal region. The recorded electrical activity is due to potential difference of the retinal pigment epithelium.

The patient in the recording shown in Figure 5.2.14 had rapid eye blinks that appeared after eye opening. On the left side of the figure is a normal posterior dominant rhythm (PDR). At the marker in the middle of the page is eye opening with the expected attenuation of the background. Two seconds later, there is onset of eye blinks.

Movement of the globe creates slow activity that is easily identifiable as ocular in origin when eye blink is vertical. However, movements can occasionally be confused with pathologic frontal slow activity. Lateral and vertical conjugate eye

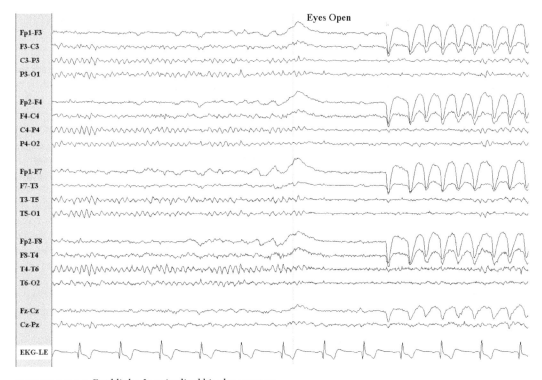

FIGURE 5.2.14 Eye blinks. Longitudinal bipolar montage.

movements produce disparate deflections on the eye leads, so that slow activity on the EEG can definitively be determined to be cerebral or ocular.

Eye movement recording is discussed in more detail in Chapter 5.3 in the section on Noncerebral potentials.

EMG electrodes are not used in most routine adult studies but are used during sleep studies for documentation of nocturnal myoclonus or other movements. EMG is a frequent contaminant of EEG recordings, especially in temporal leads, and can be mistaken for sharp activity; if needed, a non-cephalic EMG electrode may help identify muscle activity. EMG monitoring is most commonly used for determination of muscle tone in sleep recordings in neonates. It is also helpful in adults to establish the correlation between EEG activity and changes in muscle tone (as in myoclonic, tonic, or atonic activity). Two surface electrodes are placed 3 cm apart over the muscle of interest. The IFCN recommends simultaneously recording from muscles on both sides for left–right comparison and also suggests recording from antagonistic muscles when investigating negative myoclonus or atonic seizures.[4] Patterns of EMG artifact can also help distinguish epileptic from nonepileptic convulsive seizures.[5]

Respiratory monitoring can be performed in a number of ways. One is by chest transducer, essentially a strain gauge around the chest to record chest excursions. Airflow can be measured by a detector near the nares, but this has a greater possibility of disturbing the patient. Airflow meters can be used on intubated patients, but this is seldom clinically indicated.

Running the Test

There are multiple stages in the performance of the test. These begin with patient identification and verification of the study to be performed, followed by the sequence of technical and administrative events required for complete performance.

Patient Identification and Study Verification

The patient is identified just as for any hospital or office procedure, using clinic or hospital documentation, arm-band if available, and check-in ID if not.

The study is also verified, since it is possible that the wrong study has been scheduled. The technologist can verify the study intent by review of the office or hospital records pertaining to the study, particularly the designation of indication.

The technologist needs to verify the following:

- Identity of the patient,

- Correctness of the study,
- Particulars of the study so that the clinical question can best be answered.

On the recording as sent to the reading physician, the following information needs to be attached.

- Name
- Age
- Identification number of the patient
- Index number of the recording
- Time and date of the recording
- Clinical reason for the study
- Time of the last seizure, if appropriate
- Ordering clinician
- Current medications
- Sedative medications used
- Name of the technologist
- Technical summary, including activation methods and artifacts
- Technologist's observations, including regions of particular interest

Pretest Calibration and Testing

Pretest calibration and testing should be fairly standard and includes the components discussed here. The study reader should review the results of this calibration and testing since errors are not always noticed by the technologist and errors can have significant effects on interpretation.

Impedance Testing

Electrode impedance should be at least 100 ohms and usually no more than 5 kohm. Sometimes, impedance cannot be kept within this window, so if the impedance has to be higher than 5 kohm, then the impedance should at least be approximately equal for the electrodes. Impedances up to 10 kohms are acceptable with modern digital EEG equipment, provided the impedances are balanced. Excessively high impedance in one or several electrode indicates that there is a problem with the leads or fixation of the leads to the scalp. High electrode impedance increases noise, particularly if the impedances are not balanced. Unbalanced impedances may result in loss of common mode rejection, so that 60 Hz artifact or EKG may appear in the affected channels.

Excessively low impedance usually indicates smear between the electrodes and may impair visualization of electrocerebral potentials. When two electrodes are electrically connected by conductive gel/paste, they act as a single large electrode. Even in referential recordings they are a problem, limiting the sharpness of localization.

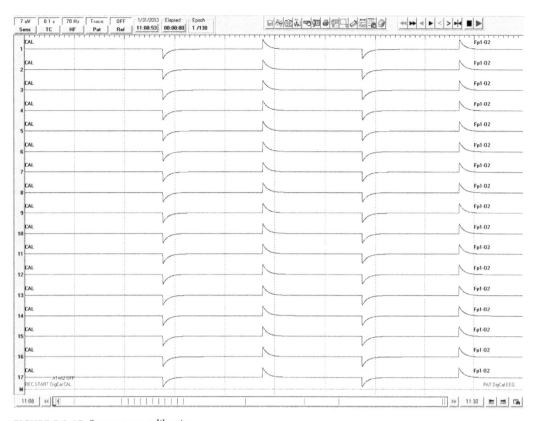

FIGURE 5.2.15 Square wave calibration.

Square-Wave Calibration

Square-wave calibration (see Figure 5.2.15) produces a typical appearance that can be compared visually from channel to channel. One or more channels that have distorted waves from square-wave calibration are an indication of either errant settings or equipment failure. Square-wave calibration is performed before and after the study.

A square-wave pulse is delivered from a waveform generator into each amplifier input. This pulse is 50μV in amplitude and is alternated on and off at 1 second intervals. The wave does not appear square because of the effects of the preset default filters.

The low-frequency filter (LFF) transforms the plateau of the signal pulse into an exponential decay. The rapidity of the decay depends on the filter setting. The lower the cutoff frequency setting, the slower the decay. Higher settings of the LFF cause the decay to baseline to occur rapidly.

The high-frequency filter (HFF) rounds off the top of the peak of the calibration recording. Lower settings of the HFF cause the peak to be blunted and of lower amplitude. Higher settings of the HFF cause the peak to be sharper and of higher amplitude.

We recommend trying different filter settings while recording square-wave calibration. The experienced neurophysiologist can determine an error in response of the system by abnormalities in the square-wave calibration. Some of these abnormalities include

- Peak too rounded,
- Peak overshoot,
- Incorrect rate of decay,
- Too low or too high amplitude of the signal.

These determinations are made in comparison with other recordings and in comparison to the recordings from the other channels. These abnormalities are highly unlikely with modern equipment.

Bio-calibration

Biological calibration (bio-calibration, or biocal) assesses response of the amplifiers and filters to a complex biological signal composed of a host of frequencies (Figure 5.2.16). In the days of paper

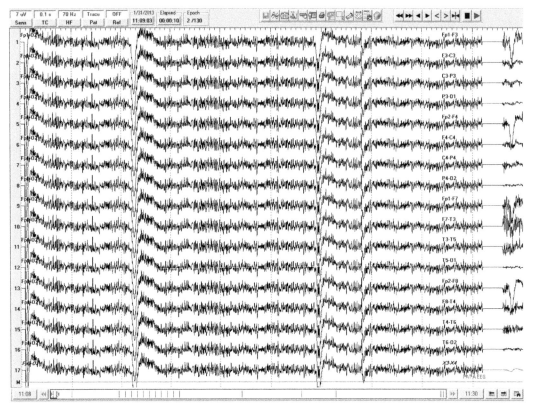

FIGURE 5.2.16 Biocal.

recordings, the montage Fp1-O2 was used for every channel, testing the integrity of the amplification system and the recording pens.

Today, digital equipment provides each channel with its own amplifier, so biocal can be each electrode against a common reference (Figure 5.2.17).

The technologist and reader should review the biocal for unexpected technical issues.

Integrity of the System

Integrity of the system is checked especially for studies where there is so little signal that recording

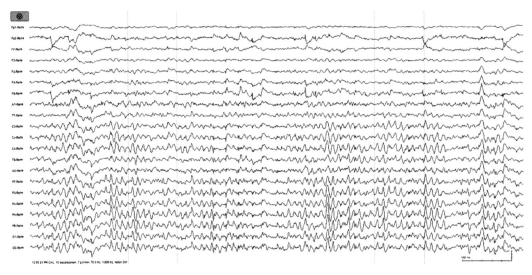

FIGURE 5.2.17 Biocal. Montage = each electrode to a common reference.

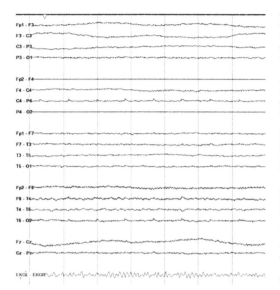

FIGURE 5.2.18 Integrity of the system: Electroencephalogram (EEG) recorded when patient was disconnected. Longitudinal bipolar montage.

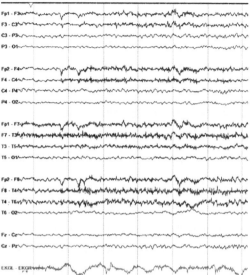

FIGURE 5.2.19 Integrity of the system: Electroencephalogram (EEG) from the same patient as in Figure 5.2.18, but connected. Longitudinal bipolar montage.

system error has to be considered. Brain death and severe encephalopathy can produce recordings that are almost flat. To test the integrity of the system, the technologist can touch the electrodes, and the resulting artifact is readily visible. For routine recordings, representative electrodes need to be touched, not necessarily each one, but for brain death recordings, each electrode must be touched.

In the example here, which caused interpreter confusion, the EEG appeared to be of low voltage (Figure 5.2.18) when in fact the patient was disconnected and had been transported elsewhere for a diagnostic test.

Fortunately, an earlier short segment (Figure 5.2.19) in the same patient showed true cerebral EEG activity.

Montage Selection

Modern digital EEG allows for montage selection by the interpreting physician rather than use of predetermined montages during recording. However, our lab still requests technologists to change montages during the acquisition of outpatient EEG recordings. Both bipolar and referential montages are used. Among the most common are longitudinal bipolar, transverse bipolar, circumferential bipolar, average reference, and ear reference. Inpatient prolonged EEGs are obtained displaying one montage, but

the reviewer can analyze segments of interest with various montages.

Filters

The LFF setting for routine EEG is a 1 Hz or lower cutoff frequency. This corresponds to a time constant (TC) of 0.16 sec. If the LFF is set higher, there is distortion and attenuation of some slow waves. The waves can have an increased number of phases and seem to be composed of faster frequencies. The technologists should be discouraged from turning up the LFF when there is an abundance of slow activity. The LFF cutoff frequency setting can be adjusted downward to improve the identification of suspected slow activity.

The HFF setting for routine EEG is 70 Hz. This is slightly higher than line power frequency. Turning the HFF to a lower frequency will attenuate electrical artifact; however, this should be discouraged because this will also attenuate physiological sharp activity.

The 60-Hertz or "notch" filter attenuates specifically line power, 60-Hz in the United States and Canada. The 60-Hz filter is often needed so that line artifact does not obscure the recording. The filter should not be used to correct focal 60-Hz artifact, which is most likely related to focally increased electrode impedance. Focal 60-Hz artifact should prompt the technologist to perform an electrode impedance check and correct electrode impedances.

Sensitivities

Amplifier sensitivity is initially set to 7 μV/mm. Increased sensitivity is used with low-voltage recordings, most common in elderly patients in the awake state, and in pathological states of electrocerebral suppression. The sensitivity is increased to 2 μV/mm for brain death studies. Reduced sensitivity is commonly used for patients with high-voltage EEGs, as in children, especially in the sleeping state, and when there are high-amplitude transients such as seizure discharges.

Sensitivities on reading need to be selected with care. Reduction in sensitivity to better view a high-amplitude event may make lower amplitude components invisible, such as a small spike component or notch. This effect is especially notable with seizure discharges: a reduction in sensitivity to view the discharges may appear to accentuate post-ictal suppression because the sensitivity is not returned to default levels.

Display Time and Page Rate

The concept of *display time* is new to digital recordings. Traditional paper EEG recordings used a paper speed of 30 mm/sec; this gave an x-axis resolution that allowed for adequate visual interpretation of the spectrum of frequencies of routine EEG, just as the standard sensitivities gave a y-axis scale that allowed for detection of most of the range of EEG amplitudes. Digital displays depend on resolution of the monitors, graphics cards, and acquisition and review software, but, in general, the display time is adjusted so that the display looks roughly similar to a paper display. For a typical 19-inch monitor, this means display of approximately 10 sec of EEG on one screen, with part of the display taken up by other data elements. But since display sizes are not standard, we cannot give fixed recommendations on display time.

Display time may be altered in a few circumstances. Display time can be shortened substantially if the reader is comparing timings with very short differences (e.g., spike onset from one hemisphere or the other). Display time can be lengthened if the reader is concentrating on EEG features such as sleep stage, where overview of much longer times is warranted.

Page rate is the rate at which the pages change. If we were to display pages at a rate concordant with the acquisition speed, reviewing each EEG efficiently would be impossible for most of us, so we page through digital EEGs faster than acquisition. Excessively fast speeds increase the risk of missing transients or other subtle abnormalities. We also commonly step back in study time to replay an event or region of interest, often with a change in montage and/or sensitivity.

Video/Audio

Video has become standard with all EEG studies. The EEG technologist should verify that both video and audio are recording correctly at the beginning of the study. Reviewing the video will help the technologist with detailing and refining annotations after the study is complete.

Annotation

Important events must be noted using annotations that are available on all modern EEG devices. Technologists need to be familiar with how to create and edit annotations and must know the preferences on the part of the reading physicians for documentation of annotation.

Among the observations that should be noted are

- Apparent state changes.
- Beginning and ending of activation procedures and comments about the performance (e.g., good effort on hyperventilation or not).
- Clinical events that might be seizures. The technologist will likely note the beginning and ending and later will have to create more detailed notes about the event, appearance, etc. Not only is a description of the seizure itself important, but so is the post-ictal period.
- Movement artifact deserves a description in the technologist's annotations (e.g., tremor or dyskinesias).
- Response to stimuli from the technologist. Our technologists usually assess responsiveness appropriate to patient condition, with a spectrum of stimuli ranging from sternal rub to questions assessing mental status.
- EEG findings that the technologist has noted and wants to bring to the attention of the reading physician.
- Artifacts identified by the technologist and noted at least the first time or two (e.g., ventilator, IV pump, or other artifact of the ICU). Similarly, electrical transients that are typical of a medical setting, such as nearby

machinery turning on and off, should be noted if visible to the technologist on the record.

- As part of the annotation, specific patient behaviors are documented.

Testing Patients During Events

Stimulation

Technologists assess the responsiveness and mental status of the patient during the study. For awake patients, this usually includes noting the response to questions such as name and location, and some additional cognitive responses (e.g., "Name a red fruit").

For encephalopathic patients, responses to verbal stimuli are noted, as are responses to tactile stimulation if there is no response to verbal stimulation. For severe encephalopathy and coma, response to sternal rub or similar somatosensory stimulation is recommended. The annotation of the stimulus not only allows the reading physician to know when an alerting response might happen but also lessens the likelihood that the mechano-electric effects of the stimulus might be misinterpreted as electrocerebral response.

Provocation of Seizures

Provocation of seizures during the study is attempted if the patient reports a stimulus likely to induce seizures. When psychogenic nonepileptic events are suspected, suggestion may be used as long as there is no deception (such as in the use of saline injection falsely described as a proconvulsant drug).

Mechanisms to provoke seizures include

- Asking the patient what provokes the event, then recreating that as best as possible in the lab; for example, standing quickly, eating or drinking, and listening to particular music have been described by patients as evoking clinical seizures.
- Induction techniques such as hyperventilation and photic stimulation, which can trigger epileptic seizures, can also be used to trigger nonepileptic events.
- Suggestion can also be used, though deception should be avoided in clinical practice.

The technologist might remark that signs of an impending seizure may be appearing. While a clinical event in response to suggestion does not rule out genuine epileptic events, this does at least make the argument for a psychological component and favor nonepileptic events.

Activation Procedures

Photic Stimulation

Photic stimulation is produced by a bright strobe, which is placed in front of the patient with the eyes closed. The flashes are bright enough to illuminate the retina even through closed eye lids.

The stimulation protocols are programmed into most modern EEG machines, but one typical protocol is the following:

- Train duration of 10 sec,
- Interval between trains of 10 sec,
- Initial flash rate of 3/sec.

Higher flash rates are subsequently delivered up to 30/sec.

Abnormal EEG activity elicited by a specific frequency should be identified by the technologist, and, subsequently, that particular frequency should be repeated at the end of the photic stimulation session to verify that the response was not coincidental.

For safety reasons, a full-fledged generalized tonic-clonic seizure should not be precipitated with photic stimulation. If a clear photoparoxysmal response (PPR) appears, the technologist should abort the stimulation train before a seizure develops. If a consistent PPR is noted at one or two consecutive stimulation frequencies, then stimulation can be resumed from the highest frequency to establish the upper limit of the photosensitivity frequency range.

A group of European experts recommended guidelines for photic stimulation that differ slightly from the common practice.[6] These guidelines should be considered in patients with suspected or proved photosensitivity or to maximize the detection of photosensitivity. Presented here is a selected list of recommendations.

- Perform photic stimulation in the waking state, preferably in the early morning, in a dimly lit room, in an upright position.
- Perform photic stimulation at least 3 min after hyperventilation, or best at the end of the recording.
- Position the lamp at a distance of 30 cm from the nasion; instruct the patient to look at the center of the lamp and to close the eyes when asked.
- Stop photic stimulation immediately as soon as generalized epileptiform discharges are noted during stimulation with any frequency to avoid provoking a generalized tonic-clonic seizure.

- Test three eye conditions with separate 5-sec trains of flashes, starting with active eye closure (closing the eyes as soon as the flashing starts, which has the lowest threshold for a PPR), eyes closed, then eyes open (which has the highest threshold for precipitating a PPR). There should be a pause of at least 5 sec between stimulations. If time is limited, stimulation is performed using the most sensitive eye condition, that of active eye closure at the beginning of each intermittent photic stimulation (IPS) train. In that case the stimulation can be for 7 sec.
- Use the following IPS frequencies in this sequence: 1, 2, 8, 10, 15, 18, 20, 25, 40, 50, and 60 Hz (not always possible since the highest frequency possible with several equipment makers is 30 Hz). If a generalized PPR is noted at a certain stimulation frequency, the stimulation at that frequency is stopped immediately, and the next stimulation is performed starting with the highest frequency, moving in the direction of decreasing frequency until a PPR is noted again. This procedure protects the patient from a convulsive seizure and defines the lower and the upper IPS frequency thresholds. When there is doubt about whether a true generalized PPR was provoked at a particular stimulation frequency, the stimulation can be repeated after a pause of at least 10 sec.

Hyperventilation

Hyperventilation is performed for 3 min on routine testing, and should be performed for 5 min if there is strong suspicion of absence epilepsy. Hyperventilation is often not performed in elderly patients or patients at risk of complications from impaired cerebral perfusion associated with hyperventilation.

The normal response to hyperventilation is diffuse slow activity with the appearance of theta and delta range activity. The slow activity is of higher amplitude in children than adults. Hypoglycemia augments the slow activity.

Hyperventilation is used predominantly to activate generalized absence seizures. In some patients, the 2.5–4 Hz spike-and-wave discharges are only seen during hyperventilation.

Sleep Deprivation

Sleep deprivation increases the possibility of seeing epileptiform activity and therefore is used for patients in whom routine EEG has not been able to identify interictal epileptiform activity. An important mechanism of activating epileptiform discharges is through facilitating sleep. However, sleep deprivation may also have a more direct activating mechanism.

Termination of the Test

Post-procedure calibration is similar to the pre-procedure calibration. This should be routine and include all of the elements of pre-procedure calibration.

Documentation begins with the technologist's worksheet, which contains most of the information required for the reader to facilitate interpretation of the test. However, this information has limitations and the reader occasionally needs to review the electronic health record.

The physician's report can be dictated or electronically generated but should be created in a timely fashion. We require outpatient studies to be read within 24 hours of completion, and inpatient recordings should be interpreted as soon as possible so that critical abnormalities are addressed.

Storage and archiving of modern digital EEGs are usually on optical disc for archive, with recordings kept on fixed disc for immediate review for a variable length of time. We recommend maintaining a record available for on-demand viewing at least until the physicians have reviewed the record and seen that patient. For hospitalized patients who may have a series of recordings, maintaining the recordings online for as long as the patient is in the hospital is recommended.

Archive is through a number of mechanisms, and many facilities keep two copies, one local and one remote. This is similar to data handling of patients' electronic medical records.

EEG ANALYSIS

Overview

EEG is performed using a variety of montages, so EEG can be assessed with a spectrum of presentations. A spike may be more visible on one montage than another. Modern digital machines have the ability to change montage while displaying the same epoch, adding extra interpretive flexibility.

Rules of Polarity

All EEG channels have two inputs. Each EEG channel represents the difference in potential between these inputs. *Input 1* is usually a single active electrode. *Input 2* may be another active electrode, summed activity of two or more electrodes, or an inactive reference.

Historically, in referential recordings the first input has been called "active" input and second input "reference" input. However, in bipolar montages and in the instance of an active reference, both inputs are active. By convention, a negative potential in the first input is seen as an upward deflection, whereas a positive potential in the first input is seen as a downward deflection. Potentials arising in the second input will have the reverse appearance.

Polarity convention of EEG display is as follows:

- Relative negativity at input 1—upward deflection,
- Relative negativity at input 2—downward deflection,
- Relative positivity at input 1—downward deflection,
- Relative positivity at input 2—upward deflection.

However, this elementary localization only applies if a signal is at one electrode and the other is at zero-potential, and this is seldom the case. The deflection of the display is the difference in potential. For example, if input 1 has a negative signal, one would expect an upward deflection, but if the field of the potential is such that input 2 has an even greater negative signal, then the deflection would be downward since input 1 is relatively positive in comparison to input 2. For bipolar montages, adjacent electrodes are usually connected in the two inputs.

In bipolar recordings, by convention, for any electrode pair comprising an EEG channel in a chain, input 1 would be the electrode either anterior or on the left of the electrode connected to input 2.

Montages

Montages are created so that viewing the EEG gives the neurophysiologist a clear picture of the spatial distribution of EEG activity across the cortex (see Figure 5.2.20). A good montage is one that can be easily imagined and remembered. It should also have equal electrode distances within each chain (unless it includes electrodes outside the 10–20 system).

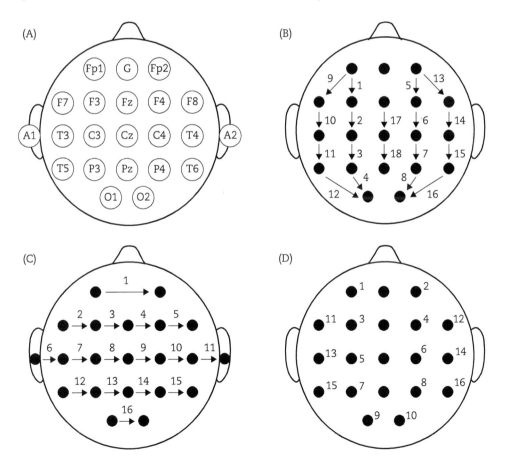

FIGURE 5.2.20 Montages. A = electrode positions; B = Longitudinal bipolar (LB); C = Transverse bipolar (TB); D = Referential montage electrode positions (Ref).

The American Clinical Neurophysiology Society has published extensive guidelines for performance of EEG, which includes recommendations for electrodes and montages.[7,8] These will be called the *Guidelines* for the rest of this text. The guidelines recommend the following:

- Record at least 16 channels.
- Use the full 21-electrode array of the 10–20 system.
- Both bipolar and referential montages should be used.
- Electrode connections for each channel should be clearly indicated at the beginning of each montage.
- Pattern of electrode connections should be made as simple as possible and the montages easily comprehended.
- Bipolar electrode connections should run in a straight unbroken line with equal interelectrode distances.
- Display of more anterior electrodes generally should be placed above those of more posterior location.
- At least some common montages should be used between laboratories for ease of comparison.

In addition, recommendations that most labs adhere to include

- Display of left-sided electrodes generally should be placed above those of right-sided electrodes.
- Although 16 channels are considered minimum, montages should be used employing the maximum number of channels of the machine to ensure adequate coverage.
- Three classes of montages should be used:
  - Longitudinal bipolar
  - Transverse bipolar
  - Referential

If sufficient channels are available, polygraphic channels are desirable. EKG is most commonly recorded and should be routine for most studies, but EMG and respiratory monitoring can be of value.

Recommended montages for routine use in adults and children after the neonatal period are shown in Table 5.2.2. Additional channels are used when available and needed. The additional channels may be used for EKG, eye movements, respirations, or EMG.

TABLE 5.2.2 MONTAGES FOR ROUTINE ELECTROENCEPHALOGRAM

Channel	Longitudinal bipolar (LB)	Transverse bipolar (TB)	Average (Ave)	Ipsilateral ear (Ipsi)	Circumferential (Circ)
1	Fp1 – F3	F7 – Fp1	Fp1 – Ave	Fp1 – A1	T3 – F7
2	F3 – C3	Fp1 – Fp2	Fp2 – Ave	Fp2 – A2	F7 – Fp1
3	C3 – P3	Fp2 – F8	F3 – Ave	F3 – A1	Fp1 – Fp2
4	C3 – O1	F7 – F3	F4 – Ave	F4 – A2	Fp2 – F8
5	Fp2 – F4	F3 – Fz	C3 – Ave	C3 – A1	F8 – T4
6	F4 – C4	Fz – F4	C4 – Ave	C4 – A2	T3 – T5
7	C4 – P4	F4 – F8	P3 – Ave	P3 – A1	T5 – O1
8	P4 – O2	A1 – T3	P4 – Ave	P4 – A2	O1 – O2
9	Fp1 – F7	T3 – C3	O1 – Ave	O1 – A1	O2 – T6
10	F7 – T3	C3 – Cz	O2 – Ave	O2 – A2	T6 – T4
11	T3 – T5	Cz – C4	F7 – Ave	F7 – A1	F3 – C3
12	T5 – O1	C4 – T4	F8 – Ave	F8 – A2	C3 – P3
13	Fp2 – F8	T4 – A2	T3 – Ave	T3 – A1	P3 – O1
14	F8 – T4	T5 – P3	T4 – Ave	T4 – A2	F4 – C4
15	T4 – T6	P3 – Pz	T5 – Ave	T5 – A1	C4 - P4
16	T6 – O2	Pz – P4	T6 – Ave	T6 – A2	P4 – O2
17	Fz – Cz	P4 – T6	Fz – Ave	Fz – A1	Fz – Cz
18	Cz – Pz	T5 – O1	Cz – Ave	Cz – A1	Cz – Pz
19	EKG	O1 – O2	Pz – Ave	Pz – A1	EKG
20		O2 – T6	EKG	EKG	
21		EKG			

The ipsilateral ear reference (Ipsi) can be replaced with the linked reference (LE) if there is prominent EKG artifact from one or both ear references. The EKG artifact tends to be of opposite polarity on the two sides, and linking the ears will usually attenuate it or eliminate it.

Localization

Localization of an abnormal potential depends on spatial mapping using the electrode positions and applied montages discussed earlier. Here, we will discuss montages and localization in more detail. Modern EEG equipment allows for changing of montage on the fly, and it allows for review of the same epoch in multiple montages for comparison. This is only part of the post-processing that can be performed on digital EEG recordings.

Referential Montages

In referential montages, a single reference or two references (as in *ipsilateral ear reference* recordings) will be the second input of each channel, while principal active electrodes are connected to the first input. In the ideal situation where the reference is neutral, potentials of interest are compared by amplitude, the largest amplitude reflecting the center of the field. However, references are often not neutral, so, just as with bipolar montages, the reader has to consider the location(s) of the reference. Digital EEG has the ability to change the reference without having to reacquire the signal; this provides the ability to reduce the effect of electrical activity near the reference electrode(s).

The *average reference* is derived from averaging the activity of all electrodes, except frontopolar electrodes, which are subject to large amplitude eye movement artifacts. Assuming that no large field synchronous activity is present, there is cancellation based on cerebral activity being out of phase in different channels. The average reference is ideal for any focal abnormality because the contribution of the focal discharge to the average is greatly diluted by the uninvolved electrodes. However, when discharges have a wide field, the average reference may become contaminated. Therefore, the average reference is not ideal for examining generalized spike-and-wave discharges and other generalized abnormalities.

The *ipsilateral ear reference* or *linked ear reference* montages are optimal for evaluation of generalized discharges, which tend to have the lowest amplitude in the temporal periphery. The ear reference is not suitable for temporal lobe discharges since the ear can be considered a lateral-basal temporal electrode. It is frequently involved in temporal lobe discharges.

The *average reference* will usually be a more appropriate reference for studying temporal lobe activity. However, if the temporal lobe activity has a wide field, the average reference could also become contaminated. This can be solved by removing involved electrodes from the average or using the midline electrodes (Cz, Fz, or Pz) if the discharge has not involved the midline. If the discharge field is anterior, Pz could be sufficiently distant to be neutral. In contrast, if the ictal discharge is predominately posterior, then Fz would be more appropriate.

Laplacian referential montage is excellent for identifying focal gradients by using a unique reference for each electrode, weighted by surrounding electrodes. This uses mathematical manipulations to at least partially attenuate volume conduction and thereby isolate regions of greater electrical interest. The Laplacian montage is excellent for pointing out small focal potentials with a steep gradient but is not appropriate for displaying generalized or widespread activity.

Localization in a referential montage is dependent on amplitude, assuming the presence of a neutral reference. The channel containing the highest amplitude will represent the center of the field.

Bipolar Montages

Bipolar montages are composed of chains linking adjacent electrodes. These chains are either longitudinal or transverse. They may also be in an arc, circle, or semicircle. The *longitudinal bipolar montage* (also called "double banana" because of the appearance on a montage diagram) can be organized in several ways. It is a general (but not universally followed) convention that anterior should be ahead of posterior and left ahead of right. In addition to the example displayed in Table 5.2.2, one acceptable alternative arrangement is left temporal, left parasagittal, midline, right parasagittal, right temporal; another arrangement is left temporal, right temporal, left parasagittal, right parasagittal, midline. There are fewer permutations in the arrangement of transverse bipolar montage.

Localization of EEG activity in bipolar montages is by reversal of polarity when the center of the field is within the center of the chain (see later discussion). Reversal of polarity will not be seen when the EEG activity is centered at the end of the chain, for example in the frontal or occipital pole in the longitudinal bipolar montage. This is where a circumferential montage may be useful.

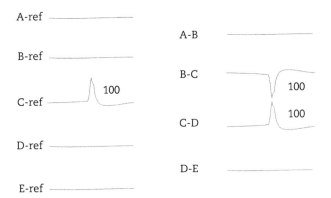

FIGURE 5.2.21 Referential versus bipolar example. Activity at electrode C seen in the two montages.

In a circumferential montage, the frontopolar and occipital electrodes are at the center of the anterior and posterior semicircular chains.

Localization in a bipolar montage is accomplished by identification of reversal of polarity. Described here are several situations and the expected pattern with each.

Potential is present in a single electrode (Figure 5.2.21): In this situation, there will be reversal of polarity between the two channels that have this electrode in common.

Two electrodes are equally involved, both contained within a chain of electrodes, and not involving the ends of the chain (Figure 5.2.22): The channel that compares the two affected electrodes would show cancellation. The reversal of polarity will be seen across that channel. One can state that there is a reversal of polarity across a zone of equipotentiality between electrodes B and C. The two channels showing a deflection will be mirror images of each other, again with equal amplitude of opposite polarity.

Two electrodes are unequally involved, each contained within the chain, with the ends of the chain not involved (Figure 5.2.23): There will be reversal of polarity seen between the two channels that contain the most affected electrode. The potential will also be seen in the channel containing the less affected electrode and the unaffected electrode adjacent to it. The amplitude in the channel with the largest deflection will be equal to the sum of the amplitudes in the two channels with smaller deflections. From this, one can conclude that, if there is a reversal of polarity that is not a mirror image, then it indicates that there is involvement of more than a single electrode.

Potential is present at the end of the chain and not involving any other electrode in the chain (Figures 5.2.24 and 5.2.25): In this instance there will be no reversal of polarity. A deflection will be seen in the first (or last) channel of the chain, where the potential is contained.

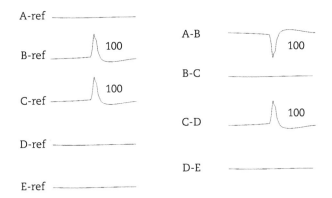

FIGURE 5.2.22 Referential versus bipolar example. Activity equal in electrodes B and C.

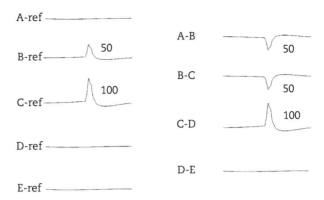

FIGURE 5.2.23 Referential versus bipolar example. Activity greater in electrode C than B.

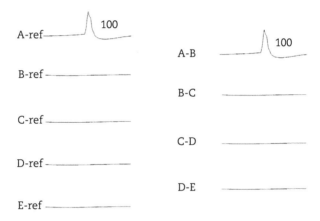

FIGURE 5.2.24 Referential versus bipolar example. Activity in electrode A.

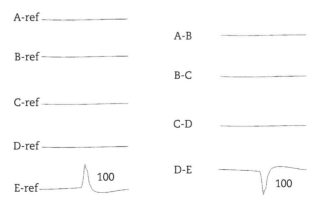

FIGURE 5.2.25 End of chain phenomenon. Activity in electrode E.

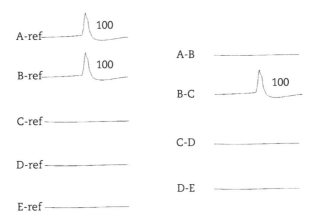

FIGURE 5.2.26 End of chain. Activity equal in electrodes A and B.

The potential involves one end of the chain and the electrode adjacent to it, equally (Figure 5.2.26): There will be cancellation in the channel that contains the two affected electrodes. The channel next to it will show a deflection. There will be no deflection in subsequent channels. There will be no reversal of polarity.

Every pattern in a bipolar montage has several potential patterns in a referential montage, assuming a neutral reference. Usually, one pattern is the most likely.

Consider Figures 5.2.27 and 5.2.28 together. The left side of each figure is a bipolar recording that is identical. The right is a potential referential recording that could correspond to the bipolar recording.

Which of these two possibilities is most likely? In these examples, the distribution shown in Solution B is less likely than that of Solution A because the Solution B distribution assumes that three electrodes are all equally affected, an unlikely distribution.

Although a bipolar montage can be used to suspect asymmetries in widespread activity, these asymmetries have to be confirmed in a referential montage. The main reason for this is that each bipolar channel is an arithmetic subtraction of adjacent active electrodes. There will be a low amplitude if adjacent electrodes are equally affected. The presence of a high-amplitude signal depends on a sharp gradient between adjacent electrodes. Fortunately, most potentials have the highest gradients near the center of the field, but this is not always the case. The examples in Figures 5.2.29 and 5.2.30 display the unlikely scenario where the side of higher voltage has a lower gradient so that there will be cancellation in a bipolar montage.

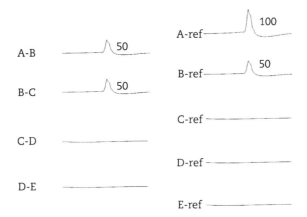

FIGURE 5.2.27 Bipolar versus reference localization example. Solution A: Referential recording on the right could produce the bipolar recording on the left.

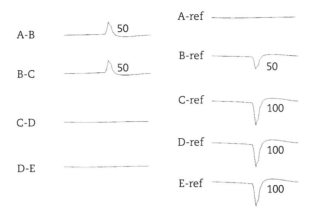

FIGURE 5.2.28 Bipolar versus reference localization example. Solution B: Referential recording on the right could produce the bipolar recording on the left but would be less likely than the solution in Figure 5.2.27.

Special Considerations

Average Versus Ear Reference: Contamination of the Average

Presented here are some examples of how the same activity may have a different appearance in the ipsilateral ear reference montage versus the average reference montage. The example in Figure 5.2.31 shows the posterior dominant alpha, which is clear in the right side of the figure in this ear reference epoch.

Figure 5.2.32 is of the same epoch but with an average reference. The posterior dominant rhythm is evident, but also appears in the frontopolar leads because the posterior dominant rhythm contaminates the average.

End-of-Chain Phenomenon

Bipolar montage will not demonstrate reversal of polarity for discharges maximally involving the end of the electrode chain, as was illustrated in the previous diagrammatic examples. Figures 5.2.33 through 5.2.35 show this for a real patient. The patient recorded in Figure 5.2.33 has right frontal sharp waves without reversal of polarity. The ear-reference montage for the same epoch (Figure 5.2.34) shows that the right frontopolar region is maximally involved. Bipolar circumferential montage shows reversal of polarity across the Fp2 (Figure 5.2.35) to localize the discharge.

EEG Review and Analysis
Overview

EEG performance and interpretation should be a systematic process, with the following elements:

- Understand the clinical snapshot of the patient, including reason for the study, age, and conditions that affect interpretation.

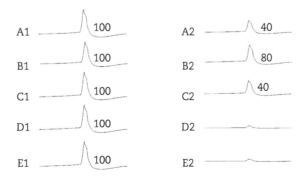

FIGURE 5.2.29 Localization with a referential montage. Hypothetical scenario of greater signal on the left electrodes than on right. For comparison with Figure 5.2.30.

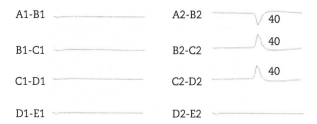

FIGURE 5.2.30 Localization with a referential montage. Bipolar solution to the scenario in Figure 5.2.29. This is for illustrative purposes: the field described would be extremely improbable.

- Review the study for background patterns in the context of state.
- Look for changes in state.
- Look for transients and rhythms that may be abnormal.
- Assess response to stimulation and activation methods.
- Synthesize an impression that places the EEG findings in the context of the clinical snapshot.

This section discusses some specifics of the basic interpretation of EEG.

Terminology

Rhythmic: Term used to describe ongoing EEG activity composed of recurring waves of equal duration. The waves need not be identical, but they usually resemble each other. Cerebral activity is never perfect, and slight variation should be allowed. For example, the activity in Figure 5.2.36 is rhythmic, but some individual waves are slightly shorter or longer than others, as demonstrated in Figure 5.2.37.

Rhythm: EEG activity composed of recurring waves of approximately equal duration. A rhythm is often characterized by its frequency.

Frequency: The number of waves of a specified rhythm per second, or 1/wavelength. Frequency is measured in Hertz or Hz, meaning cycles per second. Wavelength is measured in milliseconds or seconds. Frequency can be applied to single waves as well as to a rhythm. If applied to a single wave, inferred frequency is 1/wavelength. For a rhythm,

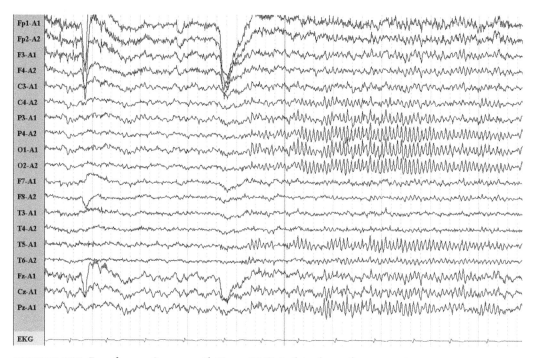

FIGURE 5.2.31 Ear reference. Compare with Figure 5.2.32. Ipsilateral ear reference montage.

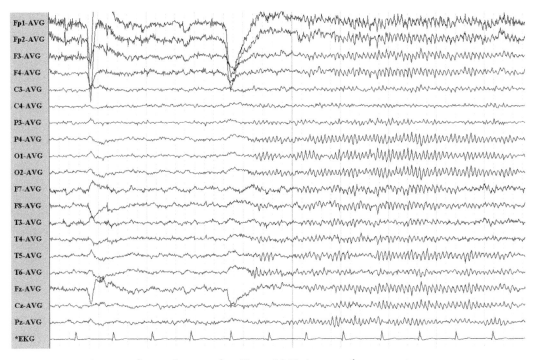

FIGURE 5.2.32 Average reference. Same epoch as Figure 5.2.31. Average reference montage.

the frequency will express how many waves will fit in 1 sec. In the example of Figure 5.2.37, nine waves can be counted between the two 1-sec marker lines.

Regular: Activity that is uniform in frequency, with individual waves having fairly consistent shape

in addition to fairly consistent duration. Regular rhythmic activity of stereotyped appearance is sometimes referred to as *monomorphic*. Sinusoidal activity is a good example of regular activity

Irregular: Activity that is not uniform (see Figures 5.2.38 and 5.2.39). It is theoretically

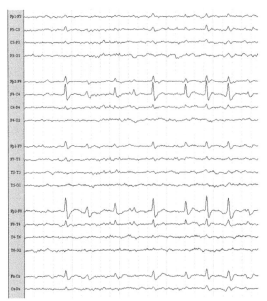

FIGURE 5.2.33 End-of-chain; right frontal sharp waves. Longitudinal bipolar montage.

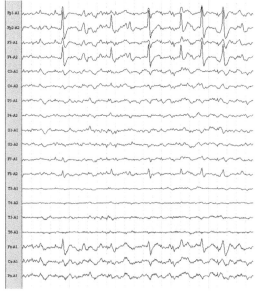

FIGURE 5.2.34 End-of-chain; right frontal sharp waves. Ipsilateral ear reference montage.

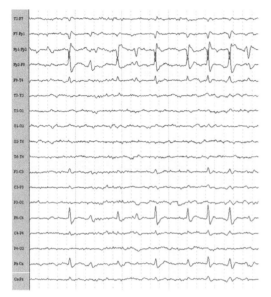

FIGURE 5.2.35 End-of-chain; right frontal sharp waves. Bipolar montage across the front.

possible for rhythmic activity to be irregular, but that is uncommon.

Arrhythmic: Term used to describe ongoing EEG activity composed of waves of unequal duration. Figure 5.2.39 shows an example of arrhythmic activity. In this activity, individual wave components have differing wavelengths.

Arrhythmic activity is also *irregular*. Note that individual waves not only have unequal duration, but also unequal shape and unequal amplitude. This is often called *polymorphic* if it is persistent. Activity such as that shown in Figures 5.2.38 and 5.2.39 can be continuous or intermittent. If the activity is intermittent, it can be described as rare, occasional, frequent, very frequent, or almost continuous.

Transient: A wave or combination of waves that stands out from the surrounding background. A transient can be normal or abnormal.

Complex: Combination of two or more waves. This combination will usually be consistent when the complex recurs. Figures 5.2.40 and 5.2.41 show a polyspike-and-wave complex that includes a series of three spikes followed by a high-voltage slow wave. Figures 5.2.42 and 5.2.43 show a series of spike-and-wave complexes, demonstrating that complexes look fairly consistent when they recur.

Periodic: Term used to describe transients or complexes that recur, but with intervening activity between them. The rate of recurrence of periodic transients is less than the frequency of this transient, determined as 1/wavelength. Figure 5.2.44 demonstrates the difference between rhythmic and periodic discharges. The bottom line shows a single transient. The top line shows the same transient recurring as a periodic discharge. The middle line shows the same transient recurring as a rhythmic train.

Differentiation of a Periodic Pattern from a Rhythm

The *period* is the time from the beginning of one discharge to the beginning of the next. The *wavelength* is the duration of the discharge. A periodic pattern has a period longer than the wavelength. A rhythmic pattern has a wavelength that is immediately followed by the next wave. The periodicity is expressed as cycle per second (cps), while frequency is expressed as Hertz (Hz).

Spatial distribution: The electrodes involved with a discharge and the degree of their involvement determines the field. Discharges can be described as *focal*, *regional*, *lateralized*, or *generalized*. *Focal* discharges are restricted to a few

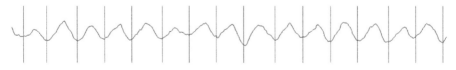

FIGURE 5.2.36 Rhythm of a specified frequency.

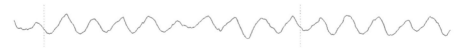

FIGURE 5.2.37 Same activity as Figure 5.2.36 without vertical lines demarcating each wave. The only vertical lines mark 1 sec.

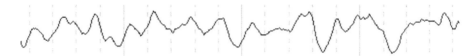

FIGURE 5.2.38 Irregular electroencephalogram (EEG) activity.

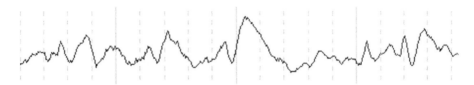

FIGURE 5.2.39 Irregular electroencephalogram (EEG) activity.

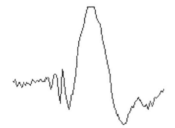

FIGURE 5.2.40 Polyspike-and-wave complex.

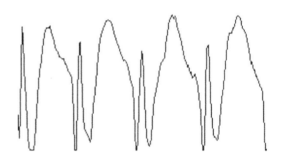

FIGURE 5.2.42 Rhythmic spike-and-wave activity.

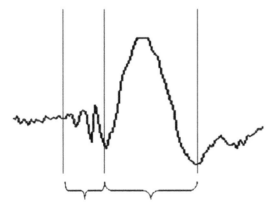

FIGURE 5.2.41 Analysis of the polyspike-and-wave complex, from the previous figure, showing the polyspike component followed by the slow wave component.

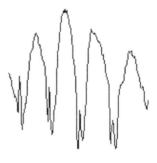

FIGURE 5.2.43 Rhythmic spike-and-wave activity.

electrodes on one side. The term *regional* can be applied to a discharge that involves more than a few electrodes. If electrodes on one side are all affected, the discharge can be considered lateralized. *Generalized* discharges affect all electrodes, on both sides. It is almost never the case that all electrodes are affected equally. Many generalized discharges have voltage predominance anteriorly, but there can be voltage predominance in a variety of regions. The terms "diffuse" and "widespread" are sometimes used synonymously with generalized, but these terms indicate a less clearly generalized field. For focal and regional discharges, a field can be designated with isopotential lines that join equally affected regions. Figure 5.2.45 shows an example of a field. The center of the field is at

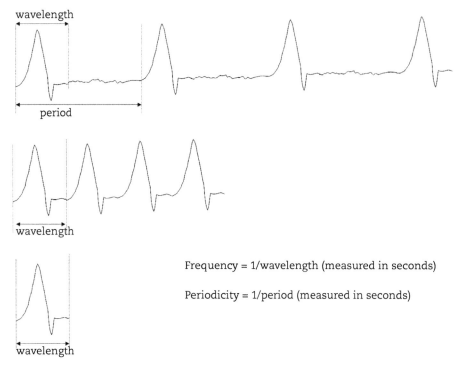

Frequency = 1/wavelength (measured in seconds)

Periodicity = 1/period (measured in seconds)

FIGURE 5.2.44 Periodic pattern versus rhythmic pattern. *Top*: Periodic discharge. *Middle*: Rhythmic discharge. *Bottom*: Single discharge.

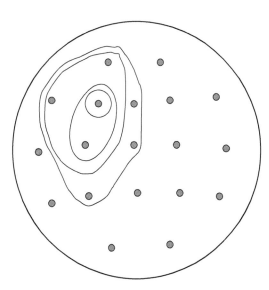

FIGURE 5.2.45 Spatial distribution of a potential represented with isopotential lines on diagram with standard 10–20 electrode placement. The center of the field is at F3, followed by C3 then Fp1 and F7, then Fz, Cz, and P3.

F3, then C3 is a bit less involved, followed by Fp1 and F7, then Fz, Cz, and P3.

Timing

When discharges are seen in several locations, then the temporal relationship of the activity in these different regions can be described with the terms *synchronous*, *asynchronous*, and *independent*.

Synchronous: Occurring in two regions simultaneously. To indicate that a discharge is occurring on the two sides simultaneously, the terms *bisynchronous* or *bilaterally synchronous* are frequently used. Figure 5.2.46 shows a bilaterally synchronous spike-and-wave discharge.

Asynchronous: Describes transients or other activity that is seen in several regions, but not simultaneously.

Independent is often applied to a more extreme situation where discharges occur at different times in two or more regions, or on the two sides. The circled discharges in Figure 5.2.47 are occurring independently on the two sides and in

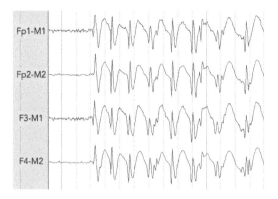

FIGURE 5.2.46 Synchronous spike-and-wave discharge. Ipsilateral ear reference.

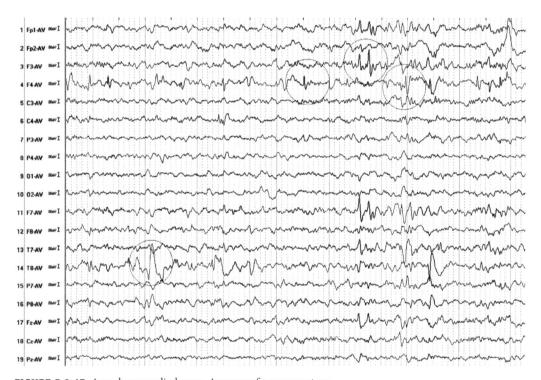

FIGURE 5.2.47 Asynchronous discharges. Average reference montage.

different regions on the same side. The recordings in Figure 5.2.48 show both independent and bisynchronous discharges.

Synchronous activity can be *in-phase*, indicating a perfect correspondence in time and polarity, or *out-of-phase*, indicating a small delay on one side in comparison with the other and different polarity. When there is a horizontal dipole, with negativity in one region and positivity in another, the discharge is out of phase in these two regions.

Basic EEG Analysis

EEG analysis consists of characterization of rhythms and transients. EEG rhythms are divided into frequency bands for descriptive purposes (see Table 5.2.3). Each frequency band can be seen in normal or abnormal settings, and the interpretation depends on the context. For example, alpha activity in the occipital region is normal in an awake patient with eyes closed. The same frequency of activity is very abnormal when diffusely distributed in a comatose patient.

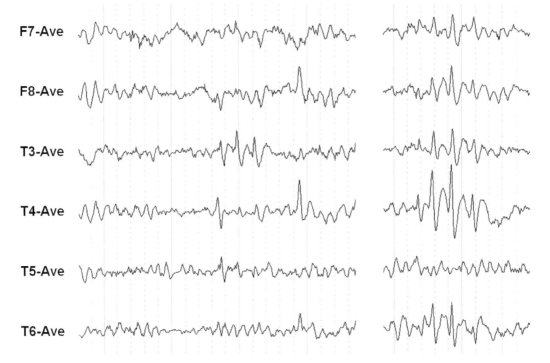

FIGURE 5.2.48 Independent and bisynchronous discharges. Average reference montage.

TABLE 5.2.3 ELECTROENCEPHALOGRAM (EEG) FREQUENCY BANDS IN CLINICAL EEG

Rhythm	Frequency	Normal and abnormal examples
Alpha	8–13 Hz	Waking posterior rhythm in older children and adults. Mu rhythm. Alpha coma. Seizure activity in the alpha range.
Beta	>13–25 Hz	Drowsiness. Drug-induced. Breach rhythm over a skull defect. Seizure onset.
Gamma	25–80 Hz	Physiological activation. Seizure onset.
Theta	4–7 Hz	Drowsiness, young children; temporal theta in the elderly. Structural lesion. Encephalopathy.
Delta	<4 Hz	Sleep, posterior slow waves of youth. Focal structural lesion. Encephalopathy.

In addition to the preceding bands, there are higher frequency bands that are not usually captured with routine clinical EEG but may become important in the future (Table 5.2.4). The evaluation of these faster frequencies requires modified sampling rate and filter settings.

Fundamental Frequency Bands

Alpha rhythm is 8–13 Hz. It is most commonly seen in normal patients from the occipital regions in the awake state with eyes closed. When the eyes open, the alpha rhythm is attenuated. Because the occipital rhythm is in the alpha range, the term *alpha rhythm* is sometimes used for the *posterior dominant rhythm*. Therefore, one needs to keep in mind the dual use of this term. There are other EEG activities in the alpha range: the *mu rhythm*, which is the resting rhythm of the Rolandic region, and the *third rhythm*, which is seen at times in the temporal region.

Beta rhythm is 13.1–25 Hz and is most often seen in patients who have been sedated with benzodiazepines and barbiturates. Beta activity should be commented on during interpretation of the record, and an association with concurrent medications should be considered.

Theta rhythm is 4–7.9 Hz and is seen most commonly in normal drowsiness and in children.

TABLE 5.2.4 HIGHER FREQUENCY BANDS

| Ripples | 80–250 Hz | May be physiological or pathological |
| Fast ripples | 250–500 Hz | Usually pathological, associated with epilepsy |

Theta is most likely to be abnormal if it is the posterior dominant rhythm in a waking adult, or if it is focal.

Delta activity is less than 4 Hz and is most commonly seen in sleep. There is a gradual increase in the amount of delta activity as the patient progresses from stage 2 to deeper sleep. Focal delta activity develops in patients with acute focal structural lesions. Irregular and persistent delta activity is often called *polymorphic delta activity*.

Transients

Spikes and Sharp Waves
Spikes and sharp waves are abnormal sharp transients suggestive of epilepsy. Spikes and sharp waves are also referred to as *interictal epileptiform discharges*. Spikes have a duration of less than 70 msec, and sharp waves have a duration of 70–200 msec, therefore appearing less sharp than spikes. Combinations of spikes, sharp waves, and slow waves are also epileptiform discharges (see Table 5.2.5).

Spikes and sharp waves generated at the crown of a gyrus are usually surface-negative, with the positive end of the dipole deep to the cortex. However, some spike foci have a horizontal dipole, where both the positive and negative poles are seen on surface recordings. One notable example is Rolandic epilepsy, in which the positive end of the dipole can be seen anteriorly. This is discussed in greater detail in Chapter 6.3.

There are a number of features that distinguish spikes and sharp waves from nonepileptiform sharp transients.

- Epileptiform discharges are different from the surrounding activity.
- Epileptiform discharges tend to be of high voltage.
- Epileptiform discharges are usually asymmetrical with a longer and larger second half in comparison with the first half.
- Epileptiform discharges tend to have more than one phase.
- Epileptiform discharges tend to have an after-going slow wave.
- Epileptiform discharges are more convincing if they arise from an abnormal background.
- Epileptiform discharges should be different from normal sharp activity (such as vertex waves) in their fields and in the states of arousal of the patient.

Figure 5.2.49 shows some of the elements of an epileptiform discharge. These include high voltage, asymmetrical shape, more than one phase, and after-going slow wave.

TABLE 5.2.5 EPILEPTIFORM TRANSIENTS

Transient	Duration	Variants
Spike	25–70 msec	Spike-and-wave complex polyspike complex Polyspike-and-wave complex
Sharp wave	70–200 msec	Sharp-and-wave complex; multiple sharp-and-wave complex
Sharply contoured slow wave (may be seen with epilepsy, but not strictly epileptiform)	>200 msec	

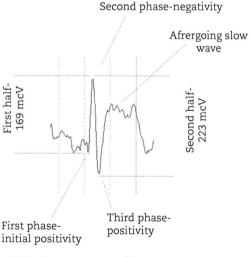

FIGURE 5.2.49 Analysis of the spike-wave complex. The complex is divided by the vertical markers into fundamental components.

Sharp potentials that are normal are frequently a source of overinterpretation. Sharp potentials that are often misinterpreted include benign variants such as wicket spikes; sharp physiologic activity, as is seen with skull defects; EMG potentials; and artifact. Differentiation of spikes and sharp waves from nonepileptiform potentials may also take into consideration the consistency of appearance of epileptiform discharges. Figure 5.2.50 shows a nonepileptiform sharp activity that looks symmetrical and is similar to surrounding activity except for higher amplitude and sharpness. Figure 5.2.51 demonstrates lateral rectus spikes, or EMG potentials from the lateral rectus that could be misinterpreted as epileptiform discharges.

Epileptiform discharges do not consistently indicate epilepsy. Caution should be used in the interpretation of pediatric EEGs with occipital or Rolandic sharp waves. Caution should also be exercised in the final interpretation if only a single spike is recorded during the entire EEG. Figures 5.2.52 through 5.2.56 show examples of spikes and sharp waves.

Sharply Contoured Slow Waves

These are transients that could have been sharp waves had they not been longer than 200 msec. Such discharges have a weaker association with epilepsy and should not be called epileptiform.

Slow Waves

Slow wave transients can be in the theta or delta range and stand out from the background. Focal slow activity can occasionally be the only abnormality seen in association with focal epilepsy.

Clinical Analysis and Interpretation
Review of Routine EEG

Some neurophysiologists begin with a review of the EEG before any of the clinical information is reviewed. However, most of us prefer to know some clinical details, including the age of the patient, reason for the study, current medications, and the technologist's impression of the state.

Review includes determination of the following:

- Background rhythm,
- Topographical organization of the background activities,
- Transients,
- State changes,
- Response to activation methods.

Particular attention is paid to the following:

- Ictal activity,
- Sharp waves or spikes,
- Focal and generalized slow activity,
- Inappropriate response to stimuli,
- EEG correlates to changes in state or behavior.

It is often best to proceed with one uninterrupted rapid review of the recording before returning to it for a more detailed and in-depth assessment. The reason for this is that there may be a prominent abnormality later in the recording that would alter the approach to the interpretation of the preceding part of the study.

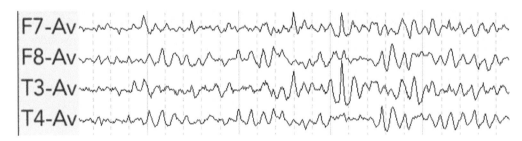

FIGURE 5.2.50 Spike-like potentials that are not epileptiform.

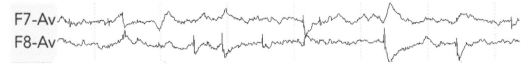

FIGURE 5.2.51 Lateral rectus spikes.

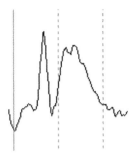

FIGURE 5.2.52 Spike potential. The duration of the discharge is 69 msec. It qualifies as a spike. The dotted vertical lines are at 200 msec intervals.

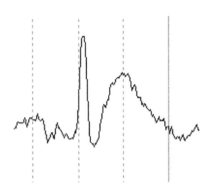

FIGURE 5.2.53 Sharp wave. The discharge has a duration of 95 msec, and therefore is a sharp wave.

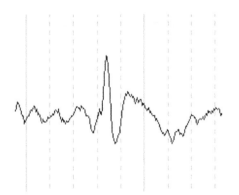

FIGURE 5.2.54 Sharp wave. This discharge is also a sharp wave. Even though it has an after-going slow wave, it is not called a sharp-and-slow wave complex unless the slow wave has an amplitude at least as high as the sharp wave.

Review of Video-EEG

Video-EEG is initially reviewed by the EEG technologist. It is unrealistic for the neurophysiologist to review the entire video-EEG in real time, but the epochs focused on include those thought to be of interest to the technologist and ones that

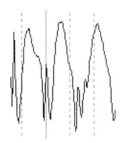

FIGURE 5.2.55 Spike-wave complexes.

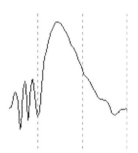

FIGURE 5.2.56 Polyspike-and-wave complex.

were noted by the event marker. For most EEG devices, a spike and seizure detection function identifies suspected seizures as well as spikes and sharp waves. In addition quantitative EEG displays help identify regions of interest. Also, the patient, patient's family, and nursing personnel are instructed to push an event marker button, which highlights the particular epoch of the EEG recording. Ideally, the technologist reviews all the patient events and computer seizure detections and marks all the seizures as well as suspected ictal discharges, but this is not standard in all institutions. The electroencephalographer reviews these segments closely, analyzing both the EEG discharges and the clinical seizure semiology.

Review of Activation Method Segments
Hyperventilation

Hyperventilation is used predominantly to activate the generalized spike-and-wave discharges in absence epilepsies. In some patients, the discharges are only seen during hyperventilation. The normal response to hyperventilation is increased generalized theta and delta activity. This is more prominent in children than in adults. An excessive amount of slow activity can be seen in patients with hypoglycemia. At times, hyperventilation can bring out focal slow abnormalities that are subtle at other times.

Photic Stimulation

Responses to photic stimulation can be normal, abnormal, or artifactual. These are

- Normal:
  - *Visual evoked response*: This is the same potential that is recorded during flash evoked potentials. This has a major positive component from the occipital leads O1 and O2; it occurs approximately 100 msec after each stimulus. It is seen at flash frequencies of 5/sec and less.
  - *Driving response*: The driving response appears with faster flash frequencies, 7/sec and higher. It is time-locked to the stimulus.
- Abnormal:
  - *PPR*: The photoparoxysmal or photoconvulsive response is a marker for seizure tendency. The discharge typically starts later than the onset of the flash and may or may not terminate when the flash train does. It is most often generalized and suggestive of idiopathic generalized epilepsy. Less often, it may occur with focal epilepsy, mainly occipital lobe epilepsy.
- Artifactual:
  - *Photomyoclonic response*: The photomyoclonic response is EMG activity in the frontal scalp muscles induced by the flash. Only susceptible individuals will show this rhythmic activity. There is about 50–60 msec between the flash and the EMG activity
  - *Photoelectric artifact*: The photoelectric artifact is produced by light from the photic strobe interacting with the electrode-gel complex. This is a chemical charge movement and not physiologic. It is noncerebral and is not EMG.

EEG Reports

The EEG report should reflect the approach to interpretations and include the following sections:

- Preamble:
  - Includes background information that could influence interpretation and reason for study.
- EEG description:
  - Description of background, state changes, and presence and absence of normal and abnormal rhythms or transients, including epileptiform and focal abnormalities, abnormal responses, or absence of response.
  - Should be purely descriptive, avoiding interpretive terms.
  - Abnormalities should be numbered.
  - Give details, including regions and electrode names; list electrodes in order of involvement, with the most involved electrode first.
- EEG diagnosis:
  - List the key abnormalities briefly, without detail (electrode names optional).
  - Number EEG diagnoses, starting with the most important.
- Clinical interpretation:
  - Identify the clinical correlate of the findings: may include a small discussion of the most likely and less likely possibilities.
  - Clinical interpretation should take into account the clinical information that was provided. This information can be quite limited, thus restricting the utility of the interpretation. A review of the electronic medical record for clinical and imaging data can improve the value of the EEG.
  - As with all neurophysiologic interpretations, the EEG report represents a type of consultation. The clinical interpretation should be tailored to the question asked. For example, if the clinical question is "rule out status epilepticus," it would be helpful for the clinical interpretation to add "there was no seizure activity." The clinical interpretation should not only be descriptive but also clinically useful.

It is acceptable to summarize the findings under "*Impression*," including a summary of the key findings under *EEG Diagnosis*, then clinical interpretation, as shown here.

EEG Diagnosis: Abnormal study because of:

1. Generalized asynchronous theta and delta activity intermingled in the background
2. Slow posterior dominant rhythm

Clinical Interpretation: This EEG consistent with a mild nonspecific cerebral dysfunction. No seizures or interictal epileptiform discharges (seizure tendency) were noted.

Epilepsy monitoring unit (EMU) reports follow the same guidelines. In our center, the report includes, in addition to identifying information, the following:

- *A preamble summarizing the background information and the reason for the study;*
- *A description of the baseline EEG (this is like a standard EEG with hyperventilation and photic stimulation, performed within the first day of admission);*
- *A daily description of clinical seizures and their electrographic correlate;*
- *A daily description of the interictal abnormalities;*
- *EEG diagnosis summarizing the key abnormalities, starting with ictal discharges (focusing on localization at onset), then interictal epileptiform discharges, then nonepileptiform abnormalities;*
- *Clinical interpretation. In this section, the clinical seizure description is provided first, with a statement about the localizing and lateralizing value of the seizure signs, then a statement about how the semiology agrees (or not) with the EEG ictal onset and other EEG abnormalities, and then a summary synthesis of all the findings to provide a seizure diagnosis, classification, lateralization, and localization, together with the degree of certainty of these determinations.*

VIDEO-EEG AND LONG-TERM EEG MONITORING

EEG monitoring and prolonged EEG recordings are most effective when video is included. These techniques were once the arena only of academic institutions, but with improvements in technology, video-EEG is available in most hospitals and office practices. Types of monitoring include

- *Short-term video-EEG. This is typically performed in the hospital or office for one or more hours, usually lasting up to a working day.*
- *Long-term video-EEG. Long-term video-EEG is often performed in hospital rooms and in the ICU. Several companies are now offering home video-EEG; this is appropriate for patients with frequent events who are not taking anti-seizure medications (ASMs), particularly if admission to an EMU is denied by insurance.*

- *Ambulatory EEG. This is usually obtained without concomitant video, usually for 24 hours, though it can be extended for 2–3 days. It is cheaper and less disruptive and restrictive than video-EEG monitoring and allows for more freedom of movement.*

Clinical Indications for Video-EEG

Video-EEG is used for direct correlation of clinical events with EEG. This is especially of use when patients are having events that might be seizures. Prolonged video-EEG monitoring was developed for more direct evaluation of seizures. The 20-min "routine" EEG is only an indirect assessment in patients with seizures and spells of an unknown nature. It may record interictal abnormalities to help the diagnosis, but it is unlikely to record seizures. The most solid clinical diagnosis requires the ability to capture and analyze a typical seizure and its EEG correlate. The technology of video-EEG allows the electroencephalographer to replay seizures an unlimited number of times for detailed analysis of the clinical signs and the corresponding EEG changes.

The main indications for video-EEG monitoring are

- *Diagnosis of atypical seizures or spells of unknown nature. The need for video-EEG could arise because events are atypical for seizures, because there has been absence of evidence for epilepsy by history and by tests, because there has been no response to ASM therapy, or because a patient with known epilepsy started having new or "different" spells.*
- *Accurate classification of seizures for optimal choice of medical therapy. This situation applies to individuals with documented epilepsy in whom there may be incomplete or contradictory clinical and EEG data for classification purposes. An example of this would include an adolescent with staring spells and an EEG that shows both focal and generalized discharges. The seizures could represent generalized absence seizures, in which case the most appropriate therapy could be ethosuximide, or focal impaired-awareness seizures, in which case ethosuximide would be ineffective and a medication more appropriate for partial seizures could be best suited.*
- *Localization of the epileptogenic zone for possible surgical resection. There is evidence to suggest that after failure of two anti-epileptic*

drugs, the chances of seizure freedom with another agent decreases markedly. Patients refractory to medical therapy should be investigated for the presence of a surgically remediable epileptic syndrome.

Additional indications for video-EEG monitoring include:

- *Quantification of seizures*. Advanced EEG analysis can produce valuable data regarding seizure and discharge quantification. Some seizures are more easily counted than others, such as generalized absence seizures.
- *Quantification of response to treatment*. The most common situation is checking the efficacy of therapy of absence seizures in childhood absence epilepsy. In this syndrome, seizures are frequent, and the response can be quantified with a 24-hour monitoring study. This is also frequently a research application.
- *Studying seizure precipitants described in the history*.
  - *Reflex epilepsy*: Video-EEG monitoring can easily record seizures if the reflex precipitant can be reproduced.
  - *Self-induction*: Some patients have resistant seizures because of auto-induction. Video-EEG monitoring can document the occurrence of auto-induction in this situation.
  - *Situational factors*: When situational factors are reported to precipitate seizures, they may potentially be reproduced in the setting of the EMU.
- *Documentation of ictal and interictal discharges during circadian rhythms*. This is frequently a research application.
- *Clinical correlate of EEG discharge*. Some patients have EEG discharges that could be ictal in nature. The presence or absence of clinical changes may be necessary for counseling regarding driving or other restrictions. Simultaneous video with the EEG allows testing and demonstration of changes in responsiveness or cognitive functions in conjunction with the EEG discharge.
- *Transitory cognitive impairment*. This is predominantly a research application. Very sensitive testing has allowed the demonstration of subtle dysfunction in association with interictal epileptiform discharges.
- *Finding interictal evidence for epilepsy*. This application does not necessarily require the video component.

Methods
Inpatient Long-Term EEG Monitoring

Inpatient long-term monitoring is performed in a fixed EMU. In this setting, the most up-to-date equipment uses cameras fixed in the patient's room. Two cameras with different angles and zoom settings are possible but not mandatory. The electrodes attached to the patient's head are connected to a head box. Signals are amplified and transmitted through a cable to a computer that records the digitized EEG signal. The video signal is similarly digitized and synchronized.

Most EMUs currently use seizure and spike detection paradigms. These can help identify seizures that patients are not aware of, but they have a very high false-positive detection rate so that every detection has to be reviewed to determine its validity.

Patients are typically admitted for several days. If they have been on ASMs, these are reduced or discontinued to facilitate the recording of seizures. Some medications have to be withdrawn carefully as they can be associated with particularly severe withdrawal seizures. In particular, this has been demonstrated for carbamazepine and oxcarbazepine. Identification of seizures can be performed in several ways.

- An event marker button that the patient or patient's family can push if a suspected seizure occurs,
- Automatic seizure detection program,
- Seizure log/diary kept by the patient/family/caretaker,
- Review of quantitative EEG displays for changes that could be consistent with seizures,
- Screening the EEG or video.

Using a combination of all of these, long-term video-EEG monitoring in the EMU is successful in the majority of patients in recording epileptic seizures for analysis.

Repeated Admissions

Occasionally, admission has to be repeated. If a second admission fails to record seizures, the approach to video-EEG monitoring may have to be modified. One of the factors that contributes to the failure of video-EEG monitoring is the elimination of daily life stressors when patients are admitted. These stressors may be necessary to precipitate seizures.

Some patients have cyclical seizure patterns, and the video-EEG monitoring session will have the highest yield if scheduled at the next expected cycle. This is most commonly encountered in women with catamenial epilepsy in whom seizures are most likely just before or during the menstrual period. In other women, seizures are also more likely around the time of ovulation. Even men may have cyclical seizure precipitation, and video-EEG monitoring could have a higher yield taking these into consideration.

Monitoring for Differentiation of Epileptic from Nonepileptic Events

If the purpose of monitoring is to determine whether an event is epileptic or nonepileptic, the recording of a highly typical nonepileptic event could be sufficient for the purposes of monitoring. However, there are potential pitfalls, and one should be extremely careful in the analysis of data. For many patients, recording additional events is advisable and continuing to record until ASMs have been cleared would provide further assurance. Some patients may have had epilepsy but new spells may be nonepileptic. The recording of a characteristic new spell that is nonepileptic does not necessarily eliminate the possibility of persistent controlled epilepsy.

The use of suggestion techniques has been controversial. Suggestion is acceptable only if it does not involve deception. Nonepileptic events are often provoked by suggestion early in the study, whereas epileptic seizures will often appear at a latency, as ASMs are cleared. Some patients may erroneously identify an event as a typical seizure because they do not know what happens during a typical event.

Not only can some patients with epilepsy be suggested to have a nonepileptic event, but others may spontaneously have an atypical psychogenic nonepileptic event in the charged environment. It is essential for a patient's family member to identify an event as typical. If typical events are recorded and are deemed psychogenic and nothing different happens after ASMs have been cleared, then the possibility of pure psychogenic nonepileptic events is most likely. One can be most secure in this diagnosis when the onset of episodes is recent and it can be clearly confirmed that no events other than typical recorded ones have occurred in the past.

Monitoring for Classification of Seizure Type

If the purpose of the video-EEG monitoring is to classify the seizure type, then recording of a single seizure may be sufficient if that recorded seizure has a clear focal onset and seizure semiology that agrees with the EEG localization. In other instances, however, one cannot be so certain with a single recorded seizure. In some patients, the seizure onset may appear generalized but the clinical seizure pattern may suggest a focal origin. In these instances, it may become necessary to record more than one event, in addition to interictal epileptiform activity.

Monitoring for Presurgical Localization

Inpatient video-EEG is the only appropriate test for patients who are being evaluated for the possibility of epilepsy surgery. If video-EEG monitoring is scheduled for the purpose of presurgical seizure localization, then recording of 3–6 seizures is usually required. In the presence of conflicting data, a larger number of seizures may be needed to resolve the conflict and increase certainty.

Some patients have independent left and right temporal seizure onsets, and these patients may still be candidates for surgery if more than 80% of seizures arise in one focus or if only clinically insignificant seizures arise on one side and all clinically significant seizures arise on the other. In complicated cases, a larger number of seizures may be needed for accurate classification.

In some patients with independent interictal epileptiform discharges arising on both sides, a particular cluster of seizures may come from one of the two foci. In these patients, seizures cannot be recorded solely from a single cluster. Repeat monitoring at a different point in time may be advisable to record a separate cluster of seizures.

Baseline EEG Recording

Ideally, every session of video-EEG monitoring should be preceded by a baseline EEG. This baseline EEG provides the opportunity to record clean activity while the patient is relaxed and inactive. The posterior background rhythm can be recorded and its reactivity tested to eye opening and closure. Hyperventilation and photic stimulation should be a component of that baseline EEG if not contraindicated.

Provocation of Epileptic Seizures

Withdrawal of anti-epileptic drugs is the main method used in the monitoring unit for precipitating epileptic seizures. However, other techniques can be added, particularly *sleep deprivation*. This is most effective for generalized epilepsy, particularly juvenile myoclonic epilepsy. In that condition, seizures sometimes occur only in the setting of sleep deprivation and usually after arousal from premature awakening. In focal epilepsy, sleep deprivation may be less effective. In patients whose seizures are predominately in sleep, particularly patients with frontal lobe epilepsy, sleep deprivation is useful only as far as making seizures more likely with the next session of sleep. It is best in these instances to alternate sleep deprivation and full night's sleep. Using sleep deprivation on consecutive nights and days may not be justified or fruitful. If an ictal single-photon emission computed tomography (SPECT) is planned during the session of video-EEG monitoring, sleep deprivation at night can be followed by allowing the patient to sleep during the daytime when the ictal SPECT injection is possible. This is most useful for patients whose seizures typically occur in sleep.

If a patient or family has noted a possible provoking experience, then this should be reproduced in the EMU as closely as possible. For example, rare patients have seizures induced by reading, music, smells, or other experiences.

Withdrawal of some ASMs can unmask some discharges that would be not seen otherwise (e.g., levetiracetam, valproate, and benzodiazepines). In addition, withdrawal of ASMs can result in a greater tendency to have the seizure spread over the cortex, making it easier to see on scalp EEG.

Observation During the Study

Technologist observation during the study should be an active encounter. There are events that might occur during a study which deserve some intervention by the technologist. For example, if a seizure discharge is noted during a recording, the technologist should give a command to the patient or otherwise try to ascertain responsiveness. One command might be "Hold up two fingers" and note whether the patient makes a correct, incorrect, delayed, or no response. If the patient is unresponsive the technologist can then give a different command. When the seizure is over the patient can be tested for memory of the commands given.

Testing Patients During Events

In EMUs where patients are observed continuously and in any short-term video-EEG monitoring where an EEG technologist is present, the testing of patients during events is of great clinical utility.

Testing is aimed at the following:

- Establish if the patient is unresponsive,
- Determine if there is impairment in specific areas,
- Determine if the patient has recollection for items given during the spell or for events that occurred during the spell.

The patient's ability to follow commands and to name items should be tested at baseline. Should a suspicious ictal EEG activity appear or any behavioral changes occur that are suggestive of a seizure, then the patient should be given a command, the response to which can be assessed visually on video review. For example, the patient could be asked to point to the ceiling, touch his or her nose, or clap his or her hands. The patient can then be given items to name and remember.

One study used a sentence from the Boston Diagnostic Aphasic Battery, "I heard him speak over the radio last night," to assess reading abilities post-ictally.[9] Patients with left temporal seizures usually required more than 1 min from the termination of the seizure to read the sentence correctly. Patients with right temporal lobe seizures were able to read the sentence within 1 min from seizure termination.

When the patient has fully recovered, memory can be tested by asking for items given during the seizure as well as for events during a seizure. For example, it is not uncommon for patients with right temporal lobe seizures to produce spontaneous sentences (often with a twinge of fear) and respond almost normally to commands or other verbal stimuli. Once the seizure is over, it is quite common for these patients not to remember the conversation.

End of the Study

When Should the Study End?

The video-EEG monitoring study ends once a sufficient number of events have been recorded and the patient has been stabilized. In patients who develop a cluster of seizures or who have tonic-clonic seizures during the monitoring session, 1 day without seizures would be advisable before discharge. Certainly, the safety of discharge also depends on many individual factors, such as whether the patient lives alone and how far the patient lives from the medical center or from an emergency department. A patient who lives alone requires a greater evidence of stability prior to discharge.

Medications upon Discharge

The admission to the EMU presents an opportunity to make medication changes for many patients. For patients with documented epilepsy, the admission could be an opportunity to withdraw a medication such as carbamazepine that would be difficult to withdraw on an outpatient basis. The inpatient setting allows a faster withdrawal and treatment of consequences with intravenous or oral medications on an as-needed basis.

For patients with psychogenic nonepileptic events and no evidence of epilepsy, it is most appropriate to discontinue ASMs prior to discharge. As a component of the treatment of patients with nonepileptic events, withdrawal of ASMs helps remove the ambiguity about the diagnosis so that effective treatment can be pursued with psychotherapy or psychiatric medications as needed.

Long-Term Home Video-EEG Monitoring

Home video-EEG is less expensive than inpatient video-EEG monitoring. This modality is appropriate for patients having frequent events suspected to be nonepileptic in nature, without ASMs on board. This is also an option when hospital admission is not approved by insurance. Home video-EEG can be continued for multiple days or until the recording of a certain number of events. Medication changes during home video-EEG are not appropriate. The companies providing this service usually provide remote monitoring of patients and monitor impedances. The monitoring technologist can remotely control the camera and may dispatch an on-call technologist to the patient's home to fix problems if needed.

Short-Term Video-EEG Monitoring

This form of video-EEG monitoring, which is performed for 2–8 hours, avoids the need for hospital admission. It is the preferred form of monitoring for children and adults who have very frequent attacks or for patients in whom attacks can be reliably precipitated. For example, a variety of reflex epilepsies can be diagnosed on outpatient video-EEG. Examples could include photosensitive epilepsy, startle epilepsy, reading epilepsy, eating epilepsy, and musicogenic epilepsy.

It is usually impractical and inappropriate to make medication changes during short-term video monitoring sessions. An exception could be the individual who reports that missing a single dose of medication reliably brings on attacks or the individual who has only very mild events that would not present a risk. If the short-term video monitoring session fails to record an attack despite the use of appropriate activation techniques, then prolonged inpatient monitoring can be performed.

Ambulatory EEG Monitoring

Ambulatory EEG has the advantage of keeping the patient in an environment that includes the usual stressors. Most commonly, this technology is applied without the video component. The use of video in conjunction with ambulatory EEG is provided by some manufacturers. This concomitant video use is possible when the patient is stationary, for example working at a desk, sitting on a sofa, or sleeping. In the absence of video, interpretation of ambulatory EEG presents many challenges. It is well-known that artifact can imitate any EEG abnormality, and without knowing the concomitant behavior one cannot exclude the possibility that movement or other patterns of muscle activity and behavior could be responsible. Similarly, EEG discharge can be misread as movement or other artifact without video or other observational correlate.

Ambulatory EEG alone would be most helpful in major attacks that involve loss of consciousness or complete loss of awareness. In these instances, the persistence of a normal EEG strongly suggests a nonepileptic etiology. Ambulatory EEG can be an excellent option to assess efficacy of treatment against generalized absence seizures. Ambulatory EEG becomes less appropriate for subtle events, in particular events that do not involve alteration of awareness. Ambulatory EEG is required by some insurance companies before approval of inpatient video-EEG monitoring. It is also an option for patients who do not have seizures in the EMU but only in their normal outpatient environment, including their work environment.

EEG Review by Technologist

Review by the technologists is performed daily on patients admitted for prolonged monitoring. The review includes evaluation of burst detections. Any potentially abnormal pages are reviewed for

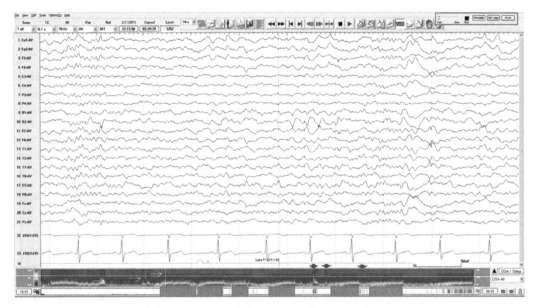

FIGURE 5.2.57 Electroencephalogram (EEG) with density spectral array (DSA). Average reference montage.

characterization. Density spectral array (DSA) is reviewed for change in spectral power, which may suggest a seizure (Figures 5.2.57 and 5.2.58). Clinical seizures as documented by staff, patient, and/or family are reviewed in detail.

Technologists create the technical note based on this initial review. This is an aid to the reading physician, guiding where to look in a long recording for abnormal electrocerebral activity or clinical events. The video is reviewed for every seizure starting approximately 30 sec before the reported seizure onset. The first clinical change is noted. The analysis of the seizure should focus on early manifestations, particularly ones that have lateralizing or localizing value. While the video is reviewed, a cursor points out the exact timing of every clinical feature in relation to the EEG (see Figure 5.2.59). The vertical line on the figure demonstrates the exact time on the EEG corresponding to the video image.

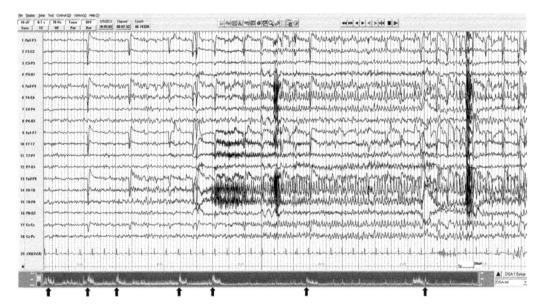

FIGURE 5.2.58 Right temporal ictal discharge. Longitudinal bipolar montage.

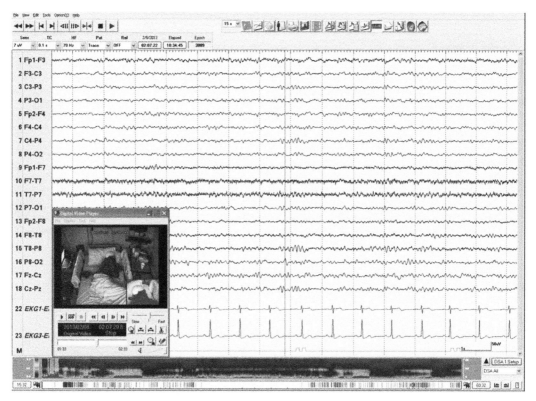

FIGURE 5.2.59 Electroencephalogram (EEG) with video inset. Longitudinal bipolar montage.

Figure 5.2.60 provides an example of annotations entered on the EEG to describe clinical as well as EEG features during a seizure. These annotations can be exported to the EEG report with their corresponding times.

Clinical annotations are entered at the cursor, making sure that the timing corresponds (see Figure 5.2.60). The end of the clinical seizure is also annotated. In some cases, it is of value to review post-ictal manifestations, particularly the presence of aphasia. After annotating the clinical manifestations, the EEG reader should review the corresponding EEG, focusing on the initial EEG changes. The EEG recording is annotated with descriptions of EEG features/patterns according to the time of occurrence of each feature. Annotation should include features of known clinical value, for example 5 Hz or faster rhythmic activity in a temporal electrode within 30 sec of seizure onset, which would favor a mesial temporal origin. Seizure termination should also be annotated. These annotations can be exported to the report along with their timing.

Safety in the Epilepsy Monitoring Unit

Safety in the EMU is a major concern because seizures are being provoked, with their associated risks. In addition, some potential risks, such as falls, are of particular sensitivity to healthcare institutions, so we must be attentive to the risks without being so overprotective that we lower patient satisfaction or reduce the diagnostic sensitivity of the study.

Events can be separated into epileptic and nonepileptic events. They are considered individually.

Serious Seizure-Related Events that May Occur in the EMU

Severe seizures: Seizures are usually not associated with serious injury, but they can be. After withdrawal of ASMs, seizures are not only more frequent but are more likely to be prolonged and more severe.

Status epilepticus (SE): SE is more likely after withdrawal of ASMs. Standard therapy for status epilepticus should be available, along with rapid

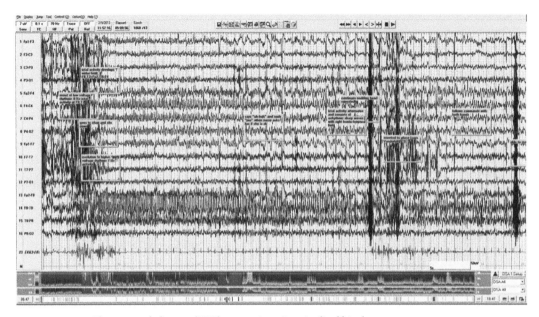

FIGURE 5.2.60 Electroencephalogram (EEG) annotations. Longitudinal bipolar montage.

access to clinicians who can activate the protocols. Vanderbilt University Hospital has a protocol for SE that is reproduced in Chapter 8.3. EMUs should have protocols for the management of severe seizures and SE.

Sudden unexpected death in epilepsy (SUDEP): The risk of sudden unexplained death is increased in epilepsy, more than 20 times that of controls when considering the age group of 20–40 years. SUDEP is responsible for 1–2 deaths per 1,000 patient-years. This is more common in patients with generalized tonic-clonic seizures, males, early age of seizure onset, longer duration of epilepsy, and multiple ASMs. SUDEP is most often seen in the setting of a seizure, usually a generalized tonic-clonic seizure, but it can occur without a clinical seizure.[10]

Methods to reduce the incidence of SUDEP are uncertain. It is believed that better seizure control, even surgical if needed, is helpful. There is evidence that complete seizure control essentially eliminates the risk of SUDEP.[11] Nocturnal supervision, whether in-person or by listening device, may not be helpful.[12] Breakthrough seizures related to poor compliance are a risk factor for SUDEP.

Most neurologists do not discuss SUDEP with their patients so as not to cause undue anxiety. However, many bereaved family members feel that patients should have been counseled about SUDEP risk and that fear of SUDEP would have

improved compliance. Physicians should consider counseling select patients who are at high risk of SUDEP due to frequent uncontrolled generalized tonic-clonic seizures. Patients with mild seizures and patients with well-controlled epilepsy need not be educated about SUDEP.

Aspiration is a common risk with seizures, especially bilateral tonic-clonic seizures. Maintenance of adequate airway and suctioning as needed are warranted. This is not usually an issue with focal seizures that do not evolve to bilateral tonic-clonic activity.

Falls during seizures: Significant head or other bodily injury can occur with seizure-associated falls.[13] Measures to reduce falls include bed side rails, bed and chair alarms to alert nurses that the patient is up, monitor tech observation to alert a nurse if the patient is not in bed, targeted toileting by a nurse or care partner (e.g., every 2 hours), and mandatory escort to and from bathroom by nurse or care partner.

Post-ictal psychosis occurs in about 4% of individuals with epilepsy, more often in those with bitemporal independent epileptogenic foci. It typically occurs after a cluster of seizures, as a delayed post-ictal manifestation, after a lucid period of 12 hours to several days. The psychosis is often preceded by insomnia and restlessness. Early treatment of these symptoms may prevent the post-ictal psychosis. Psychotic symptoms include paranoid and religious delusions, referential thinking, and auditory and visual hallucinations. Post-ictal psychosis is a self-limited condition that can be treated with antipsychotic agents such as risperidone until symptoms resolve. Prophylactic treatment after a cluster of seizures can be used in individuals with prior history of post-ictal psychosis.

Ictal asystole: Arrhythmia including asystole associated with a seizure—ictal asystole—is uncommon, having an estimated incidence of 0.27% of patients evaluated in the EMU.[14,15,16] Syncope will usually occur after 6 sec of asystole.[17] Ictal asystole is usually self-limited, but pacemaker implantation may be needed to avoid injuries from the associated syncope and falls.

Nonepileptic Serious Events

Cardiac arrhythmias are more common in patients with epilepsy, including atrial fibrillation or atrial flutter.[18] Fainting spells could be of cardiac origin. Cardiac telemetry should be considered as an adjunct to video-EEG monitoring when attacks of an unknown nature could be of cardiac origin.

Hypoglycemia can cause paroxysmal alteration of consciousness and is on the differential diagnosis of attacks of unknown nature. Hypoglycemia can also trigger seizures in a patient without epilepsy.[19]

Presyncope and syncope are on the differential diagnosis of fainting spells of unknown nature and may occur in the EMU.

Clinical Interpretation of Video-EEG Reviewing Studies

In reviewing video-EEG studies, the interpreter places the greatest emphasis on ictal clinical events. There are clinical and EEG features to each of these events.

Clinical features to be assessed are:

- Time of occurrence;
- Activity the patient was engaged in;
- Apparent precipitation;
- Time of first clinical change and the nature of the first clinical change;
- Evolution of clinical activity and a description of activity at each phase and its evolution, focusing on localizing and lateralizing signs;
- Apparent end of the clinical event;
- Duration of the clinical seizure and the nature of post-ictal behavior including interaction with examiners;
- Time of return to normal functioning, if known.

EEG features to be assessed are:

- State of the patient at the time the event started (e.g., waking vs. sleep);
- First change in the EEG, including attenuation or disappearance of previous interictal epileptiform activity and attenuation of previous background activity; if the attenuation is focal, this can be a useful localizing finding;
- First definite rhythmic activity and its localization, its evolution and pattern of spread, and the time of its termination;
- When ictal activity ends in one hemisphere or in the whole brain except one region;
- Time of complete termination of the ictal discharge;
- Post-ictal EEG pattern (e.g., generalized attenuation or lateralized or focal attenuation, or lateralized or focal irregular slow activity).

Filtering

The reviewer must look at the EEG unfiltered. Reviewing the ictal EEG in a filtered state first could result in misinterpretation of muscle and movement artifact as cerebral in origin because they have lost some of their characteristic hallmarks as a result of the filtering. The pattern of muscle artifact during a seizure can be greatly helpful. For example, generalized tonic and generalized clonic motor activity both produce typical myogenic patterns on the EEG. Subtle focal clonic activity in the face can be recognized on EEG but not clinically, and chewing and swallowing artifacts can also be recognized on the EEG.

Montages

For purposes of localization and classification, seizures may need to be viewed in more than one montage. Using an initial bipolar montage, one can suspect the center of the field based on reversal of polarity or phase reversal. The seizure can then be viewed in a referential montage, choosing a reference that is least likely to be involved in the seizure activity. For example, the ipsilateral ear is an inappropriate reference for an anterior-inferomesial temporal seizure origin; the ear ipsilateral to the seizure origin is frequently involved in the ictal discharge. The average reference can be appropriate but may need to be manipulated to exclude the most clearly involved electrodes. Thoughtful consideration must be applied to select the montage that likely provides the highest fidelity.

Video-EEG Diagnosis of Psychogenic Events

The simplest diagnosis of psychogenic nonepileptic events occurs in the absence of motor activity in patients who become unresponsive. In these patients, the presence of a completely normal EEG background during the event would be diagnostic of psychogenic etiology.

A positive diagnosis of psychogenic nonepileptic events becomes more difficult in the presence of associated motor activity. In many instances, movement and muscle artifact can dominate the EEG, rendering its analysis impossible. In such instances, analysis of the video component becomes the predominant basis for diagnosis. That could be potentially misleading, as epileptic seizures can be very bizarre in their manifestations, with minimal associated EEG change when they arise from the mesial frontal or orbitofrontal region.

The video analysis of psychogenic events should also take into consideration that no single feature or even combination of features is totally specific. It is not uncommon for rhythmic movement to be associated with a rhythmic motion artifact that could mislead into a diagnosis of seizure activity. Clues to the diagnosis could come from brief quiet periods that still include unresponsiveness or from the immediate post-ictal state when the patient is still unresponsive but quiet, allowing for a perfectly normal EEG to show through. When such periods are absent, the pattern of artifact can be helpful.

The rhythmic activity of epileptic seizures will usually evolve or at least wax and wane in its frequency, morphology, and amplitude. The rhythmic activity associated with nonepileptic events is either constant or includes irregularities that reflect on the EEG artifact. The occurrence of seizures immediately out of sleep is strong evidence against a psychogenic basis. Some patients with psychogenic events report that attacks occur out of sleep, but the EEG will usually demonstrate a waking background at onset.

Physician Interpretation and Reports

The video-EEG report should start with identifying information, duration of study, a preamble that includes the reason for the study and background clinical information of relevance, medications, seizure medication changes during the study, and electrodes used (for example 10–20 system, sphenoidal electrodes, T1/T2, etc.).

The current reimbursement favors a separate report for every day of recording, which can be brief, summarizing the activity for the past 24 hours. However, it is best to have a unified final report that includes a section for every day of recording, identified by date and times. Typically the first day includes a baseline EEG, which is a 20-min recording that cycles through standard montages (longitudinal bipolar, average reference, ear reference, transverse bipolar, circumferential) and includes hyperventilation and IPS.

For every day, the report should include a description of seizures, starting with clinical features by time of occurrence and then EEG features by time of occurrence, as well as a description of interictal EEG including waking and sleep patterns as well as epileptiform, slow-wave, and amplitude abnormalities.

After the last day of recording, an "EEG Diagnosis" paragraph summarizes the key EEG findings by number, starting with ictal discharges, then interictal epileptiform abnormalities, then slowing and amplitude abnormalities, and posterior rhythm.

The final part of the report is "Clinical Interpretation," which is a synthesis of clinical and EEG data. We recommend starting with a summary description of the clinical features of the seizures, their lateralizing and localizing significance of the overall features, and how this is supported by ictal onset and interictal epileptiform and nonepileptiform abnormalities. There follows a summary statement. The following are examples of EEG diagnosis and clinical interpretations based on a variety of scenarios.

Scenario A: A Patient with a Psychogenic Event and Normal EEG

EEG Diagnosis:

- This EEG is normal in waking, drowsiness, and sleep.
- There was no EEG change in association with one typical event, other than muscle and movement artifact.

Clinical Interpretation:

This study recorded one of the patient's typical events. The main features were (mention the most prominent features, stressing the ones that point to a psychogenic origin).

There were no associated EEG changes other than muscle and movement artifact (if present).

By both EEG and clinical criteria, this event was nonepileptic, most probably psychogenic in nature. In addition, due to the absence of interictal EEG abnormalities, this study fails to provide support for coexistent epilepsy.

Scenario B: Psychogenic Event Plus Epileptiform Abnormalities on the EEG

EEG Diagnosis:

- Frequent left anterior temporal sharp waves
- Intermittent irregular slow-wave activity recorded from the left temporal lobe.
- There were no EEG changes (other than muscle and movement artifact) in association with one of the patient's typical events.

Clinical Interpretation:

This study recorded one of the patient's typical events. Its main clinical features were. . . . The EEG showed no change (other than muscle and movement artifact). By both clinical and EEG characteristics this event was nonepileptic and most probably psychogenic in origin.

On the other hand, the interictal EEG recorded left anterior temporal sharp waves and suggested potential epileptogenicity in the left anterior temporal region.

Scenario C: Predominantly Subjective Episodes Without Definite Altered Awareness or Responsiveness with a Normal EEG.

EEG Diagnosis:

- This is a normal video-EEG study.
- Subjective clinical events were not associated with EEG changes.

Clinical Interpretation:

This study recorded two episodes that were predominantly subjective. There were no associated EEG changes. This study does not support an epileptic nature for these attacks. However, since most focal aware seizures are not associated with scalp EEG changes, the possibility of focal aware seizures is not ruled out.

Scenario D: No Events and Normal EEG

EEG Diagnosis:

- This is a normal 3-day video-EEG study.

Clinical Interpretation:

No events were recorded. This normal study fails to provide support for the diagnosis of epilepsy but cannot rule it out, particularly in the absence of recorded attacks.

Scenario E: No Events but with Interictal Epileptiform Discharges and Slow Activity

EEG Diagnosis: This 4-hour video-EEG study is abnormal because of

- Frequent left anterior temporal epileptiform discharges;
- Left anterior temporal intermittent irregular delta activity.

Clinical Interpretation:

- This study is most consistent with the interictal expression of focal epilepsy with a left anterior temporal potential epileptogenic zone.

Scenario F: Examples of Recorded Seizures with Totally Congruent Data

EEG Diagnosis: This 7-day video-EEG study recorded:

- Two ictal discharges associated with clinical seizures. Both had a focal onset in the left inferomesial temporal region.
- Occasional left inferomesial temporal or left inferomesial temporal predominant sharp waves, which became extremely frequent during sleep.
- Occasional left temporal intermittent rhythmic delta activity (TIRDA).
- Frequent left temporal irregular theta/delta activity.

Clinical Interpretation:

- This study recorded two focal impaired-awareness seizures. The clinical onset was with cessation of normal activity, blank stare, and chewing and swallowing movements, which favor a temporal involvement. Post-ictally, after the first event, the patient was found to be aphasic for almost 2–3 min, which favors a left temporal localization. This localization was supported by the ictal EEG onset and interictal epileptiform and slow activity that was left inferomesial temporal or inferomesial temporal predominant.

- In summary, this study is diagnostic of focal epilepsy with confident localization of the epileptogenic zone to the left inferomesial temporal region, with excellent convergence of clinical seizure pattern, ictal EEG, interictal epileptiform activity, and slow-wave activity.

Scenario G: Example of Fairly Congruent Data, Less Definitive

Example 1. Left lateral temporal
EEG Diagnosis: This 3-day video-EEG monitoring is abnormal because of

- 16 ictal discharges with associated clinical seizures. All ictal discharges started with theta activity in the left temporal region (at T7, T1>P7, F7).
- Bursts of left temporal rhythmic sharp activity in sleep (F7>T7>Fp1) lasting up to 10 sec, with some evolution raising the possibility of subclinical ictal discharges.
- Very frequent left temporal epileptiform discharges (T7 or F7 predominance).
- Left temporal intermittent irregular slow activity.

Clinical Interpretation:

- This 3-day video-EEG study recorded 16 typical focal impaired awareness seizures. Their main characteristics were sudden crying/moaning, appearing restless and scared, mild right facial twitching, head turn to the left, and bilateral limb automatisms. The early head turning to the left and right facial twitching at onset may favor a left lateral temporal localization. This localization is supported by the ictal

onset and interictal epileptiform and slow activity.

- In summary, this study is diagnostic of focal epilepsy with a probable epileptogenic zone localization in the left lateral temporal region.

Example 2. Left frontal
EEG Diagnosis: This 3-day video-EEG study is abnormal because of

- Fifteen ictal discharges associated with clinical seizures, six of which evolving to bilateral tonic-clonic activity. All 15 seizures started from the left frontal region (F3>Fp1,F7,C3); 10 of the seizures started with transitional sharp waves.
- Frequent high-frequency beta bursts recorded from the same region as above.
- Interictal epileptiform discharges from the left frontal or frontotemporal region.
- Irregular delta activity recorded from the left frontal region.

Clinical Interpretation:

- This 4-day video-EEG study recorded 15 focal impaired awareness seizures, 6 of which evolving to bilateral tonic-clonic activity.
- The seizures included early head turning to the left and hyperkinetic automatisms of the left extremities, while the right side was motionless or posturing, and versive head turning to the right and asymmetrical tonic posturing (figure-of-four) with right arm extension and left arm flexion in transition to bilateral tonic-clonic activity.
- The clinical features strongly favor a left lateralization. The initial hypermotor activity may suggest frontal lobe involvement.
- A left frontal localization was supported by the ictal EEG onset and by the interictal epileptiform and slow activity, which were consistently left frontal.
- In summary, this study is diagnostic of focal epilepsy, with strong evidence of a left frontal epileptogenic zone.

5.3

Normal EEG

BASSEL ABOU-KHALIL

OVERVIEW

The electroencephalogram (EEG) is ultimately classified as *normal* or *abnormal* or *indeterminate*. Part of the reason that EEG interpretation is so difficult is that there is a very broad range of normal, and the identification of what is normal or abnormal depends on so many factors, just some of which are age, state, and comorbid conditions. The normal EEG is defined by the absence of abnormalities. Normal EEG will be discussed in this chapter, including a discussion of artifacts. The following chapters will discuss abnormal EEG.

NORMAL ADULT EEG

Waking State

The occipital leads show a rhythm in the alpha range in waking with eyes closed. Frontal and central leads show faster activity. The posterior dominant alpha rhythm is present in relaxed wakefulness and attenuates with eye opening and disappears as the patient falls into drowsiness and sleep.

Some adults have a very low-voltage posterior rhythm that requires increased sensitivity to be visualized. Similarly, patients who have difficulty relaxing may never get into the relaxed wakefulness that allows for the posterior dominant alpha rhythm. Absence of this posterior rhythm is not abnormal unless unilateral.

Routine EEG (Figure 5.3.1) usually begins with the patient awake with the eyes closed. The technologist asks the patient to open and close the eyes to assess the posterior background rhythm and its reactivity.

If hyperventilation is used, it is performed during the initial segment of the EEG. The patient is allowed to rest, progress into drowsiness, and possibly fall asleep.

Adults with the eyes closed have a posterior dominant rhythm (PDR) of about 10 Hz. The minimum allowable frequency is 8.5 Hz, and

12–13 Hz is usually the upper end of the range. Anterior cerebral EEG shows low-voltage fast activity. Eye movement artifact is superimposed. A frontal-predominant beta activity is seen when patients are sedated with benzodiazepines or barbiturates, but this is less prominent with chloral hydrate.

Quantitative EEG analysis shows a small amount of theta and delta during the awake state, but this is not prominent with visual analysis. Older patients have less prominent posterior dominant alpha activity.

Eye closure results in appearance of the PDR, as shown in Figure 5.3.2, and disappearance with eye opening as in Figure 5.3.3.

Drowsiness

Patients progress from waking to drowsiness, during which time there are several changes, including progressive reduction of muscle artifact, a slight reduction in the posterior rhythm frequency (usually not more than 1 Hz), anterior widening of the field of PDR, and slow horizontal eye movements. This is *Sleep Stage 1A*. With progression to *Stage 1B*, there is attenuation then loss of PDR with the appearance of theta (Figure 5.3.4).

Vertex waves may be seen in Stage 1B, but this is more of a characteristic of *Stage 2* sleep. Theta becomes more prominent. Differentiation of Stage 1A from 1B is not important for routine EEG, but is important in sleep studies, as three consecutive epochs (1 epoch = 30 sec) of Stage IB is considered the onset of sleep.

Sleep

Sleep rhythms are described in Table 5.3.1. Composition of these features and background rhythms determines the sleep stages, as described in Table 5.3.2. Non–rapid eye movement (nonREM) sleep was previously divided into four stages, but now historical Stages 3 and 4 are combined into one Stage 3.

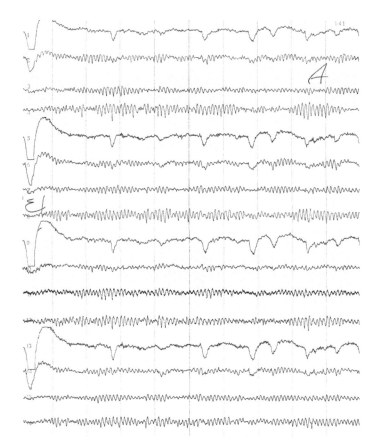

FIGURE 5.3.1 Normal waking Electroencephalogram (EEG). Longitudinal bipolar montage.

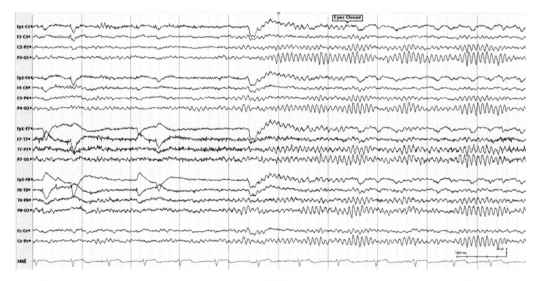

FIGURE 5.3.2 Normal waking Electroencephalogram (EEG). Posterior dominant rhythm appears with eye closure. Longitudinal bipolar montage.

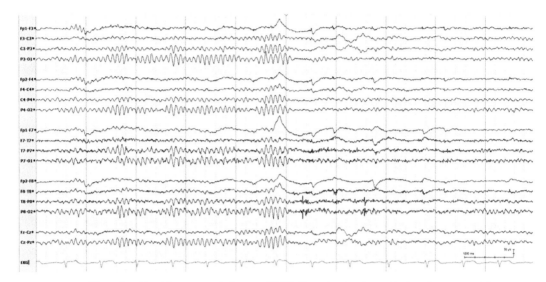

FIGURE 5.3.3 Normal waking Electroencephalogram (EEG). Posterior dominant rhythm disappears with eye opening. Same patient as in Figure 5.3.2. Longitudinal bipolar montage.

Stage 2: Sleep is most easily recognized in Stage 2 (Figure 5.3.5). Stage 2 sleep is heralded by the presence of sleep spindles, more prominent vertex waves, and K-complexes, which are longer polyphasic vertex waves associated with spindle activity. There is complete loss of the posterior dominant alpha rhythm. Since vertex waves may appear in Stage 1B, the main differentiating feature of Stage 2 is the appearance of sleep spindles. Delta begins to appear at this stage.

Stage 3: Stage 3 sleep is characterized by more delta and fewer faster frequencies. Delta

comprises more than 20% of the record. Stage 3 sleep is not commonly seen in routine office EEG (Figure 5.3.6).

REM: REM sleep is characterized by a low-voltage fast background (Figure 5.3.7). Superficially, this pattern may resemble drowsiness, but it is differentiated by rapid eye movements, hypotonia on submental electromyogram (EMG), and irregular respiratory rate.

Waking, drowsiness, and Stage 2 sleep are commonly seen in routine office EEG. The progression is from waking to Stage 1A to Stage 1B to

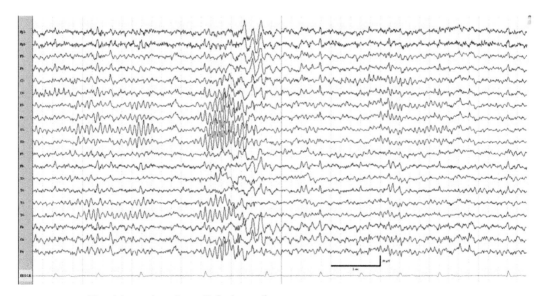

FIGURE 5.3.4 Transition to drowsiness. Linked ear reference montage.

TABLE 5.3.1 SLEEP RHYTHMS

Component	Features
Vertex wave	Negative potentials with a maximum at Cz
	Start in Stage 1B
Sleep spindle	11–14 Hz activity of 1–2 sec duration
	Maximum at C3 and C4
	Start in Stage 2
K complex	Fusion of a vertex wave and a sleep spindle
	prominent in Stage 2 sleep
Positive sharp transients of sleep (POSTS)	Positive potential with a maximum at O1 and O2
	Start in Stage 1B, but most prominent in Stage 2

Stage 2. With prolonged recordings patients may progress to Stage 3. There are three to five cycles in a night's sleep. REM sleep occurs after at least one sleep cycle and is of increased duration with later cycles.

Activation Methods

Activation methodology and response is discussed in Chapter 5.2. The responses to these activation modalities are revisited here.

TABLE 5.3.2 SLEEP STAGES

Stage	Features
Wake	Posterior dominant rhythm of 85–12 Hz
	Desynchronized background when eyes are open
Stage 1a (drowsiness)	Reduction in muscle artifact
	Anterior widening of the field of the posterior dominant rhythm
	Slow horizontal eye movements (CEM)
Stage 1b	Attenuation of the PDR
	Appearance of theta activity
	Vertex waves may appear
Stage 2	Loss of the PDR
	Sleep spindles
	Vertex waves and K-complexes
Stage 3	More delta activity (>20% of EEG)
	Fewer vertex waves and spindles
	Spindles become more anterior and slower in frequency
REM	Low-voltage fast background
	Rapid eye movements

Photic Stimulation

Responses to photic stimulation can be normal, abnormal, or artifactual. Table 5.3.3 presents the normal photic stimulation responses that may be encountered.

Photic Evoked Response

The photic evoked response is also sometimes termed the *visual evoked response* and is a positive-predominant wave seen from the occipital region approximately 100 msec after each flash (see Figure 5.3.8). This is seen at slower flash frequencies, usually less than 5/sec. With increasing flash frequency, the evoked response disappears and the driving response appears, with the transition complete by flash frequencies of 10/sec.

The photic evoked response is the same potential that is recorded during flash visual evoked potential (VEP) testing

Photic Driving Response

The photic driving response appears as the flash frequency accelerates beyond 7/sec, and the next evoked potential starts before the last evoked potential has ended. It is created by the visual evoked responses merging into each other. The driving response is usually most prominent at the frequency of the posterior rhythm, or at multiples thereof (Figure 5.3.9).

Photic driving response is time-locked to the stimulus and appears at faster frequencies than the photic evoked response. The driving response is usually seen, but absence is not interpreted as an abnormality unless unilateral or markedly asymmetric, in the absence of other abnormalities.

Photomyoclonic Response

The photomyoclonic response (Figure 5.3.10) is not cerebral in origin, but rather is electrical activity in the frontal scalp muscles, which is induced by the flash stimulus in susceptible individuals. Repeated contraction of these muscles produces EMG activity that is time-locked to the stimulus and recorded typically from the frontal leads.

The main issue with the photomyoclonic response is in differentiating this from photoparoxysmal response. Some general guidelines are discussed in Table 5.3.4.

Photoelectric Artifact

The photoelectric artifact (also called photovoltaic or photocell artifact) is a noncerebral artifact generated by the electrode–gel complex. The artifact is often caused by contamination of insecure

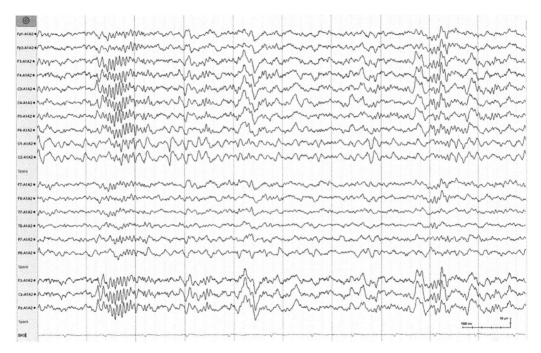

FIGURE 5.3.5 Stage 2 sleep. Linked ear reference montage.

leads with high impedance, so there is not equal representation across the forehead and a loss of common mode rejection (Figure 5.3.11).

Light produces changes in the electrode, which disturb subtle junction potentials between the electrode and gel. This potential is detected mostly in the frontal electrodes, which are directly illuminated and can be misinterpreted as a rhythmic spike potential with a frequency equal to the frequency of photic stimulation. It may be

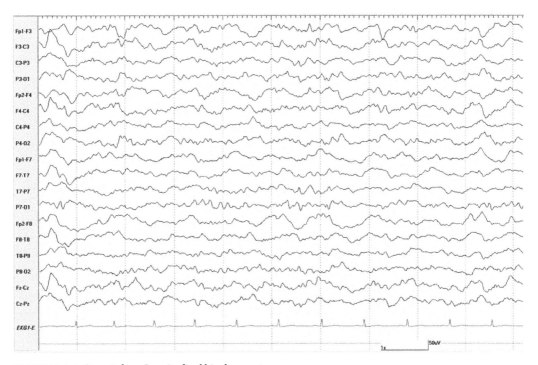

FIGURE 5.3.6 Stage 3 sleep. Longitudinal bipolar montage.

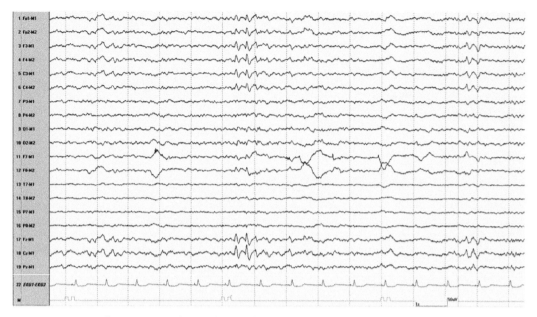

FIGURE 5.3.7 Rapid eye movement (REM) sleep. Ipsilateral ear reference montage.

difficult to distinguish from the electroretinogram (ERG) activity that records potentials from the retina. The ERG is often seen in the frontopolar electrodes as well, at high gains, when there is a paucity of electrocerebral activity.

Hyperventilation

Hyperventilation is used predominantly to activate absence seizures. The normal response to hyperventilation is generalized slow activity, both synchronous and asynchronous. The slow activity is more prominent in children than in adults.

Hyperventilation is performed for 3 min on routine testing and should be performed for 5 min if there is a strong suspicion of absence seizures. Hyperventilation is not performed in elderly patients and in those with significant vascular

disease since there may be resultant vasospasm and decreased cerebral perfusion.

Figure 5.3.12 shows generation of theta activity with hyperventilation, while Figure 5.3.13 shows generation of delta activity.

Effects of Aging

Aging results in some defined changes in EEG activity:

- Decreased voltage of the PDR;
- Slight decrease in frequency of the PDR;
- Increased theta and delta on spectral analysis;
- Increased temporal theta activity; it is suggested that the limit is 10% theta activity and 1% delta activity;

TABLE 5.3.3 PHOTIC STIMULATION RESPONSES

Type of response	Response	Description
Normal response	Visual evoked response	Occipital positive-predominant wave which peaks approximately 100 msec after the stimulus. Seen mainly at slow flash frequencies of ≤5 Hz.
	Driving response	Occipital positive-predominant wave which is time-locked to the photic stimulus. Seen mainly at flash frequencies of 7/sec and greater.
Artifact	Photoelectric artifact	Electrical activity generated at the electrode–gel interface by a flash stimulus. This is neither cerebral or muscle but rather electrochemical.
	Photomyoclonic response	Flash-induced electrical activity in the frontal muscles in response to a flash stimulus. Not a cerebral potential.

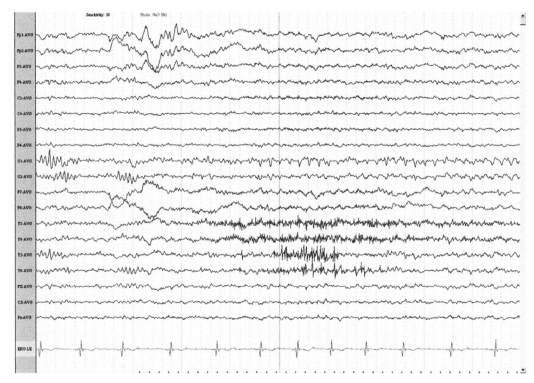

FIGURE 5.3.8 Photic evoked response. 5 Hz photic stimulation Average reference montage.

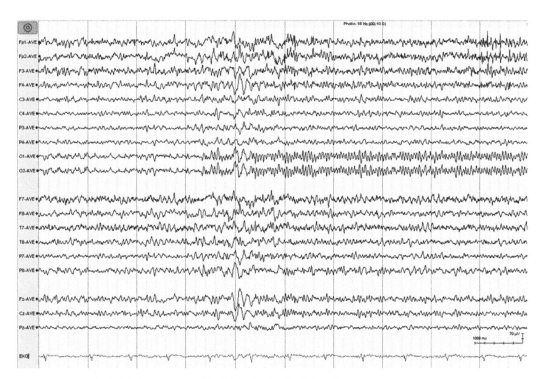

FIGURE 5.3.9 Photic driving response with 10 Hz photic stimulation. Average reference montage.

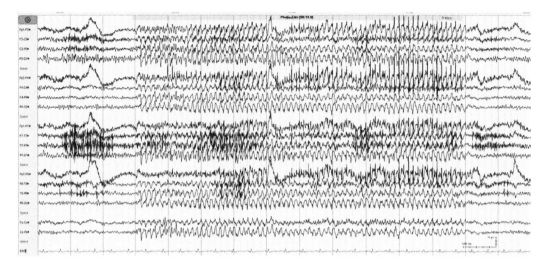

FIGURE 5.3.10 Photomyoclonic response. Longitudinal bipolar montage.

- Decreased magnitude of the responses to photic stimulation;
- Decreased response to hyperventilation.

The PDR slows slightly with normal aging, but remains at least a minimum of 8–8.5 Hz. Slowing to less than this is abnormal and consistent with encephalopathy (Figure 5.3.14).

VARIANTS AND TRANSIENTS

Overview

Variants and normal transients are a frequent accompaniment to an otherwise typical EEG (see Tables 5.3.5 and 5.3.6). Unfortunately, they can be confused with epileptiform or other abnormal EEG activity. This section describes some of the more important transients and variants that are certainly not considered pathologic. Table 5.3.7 shows the occurrence of some of these depending on state.

14 and 6 Hz Positive Bursts

14 and 6 Hz positive bursts are trains of sharply contoured positive waveforms seen mainly in the posterior temporal region but that have a wide field (see Figure 5.3.15). They appear predominantly in drowsiness and light sleep. The appearance is of a train of waves at about 14 or 6/sec, although both frequencies may rarely be seen in the same recording epoch or in the same patient. A prolonged recording may be needed to see both frequencies. The 6/sec pattern predominates in younger children, whereas the 14/sec predominates in older children.

14 and 6 Hz bursts are reported with a variety of metabolic encephalopathies,[1] in association with generalized slow activity. This should be considered a normal variant if the rest of the recording is otherwise normal. Its presence should be mentioned in the body of the report, but not necessarily in the impression.

Benign Sporadic Sleep Spikes

Benign sporadic sleep spikes (BSSS) are very small spike-like potentials that occur in the temporal or frontotemporal regions during drowsiness and light sleep (see Figure 5.3.16). BSSS is also called *small sharp spikes* (SSS) and *benign epileptiform transients of sleep* (BETS).

TABLE 5.3.4 DIFFERENTIATION OF PHOTOMYOCLONIC FROM PHOTOPAROXYSMAL RESPONSES

Feature	Photomyoclonic	Photoparoxysmal
Spatial distribution	Anterior	Posterior or generalized
Termination	End of the stimulus	May stop before the end or outlast the stimulus
Rise time of the spike	Fast (EMG) spike.	Slower, spike-and-wave complexes most common
Frequency	Same frequency as the flash	Frequency is independent of flash frequency, usually slower

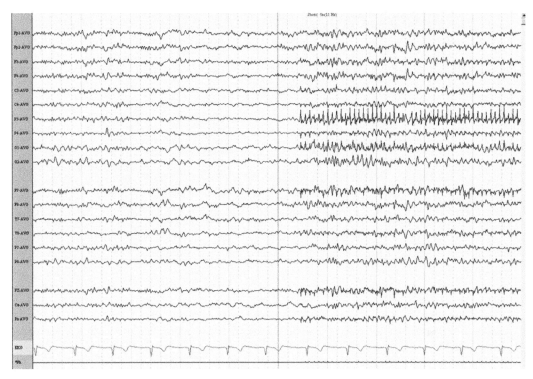

FIGURE 5.3.11 Photoelectric artifact at P3, which has a high impedance. Average reference montage.

The duration is less than 50 msec, with an amplitude usually less than 50 µV (but they may look larger in long-distance derivations). They may be monophasic, biphasic, and occasionally polyphasic. They may also have a small after-going slow wave. BSSS are usually differentiated from epileptiform spikes by small amplitude, short duration, tendency to shift from side to side, occasional oblique dipole with negativity in one hemisphere and positivity in the other hemisphere, and

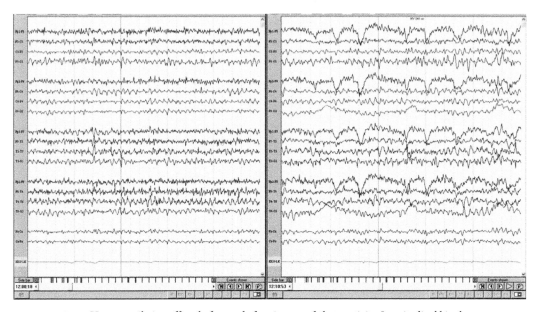

FIGURE 5.3.12 Hyperventilation effect, before and after; increased theta activity. Longitudinal bipolar montage.

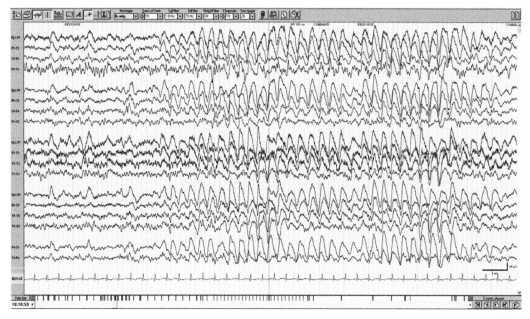

FIGURE 5.3.13 Hyperventilation effect in a 25-year-old woman; generalized rhythmic delta activity. Longitudinal bipolar montage.

otherwise normal EEG background. However, the most reliable distinguishing feature is disappearance in deep sleep, while true epileptiform discharges are usually increased in deeper sleep.

Lambda Waves

Lambda waves are positive waves from the occipital region that are present when viewing a scene or complex image (see Figure 5.3.17). The waves are blocked by eye closure. These waves resemble positive occipital sharp transients of sleep (POSTS), described later, but are differentiated in being seen only in the waking state. The pattern is completely normal. The lambda waves may be mistaken for occipital spikes; however, their positive polarity and

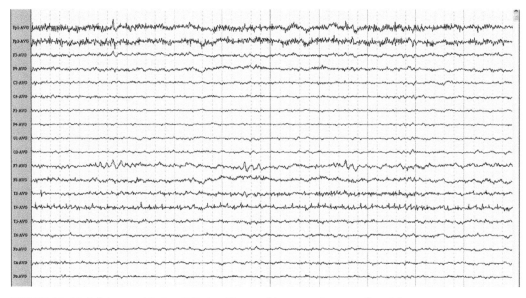

FIGURE 5.3.14 Left temporal theta activity in a 79-year-old woman. Average referential montage.

TABLE 5.3.5 NORMAL ELECTROENCEPHALOGRAM (EEG) PATTERNS AND VARIANTS: RHYTHMS

Pattern	Description
Mu rhythm	Negative arch-shaped rhythmic activity at about 8–10 Hz Attenuated by moving the contralateral arm or thinking about moving it
	Waking
Third rhythm (temporal alpha)	Alpha-range activity in the temporal region
	Seen in waking state
	Recorded only in a minority of patients
	Not clear what influences its appearance other than skull defect
Wicket pattern	Brief train of rhythmic alpha activity in temporal region
	Seen in drowsiness
Slow alpha variant	Posterior rhythm of 4–6 Hz, often notched
	A subharmonic of the posterior dominant alpha
	Seen in waking state, with eyes closed; attenuated with eye opening
Fast alpha variant	Posterior rhythm of 16–20 Hz
	A harmonic of the posterior dominant alpha
	Seen in waking, with eyes closed; attenuated with eye opening
SREDA	Periodic sharp activity which evolves into a rhythmic theta pattern Most often parietal in localization
	Most often seen in older patients in the waking state
Rhythmic temporal theta bursts of drowsiness (RTTBD)	Sharply contoured 5–7 Hz theta trains in the temporal region
	Seen in drowsiness
	Also called rhythmic midtemporal theta bursts of drowsiness (RMTD) and psychomotor variant
14 and 6 Hz positive bursts	Brief trains of sharply contoured positive waves of either frequency, occasionally combined
	Posterior predominance
	Seen in drowsiness and light sleep

blocking with eye closure make this clearly not epileptiform.

Lambda waves indicate visual exploration. Their label comes from their resemblance to the Greek lowercase letter lambda (λ). Lambda waves should be commented on in the body of the report but need not be mentioned in the interpretation.

Mittens

Mittens are seen only in sleep and consist of a partially fused vertex wave and sleep spindle. The last wave of the spindle is superimposed on the rising phase of the vertex wave (see Figure 5.3.18). This voltage summation gives the last spindle wave a faster and higher amplitude appearance, which may simulate a spike. Mittens are seen only in sleep.

The name comes from the appearance of a hand mitten, the thumb being the alpha wave and the hand being the vertex wave. Mittens are normal, but can be confused with a spike-and-wave pattern.

Mu

Mu rhythm (Figures 5.3.19 and 5.3.20) is seen in the waking state and is a negative arch-shaped rhythm of about 8–10 Hz. The potentials are most prominent at C3 and C4. Mu activity is often sharp. Its sharpness and amplitude are increased in the presence of a skull defect over the central region. In drowsiness, the mu rhythm may be broken up into fragments that can easily be over-interpreted as abnormal epileptiform activity.

Mu is very often asymmetric or even unilateral. The absence of mu activity on one side is not

TABLE 5.3.6 NORMAL ELECTROENCEPHALOGRAM PATTERNS AND VARIANTS: TRANSIENTS

Transient	Features
Mu – single transients	Fragments of the mu rhythm
	Most common in drowsiness
Positive occipital sharp transients of sleep (POSTS)	Positive waves from the occipital region
	Have a similar appearance to lambda waves
	Seen in sleep
Lambda waves	Positive occipital waves, look like POSTS
	Seen in waking, when viewing a scene or image
	Attenuated by eye closure
Wicket spikes	Sharply contoured waves from the temporal region
	May represent fragments of the third rhythm
	Seen in drowsiness and light sleep
	More common in older patients
Phantom spike-waves	Low-voltage spike-wave complexes that are single or in brief bursts
	Have a posterior usually mid-parietal predominance
	Seen in drowsiness, most often in young women
Benign sporadic sleep spikes (BSSS)	Small spike-like potentials in the fronto-temporal regions, typically shifting between the two sides
	Seen in drowsiness and light sleep
	Also known as small sharp spikes (SSS) and benign epileptiform transients of sleep (BETS)
Frontal mittens	Mitten-shaped complex formed from the fusion of a sharp alpha or theta transient with a delta wave
	Seen in sleep, especially Stage 2

TABLE 5.3.7 MOST COMMON PREVALENCE OF PARTICULAR PATTERNS DEPENDING ON STATE

State	Patterns typical of this state
Waking and drowsiness	Mu
	Third rhythm
	Slow alpha variant
	Fast alpha variant
	Rhythmic midtemporal theta of drowsiness
	14 and 6 Hz positive bursts
	Lambda waves
	Phantom spike-waves
	SREDA
	Wicket patterns and wicket spikes
	BSSS
Sleep	Mittens
	POSTS
	Wicket spikes
	BSSS

abnormal, unless there is very frequent mu activity on one side and none on the other side. The key to identification of mu rhythm is blocking by movement of the contralateral arm. Even contemplating movement can produce this change.

Phantom Spike Waves

These low-voltage 6 Hz spike-and-wave discharges can be single or in brief trains and occur typically in drowsiness. The classical benign variant has a biposterior predominance, particularly at Pz. They tend to occur mostly in young women. Figure 5.3.21 shows phantom spike waves with highest voltage at Pz.

Positive Occipital Sharp Transients of Sleep

POSTS are surface-positive potentials seen from the occipital region, maximal in derivations of O1 and O2 (see Figure 5.3.22). They look somewhat like lambda waves but are present only in sleep, whereas lambda waves are only seen in the waking state with the eyes open. POSTS are prominent

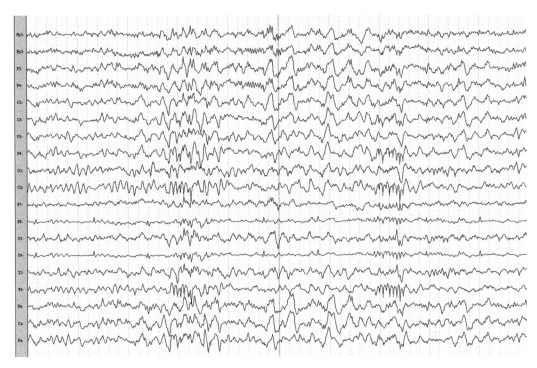

FIGURE 5.3.15 4 and 6 positive spikes. Average reference montage.

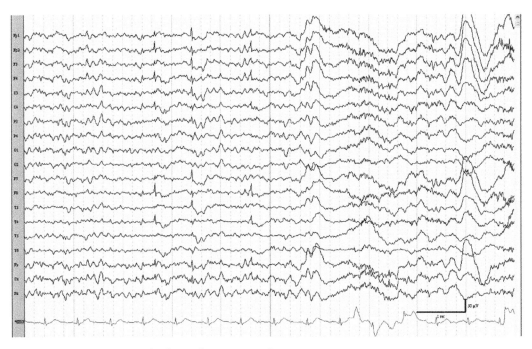

FIGURE 5.3.16 Benign sporadic sleep spikes. Average reference montage.

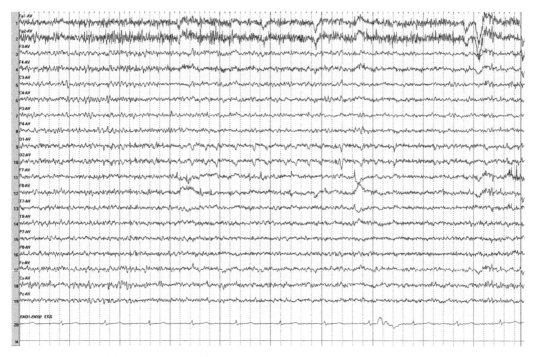

FIGURE 5.3.17 Lambda waves. Average reference montage.

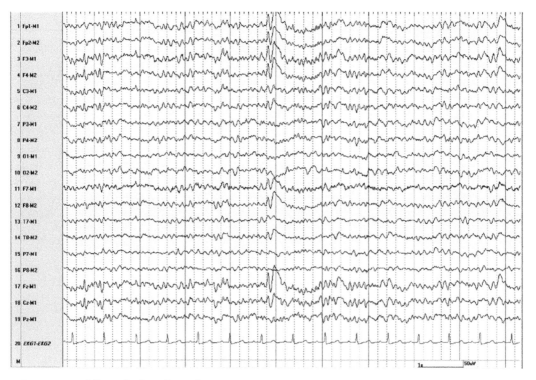

FIGURE 5.3.18 Mittens. Ipsilateral ear reference montage.

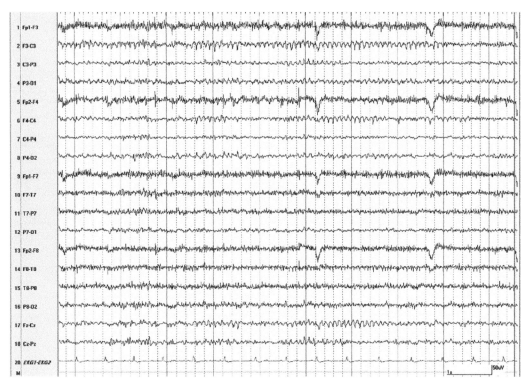

FIGURE 5.3.19 Mu rhythm. Longitudinal bipolar montage.

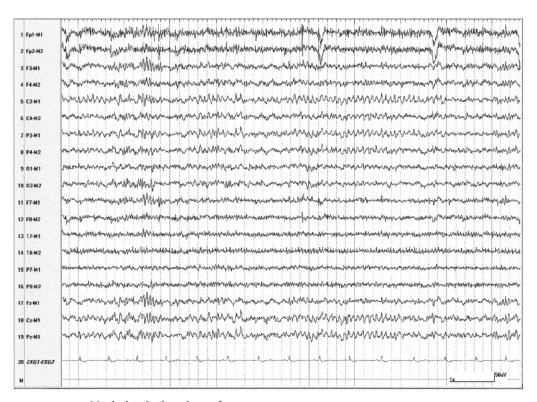

FIGURE 5.3.20 Mu rhythm. Ipsilateral ear reference montage.

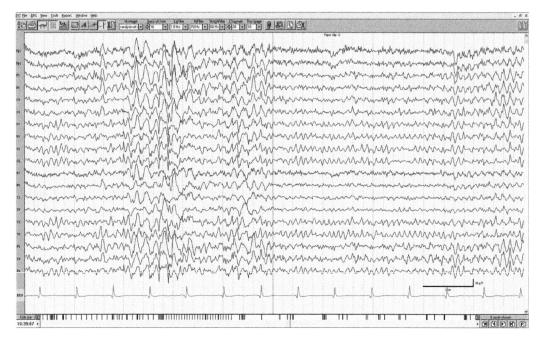

FIGURE 5.3.21 Phantom spike-waves. Linked ear referential montage.

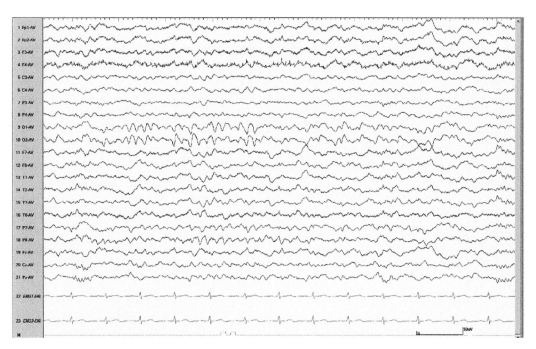

FIGURE 5.3.22 Positive occipital sharp transients of sleep (POSTS) in trains. Average reference montage.

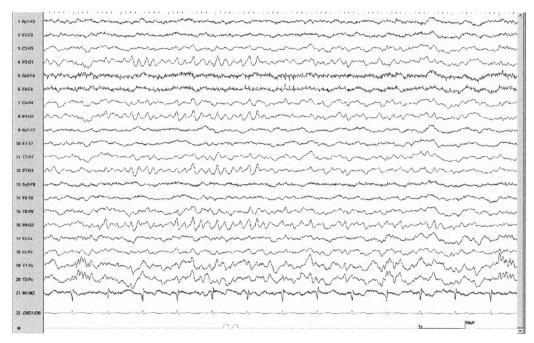

FIGURE 5.3.23 Positive occipital sharp transients of sleep (POSTS) in trains. Note that since the POSTS are positive from the second input, they produce an upgoing deflection. Longitudinal bipolar montage.

through Stage 2 sleep and disappear in deeper stages. POSTS can appear as single waves or in trains (Figure 5.3.23).

POSTS are less commonly seen in patients who are blind or who are severely visually impaired. One hypothesis is that POSTS represent a replay of visual information.

POSTS are not seen in every patient and have no diagnostic significance unless they appear only from one hemisphere. Even in this circumstance, asymmetric POSTS are unlikely to be the only abnormality on the EEG.

Rhythmic Temporal Theta Bursts of Drowsiness

Rhythmic temporal theta bursts of drowsiness (Figures 5.3.24 and 5.3.25) were once called *psychomotor variant* based on erroneous association with "psychomotor" epilepsy, but this term has been discarded. Another term, *rhythmic midtemporal theta of drowsiness* (RMTD) is also not precise because these discharges are not necessarily midtemporal predominant. This pattern consists of trains of sharply contoured notched waves in the theta (5–7 Hz, typically 6 Hz) range in the temporal region. The pattern may be bilateral but most often seems to start on one side, then within a short time develops on the opposite side.

Rhythmic temporal theta bursts of drowsiness can be distinguished from ictal activity by the following:

- Normal background before and after the rhythm,
- Absence of a progressive change in frequency that would be typical of ictal activity,
- Presence in drowsiness but not deeper sleep.

Slow Alpha Variant

The PDR in most adults is 8.5–12 Hz. In some patients, there can be a subharmonic of the posterior rhythm at 4–6 Hz. The slower frequency is typically notched. The subharmonic can be misinterpreted as a slow background in the theta range. Differentiation of a slow alpha variant (Figure 5.3.26) from a pathologically slow background can be made by the following features:

- Notched appearance of the rhythm;
- Attenuation of the rhythm with eye opening.
- Appearance of normal frequency of the PDR elsewhere in the recording, sometimes intermixed with the slow variant;
- Normal EEG activity elsewhere with slow alpha variant as opposed to

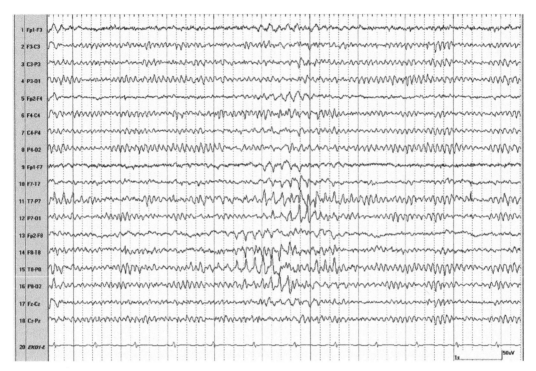

FIGURE 5.3.24 Rhythmic temporal theta burst of drowsiness with typical onset in one temporal lobe followed by the other temporal lobe. Longitudinal bipolar montage.

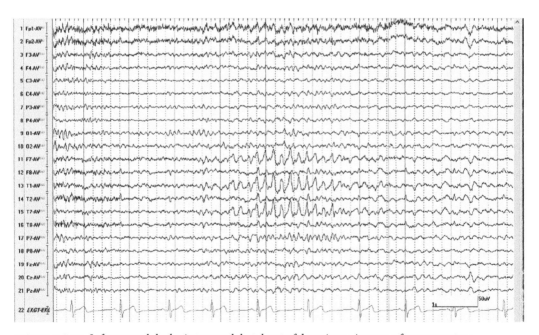

FIGURE 5.3.25 Left temporal rhythmic temporal theta burst of drowsiness. Average reference montage.

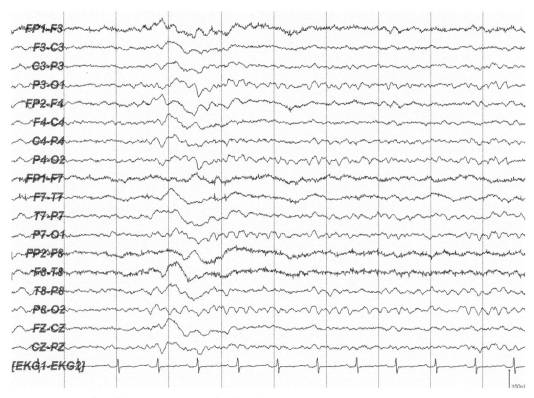

FIGURE 5.3.26 Slow-alpha variant. Longitudinal bipolar montage.

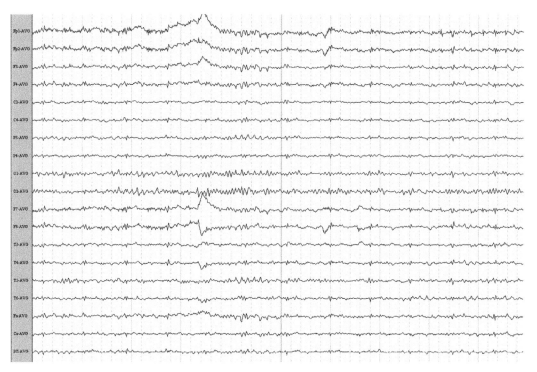

FIGURE 5.3.27 Fast alpha variant. Average reference montage.

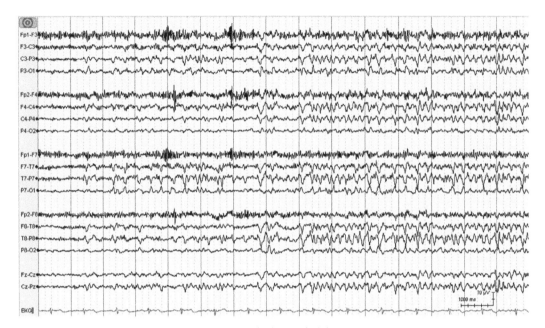

FIGURE 5.3.28 Subclinical rhythmic electrographic discharge of adults (SREDA) 1 of 3. Longitudinal bipolar montage.

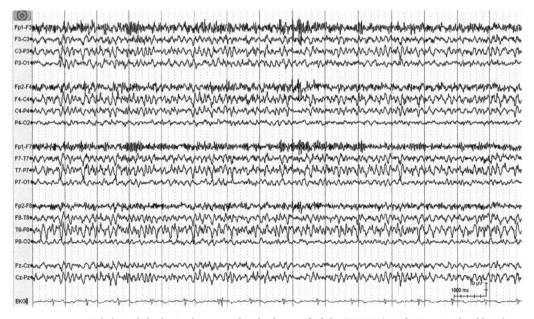

FIGURE 5.3.29 Subclinical rhythmic electrographic discharge of adults (SREDA) 2 of 3. Longitudinal bipolar montage.

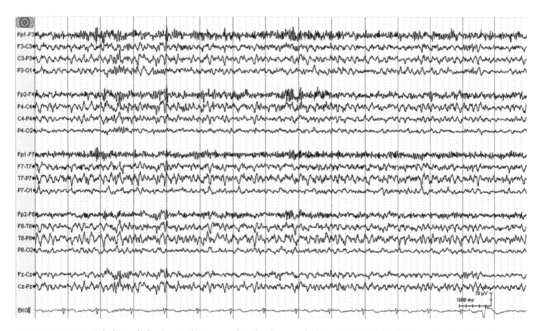

FIGURE 5.3.30 Subclinical rhythmic electrographic discharge of adults (SREDA) 3 of 3. Longitudinal bipolar montage.

generalized slow activity associated with encephalopathy.

Fast Alpha Variant

Fast alpha variant (Figure 5.3.27) is characterized by an otherwise normal PDR that appears as a harmonic of the native rhythm, appearing at twice the native frequency (16–20 Hz), which is in the beta range. The fast alpha variant is interpreted as normal.

SREDA

Subclinical rhythmic electrographic discharge of adults (SREDA) is rhythmic sharp activity that appears in some older patients in the awake state (Figures 5.3.28 through 5.3.30). Typically, periodic sharply contoured waves evolve into a rhythmic theta pattern, giving the appearance of an ictal discharge in reverse. Unlike that seen with ictal activity, SREDA may have a stuttering pattern.

Although SREDA may evolve like an ictal discharge, there is no clinical change during the discharge.

Wicket Spikes, Wicket Pattern, and Third Rhythm

Wicket spikes are sharply contoured alpha waves from temporal regions during drowsiness and light sleep. *Wicket patterns* are trains of wicket spikes. When there is persistent alpha activity in the temporal lobe, it is often referred to as *third rhythm*. Wicket spikes/wicket pattern are likely fragments of the third rhythm.

Wicket spikes can be differentiated from pathologic spikes by

- Mostly symmetrical appearance,
- Occurrence in a series of waves at 8–10 Hz,
- Absence of a following slow wave,
- Normal background activity.

Wicket spikes/wicket patterns are more common with increasing age. Figures 5.3.31 through 5.3.33 show wicket spikes/wicket patterns as well as the so-called *third rhythm*. Third rhythm was thought to be the third brain idling rhythm, in addition to the occipital alpha and the central mu rhythms.

NONCEREBRAL POTENTIALS

Artifacts can be biological or electrical. Unfortunately, electrical artifacts can predispose to enhanced perception of biological artifacts.

Biological

Biological artifacts are generated by the body but not by the brain. They can be confused with

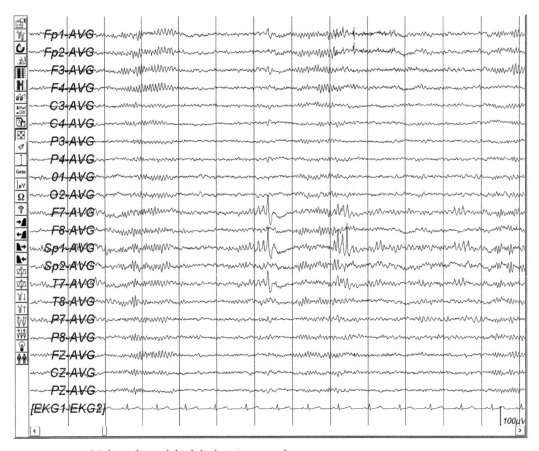

FIGURE 5.3.31 Wicket spikes and third rhythm. Average reference montage.

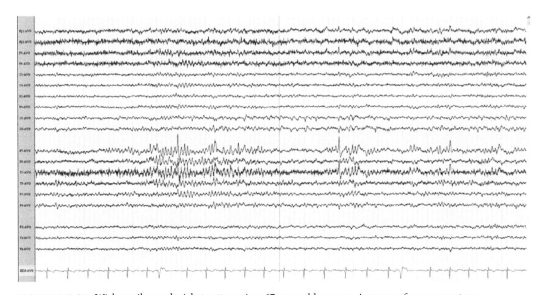

FIGURE 5.3.32 Wicket spikes and wicket patterns in a 67-year-old woman. Average reference montage.

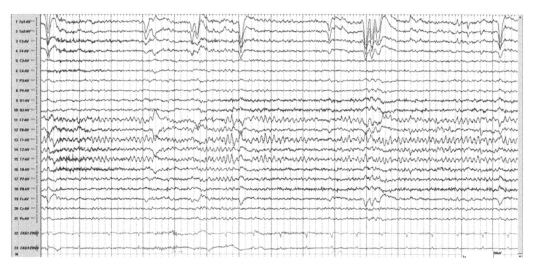

FIGURE 5.3.33 Third rhythm in an 81-year-old woman. Average reference montage.

electrocerebral activity and, if so, are frequently interpreted as slow waves or sharp waves/spikes.

Eye Movement

The eye is electrically charged, with the cornea positive relative to the fundus, so any movement of the eye results in potentials that can be recorded from anterior leads.

Vertical eye movements: Downward gaze results in the positive cornea moving away from the frontal lobe, so negativity is seen in frontal leads. The reverse is true for upward gaze. Since the eyes

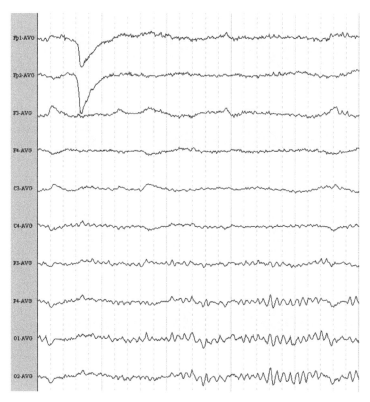

FIGURE 5.3.34 Eye closure. Average reference montage, parasagittal portion.

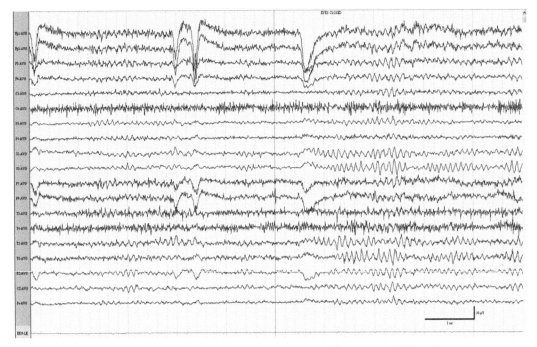

FIGURE 5.3.35 Eye blink followed by eye closure; note that the eye blink positivity is followed by a negative potential. Low frequency filter 1 Hz. Average reference montage.

move up and down together, the potentials from the two sides are synchronous. Of course, one must remember the possibility of a prosthetic eye producing unilateral eye movement artifact. Certain vertical eye movements have characteristic patterns, including eye blinks, eye opening, eye closure, and eye fluttering. These potentials can occasionally be mistaken for frontal lobe activity.

Eye closures: Eye closure results in Bell's phenomenon, an upward deviation of the eyes (Figure 5.3.34). This will be associated with a positive deflection in the frontopolar electrodes. In addition, eye closure is associated with appearance of the PDR.

Eye blink: An eye blink causes the same positive potential in the frontopolar regions, but the subsequent eye opening causes a negative deflection (Figure 5.3.35). The subsequent negative deflection distinguishes an eye blink from mere eye closure.

With eye blinks, there is a negative potential that follows the initial deep positive potential in the frontopolar electrodes. This negative potential is related to the low-frequency filter setting. If the

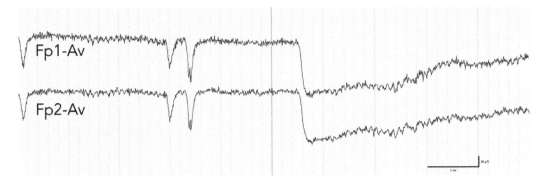

FIGURE 5.3.36 Eye blink. The tracing here is the same segment from Figure 5.3.35 with low-frequency filter turned off, showing activity at Fp1 and Fp2 with eye blinks followed by eye closure.

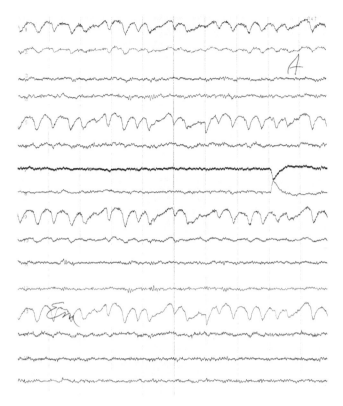

FIGURE 5.3.37 Repeated eye blinks. Longitudinal bipolar montage.

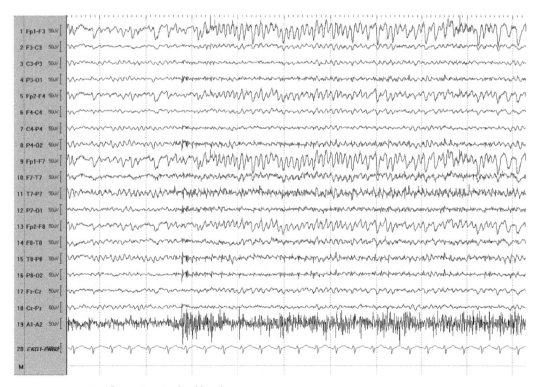

FIGURE 5.3.38 Eye flutter. Longitudinal bipolar montage.

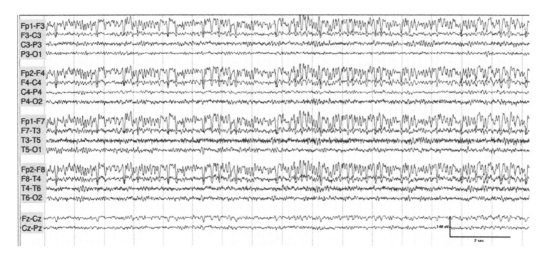

FIGURE 5.3.39 Dramatic eye flutter. Longitudinal bipolar montage.

low-frequency filter is turned off, that negativity disappears (Figure 5.3.36).

Eye blink can be more repetitive and have the appearance of frontal slow or sharp activity (Figure 5.3.37).

Eye flutter can produce artifact that is even faster than normal eye blink and can be mistaken for epileptiform activity or for frontal ictal activity (Figures 5.3.38—5.3.40).

Figure 5.3.40 shows another example of eye flutter that occurs after the patient opens eyes, in the middle of the recording epoch.

Eye opening: Eye opening results in a negative potential in the frontopolar electrodes plus

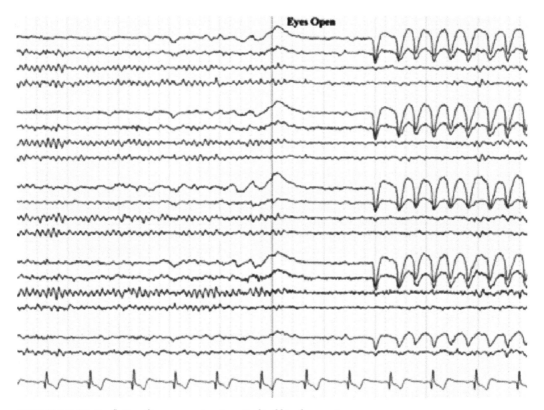

FIGURE 5.3.40 Eye flutter after eye opening. Longitudinal bipolar montage.

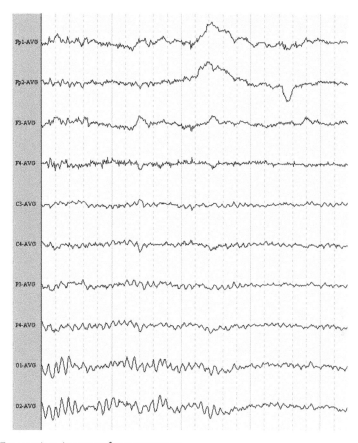

FIGURE 5.3.41 Eye opening. Average reference montage.

alteration in the posterior rhythm. The attenuation of the posterior rhythm with eye opening and reappearance with eye closing are good clues to the presence of vertical eye movements, although the technologist should indicate this phenomenon along with other patient movements. Eye closure results in restoration of the posterior rhythm. The posterior dominant frequency may be slightly faster immediately after closure. Therefore it should be measured a few seconds after eye closure.

Figure 5.3.40 shows a classic response to eye opening. Figure 5.3.41 shows a much more subtle response to eye opening with attenuation of the PDR.

Lateral eye movements: Lateral gaze results in the positive cornea moving toward the temple to the side of gaze (see Figure 5.3.42). For example, left gaze results in positivity at the F7 electrode and negativity at the F8 electrode because the right cornea moved away from it. The differential effect of lateral gaze on the two sides with opposite polarity deflections at F7 and F8 makes for easy identification of this as a lateral eye movement.

Lateral eye movements are often associated with lateral rectus spikes (Figure 5.3.43). Typical, the negative spike will be followed by a slower positive potential on the side to which the eyes moved.

Differentiating eye movement from cerebral potentials is based on some basic guidelines:

- Vertical eye movements are generally restricted to or at least markedly predominant in the frontopolar electrodes. This has resulted in the principle that slow wave activity restricted to the frontopolar electrodes is vertical eye movement artifact until proved otherwise.
- Certain eye movements such as eye blinks have a stereotypic appearance, different from frontal slow activity.
- Pathologic frontal slow activity tends to involve F3 and F4 much more than

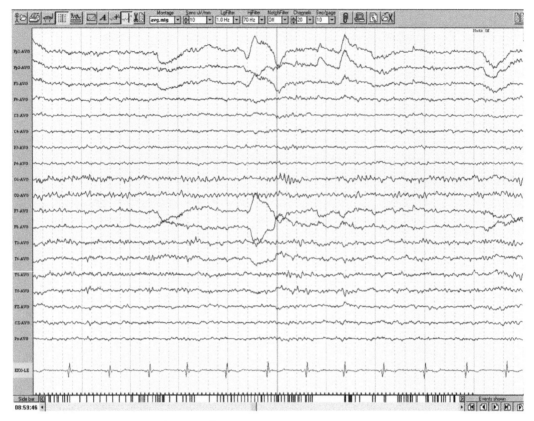

FIGURE 5.3.42 Eye movements. Average reference montage.

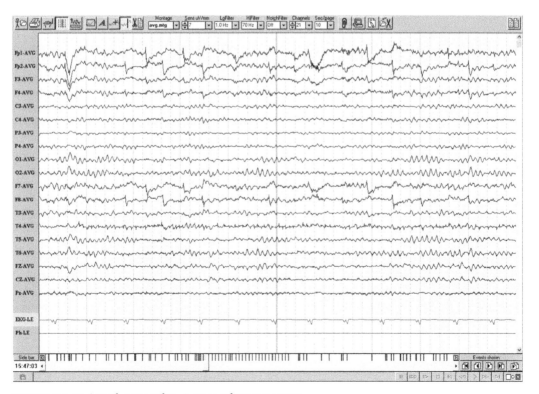

FIGURE 5.3.43 Lateral rectus spikes. Average reference montage.

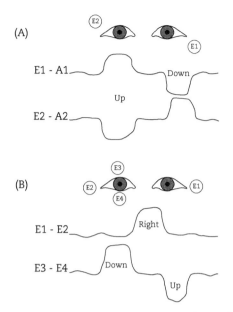

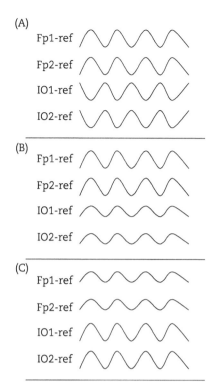

FIGURE 5.3.44 Eye movement monitoring. Some of the options for identifying eye movement and differentiation from cerebral activity.

vertical eye movements. They tend to be associated with a slow background, with activity in the theta and/or delta range. A normal background will suggest that slow activity restricted to the frontopolar region most likely represents eye movement artifact.

- Patients with marked vertical eye movements will often have prominent lateral eye movements as well, which can be easily recognized.

Eye movement monitoring: Eye movement monitoring was introduced in Chapter 5.2 and can

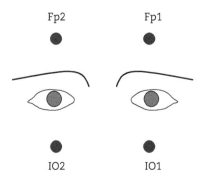

FIGURE 5.3.45 Infraorbital electrode positions for monitoring eye movements.

FIGURE 5.3.46 Comparative pattern of activity recorded from different sources with frontopolar and infraorbital electrodes. A: Vertical eye movements. B: Cerebral slow activity. C: Tongue movements.

be facilitated by periorbital positions so that eye movements can be differentiated from cerebral activity. Two arrangements that can be used are shown in Figure 5.3.44.

Infraorbital electrodes can help distinguish vertical eye movement artifact from cerebral activity, in combination with already-placed electrodes (Figures 5.3.45 and 5.3.46). Vertical eye movements will be of opposite polarity in frontopolar and orbitofrontal electrodes, while cerebral frontal slow activity will be of the same polarity, with higher voltage over the frontal polar electrodes. Infraorbital electrodes can also help identify glossokinetic potentials due to tongue movements. In this case, activity in the frontopolar and infraorbital electrodes will be of the same polarity but will be of higher voltage in the infraorbital electrodes which are closer to the tongue.

Muscle Artifact

EMG activity frequently contaminates EEG recordings, and this is prominent when patients are tense, seizing, or have other reasons for

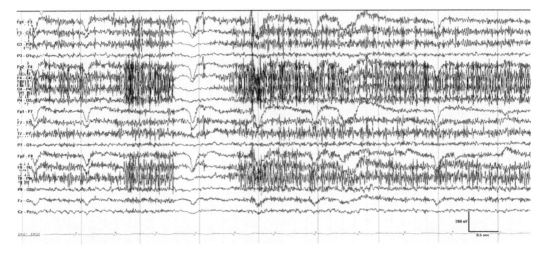

FIGURE 5.3.47 Confluent muscle artifact in a patient in the waking state. Longitudinal bipolar montage.

increased tone of scalp muscles. EMG is often prominent from the temporal leads. Frontal and occipital leads may also be prominently involved, whereas midline electrodes will usually be least affected. EMG artifact consists of short needle-like spikes. These may occur in such frequency that they become confluent and give an appearance that resembles noise. On the other hand, a single motor unit may be firing with muscle spikes recurring at a consistent frequency.

Some guidelines for differentiating EMG from epileptiform spikes are as follows:

- EMG is very fast, much faster than spikes. Activity recorded at the scalp that is shorter than 20 msec is highly unlikely to be epileptiform activity.
- EMG spikes are not followed by a slow wave.
- EMG is prominent in the waking state and disappears with sleep.

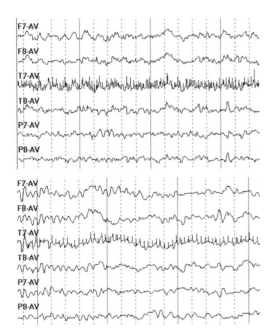

FIGURE 5.3.48 Muscle artifact from a single motor unit. Average reference montage, lateral portion.

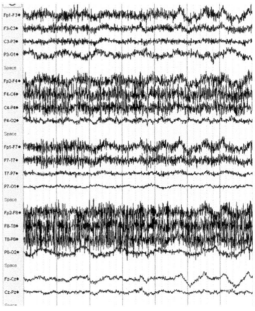

FIGURE 5.3.49 Effect of high-frequency filter on muscle artifact. High-frequency filter setting 70 Hz here, 15 Hz in Figure 5.3.50. Longitudinal bipolar montage.

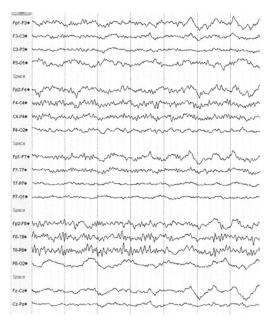

FIGURE 5.3.50 Effect of high-frequency filter on muscle artifact as in Figure 5.3.49 with filter 15 Hz. Longitudinal bipolar montage.

- EMG spikes recur at a rate that is much faster than would be seen with repetitive spikes.
- EMG is attenuated by asking the patient to relax the jaw, open the mouth, or perform another maneuver.

Figure 5.3.47 shows a typical appearance of muscle artifact. Occasionally, muscle artifact is more restricted and may even arise from a single motor unit, particularly in the midtemporal region (Figure 5.3.48).

Although muscle artifact can be filtered using the high-frequency filter, the unfiltered EEG should always be viewed first. The high-frequency filter may distort the appearance of muscle artifact such that it starts to appear cerebral in origin, as illustrated in Figures 5.3.49 and 5.3.50.

Glossokinetic Artifact

The tongue is polarized, with the tip negative in comparison to the back. Movement of the tongue is common in the waking state and can occasionally be mistaken for pathologic frontal or frontotemporal slow activity. This is potentially even more problematic in a comatose patient who is having tongue movements. Glossokinetic artifact

can be differentiated from slow activity in the following ways:

- Glossokinetic artifact is associated with activities such as speaking, chewing, and swallowing.
- Glossokinetic artifact is often concurrent with EMG artifact of the frontalis and temporalis muscles.
- Glossokinetic artifact usually disappears in drowsiness and light sleep.

If there is still doubt about identification, then electrodes can be placed below the eyes. The patient is asked to make lingual movements such as "la la la" and the potentials observed; glossokinetic artifact shows higher voltage at the infraorbital electrodes than at the frontopolar electrodes. Cerebral activity will be higher in voltage in the frontopolar electrodes. Identification of glossokinetic artifact is much better if the technologist recognizes the problem and is able to perform these maneuvers during the study.

Combinations of muscle and glossokinetic artifact produce very characteristic patterns depending on the associated activity. Some examples are displayed in Figures 5.3.51.

Figures 5.3.53 and 5.3.54 show slow waves between the bursts which are glossokinetic potentials. The EMG bursts are related to temporalis muscle contraction. Figure 5.3.54 is the same epoch but with different high-frequency filter settings, resulting in a pattern resembling polyspike-and-wave activity.

Toothbrush Artifact

During long-term monitoring a variety of artifacts are evident. When the patient is observed on video, behavioral correlates are obvious. In the absence of observation, the potentials shown in Figure 5.3.55 with brushing of teeth could be misinterpreted as seizure activity.

Mistaking this discharge for abnormal activity would be more likely if the behavior is not observed.

EKG Artifact

Electrocardiogram (EKG) artifact is seen mainly on referential montages (see Figure 5.3.56). Increased interelectrode distance predisposes to EKG artifact. Differentiation from electrocerebral artifact is most obvious if a special EKG

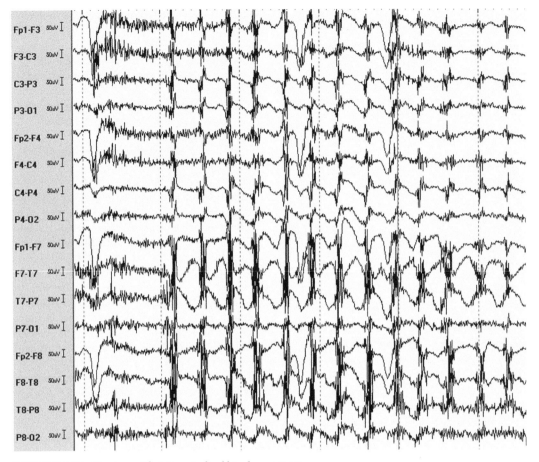

FIGURE 5.3.51 Chewing artifact. Longitudinal bipolar montage.

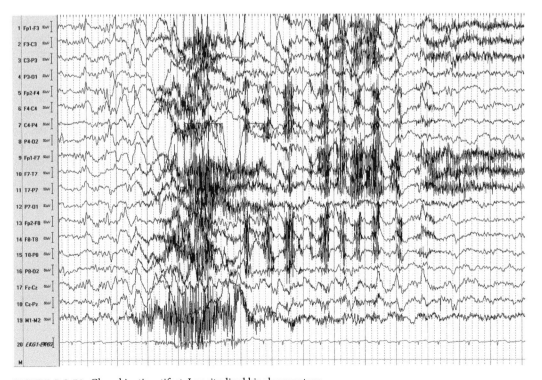

FIGURE 5.3.52 Glossokinetic artifact. Longitudinal bipolar montage.

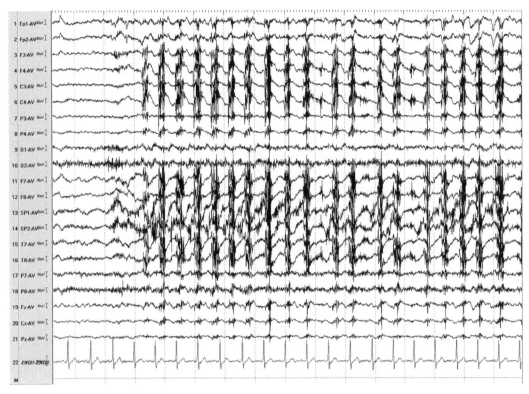

FIGURE 5.3.53 Chewing artifact. Average reference montage.

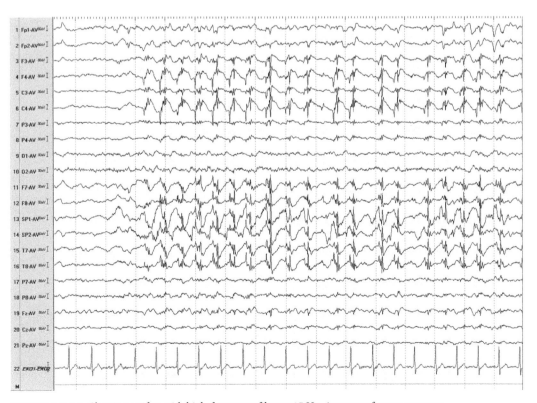

FIGURE 5.3.54 Chewing artifact with high-frequency filter at 15 Hz. Average reference montage.

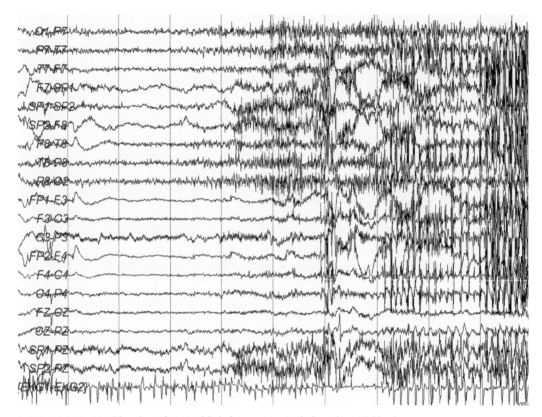

FIGURE 5.3.55 Toothbrush artifact. See labels for montage, includes sphenoidal leads.

channel is recorded, but, even in the absence of this, the regular nature of the QRS complex and the distribution of the sharp activity make the source evident. EKG artifact is most prominent in the ipsilateral ear reference montage. EKG activity can be reduced if the ears are linked (Figure 5.3.57).

EKG artifact can be harder to identify if there is intraventricular block causing the QRS complex to widen, as seen in Figure 5.3.38.

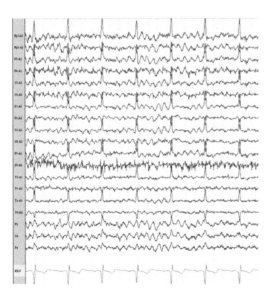

FIGURE 5.3.56 Electrocardiogram (EKG) artifact. Ipsilateral ear reference montage.

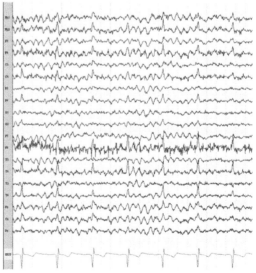

FIGURE 5.3.57 Electrocardiogram (EKG) artifact was reduced by linking the ears. Linked ear reference montage.

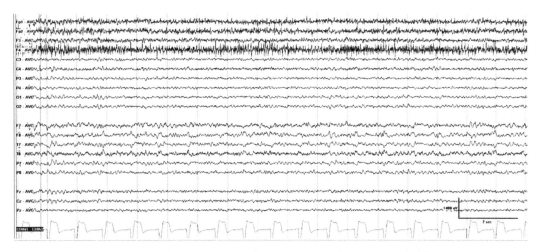

FIGURE 5.3.58 Broad electrocardiogram (EKG) artifact in a patient with intraventricular block. Average reference montage.

Pulse Artifact

Pulse artifact is due to movement of the electrode leads overlying the scalp blood vessels. Pulsation of a small artery results in movement of the electrode disc, which affects the electrode–gel connection and, if large enough, can even move the electrode leads. The appearance is an irregular delta wave that is time-locked to EKG, except that there is a delay between the QRS complex and the pulse.

Pulse artifact can be differentiated from pathological slow activity by the following features:

- The artifact usually localizes over one or two electrodes.
- The artifact is time-locked to the EKG but with a delay.
- Pulse artifact is perfectly rhythmic, unlike cerebral slow activity.

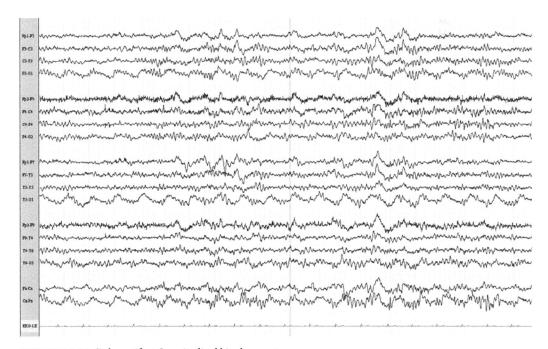

FIGURE 5.3.59 Pulse artifact. Longitudinal bipolar montage.

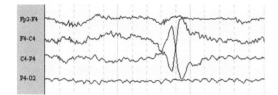

FIGURE 5.3.60 Electrode pop. Longitudinal bipolar montage, left parasagittal portion.

Initial inspection could mistake pulse artifact (Figure 5.3.59) for polymorphic delta activity, but in this situation the background is usually abnormal, with slowing and disorganization. If there is still doubt, examination of the scalp by the technologist can be revealing.

Electrical

Electrical artifact includes potentials that do not originate in the electrical activity of the body. Electrode leads can be an origin of the artifact. In addition, induced electrical current in electrode leads by nearby electric lines is a major source of artifact.

Electrodes and Leads

Electrode leads can be a source of artifact especially if there is instability in fixation of the electrode and high impedance. Movement of the electrode results in changes in the junction potential. The discharge of the junction potential results in a potential that can be mistaken for a spike discharge and is termed an "electrode pop" (Figure 5.3.60). The appearance is of a brief spike or sharp wave, followed by a gradual decay to baseline. During the spike, the responsiveness of the amplifier can be briefly impaired, so the EEG background immediately following can be transiently suppressed.

Electrode pops are reduced by having good junction between the electrode and scalp with sufficient gel. Also, stabilization of the electrode leads is helpful to minimize movement of the discs.

The example in Figure 5.3.61, obtained from the same patient as in Figure 5.3.60, shows sharply contoured slow activity that has no field, restricted to C4. This makes it likely to be artifactual.

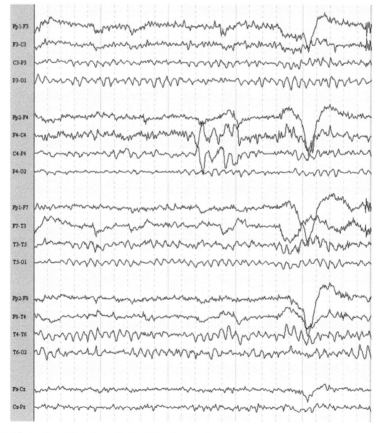

FIGURE 5.3.61 Electrode artifact. Longitudinal bipolar montage.

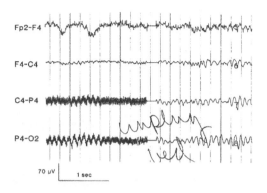

FIGURE 5.3.62 A 60 Hz artifact. Longitudinal bipolar montage, left parasagittal portion.

Machine Artifact

Machine artifact is especially prominent in the ICU. This is high-frequency stereotyped activity that is seldom confused with cerebral activity. The frequency can be the frequency of line power, but also can be at faster or slower frequencies, since mechanical devices are not time-locked to line power activity. Most mechanical devices are driven by DC power, although the power comes from AC power through a transformer; therefore, the artifact is the frequency of the motor, rather than the frequency of line power. Motors are present in ventilators, IV pumps, hospital beds, and other electrical devices.

Machine artifact can be reduced by

- Minimizing electric equipment nearby the EEG laboratory,

- Adequate grounding of the patient,
- Adequate grounding of the EEG machine.

60-Hz Artifact (Line Power)

60-Hertz interference is a result of induction from surrounding electronic circuits that are not directly attached to the patient. Movement of current through power lines produces a magnetic field that is created around the line. This magnetic field causes current to flow in electrode leads by induction, a fundamental property of electronic devices. The induced current flow will reverse at 60 Hz, since the magnetic field will also reverse at 60 Hz. Therefore, there is 60 Hz contamination in the electrode leads without any direct connection between the power lines and the EEG leads. This stray inductance is a major cause of electrical interference. It is most likely to appear when there is impedance imbalance. It is also most problematic in the ICU environment.

Figure 5.3.62 shows the right parasagittal portion of the longitudinal bipolar montage. Midway through this epoch, the air bed is unplugged and the high-frequency activity disappears. The focal nature of the 60-Hz artifact raises the possibility of high impedance at P4.

Focal 60-Hz artifact should always raise the possibility of focal high impedance (Figure 5.3.63). In this example the very fast activity at C4 without appearance in other leads suggests that this is not electrocerebral.

Phone Artifact

Telephone landlines commonly ring, especially when patients are being monitored or examined.

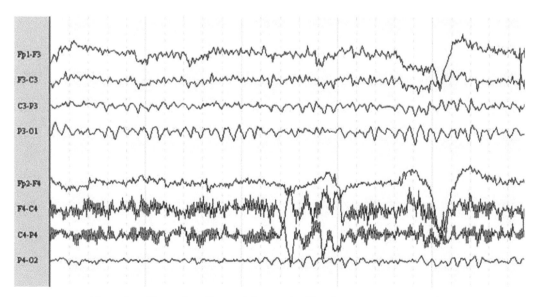

FIGURE 5.3.63 Electrode artifact with 60 Hz signal. Longitudinal bipolar montage, parasagittal portion.

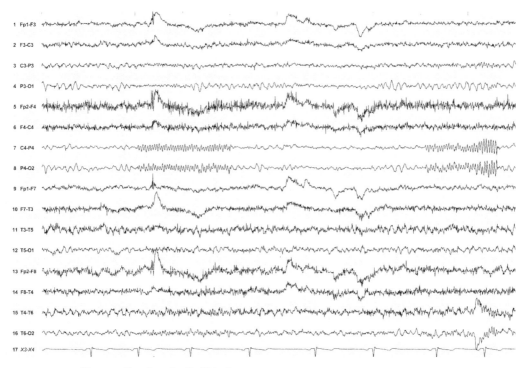

FIGURE 5.3.64 Phone artifact. Longitudinal bipolar montage.

Figure 5.3.64 is an example of the electrical artifact of the ringing of a desk phone. The stereotypic rhythmic activity lasting just a few seconds is the ringing of the phone. Cell phones typically do not produce this type of activity.

Movement Artifact

Movement artifact is due to disturbance of the electrodes and/or leads. Since electrode gel is a malleable extension of the electrode, and minor head movement produces little effect on the electrode-gel-scalp attachment, movement artifact can be minimal in a quiet patient. However, movement sufficient to disturb the connection results in charge movement between the electrode and gel and scalp, which is recorded as EEG (Figure 5.3.65). Differential amplification does not remove this artifact because the lead artifact affects the recording from a single electrode.

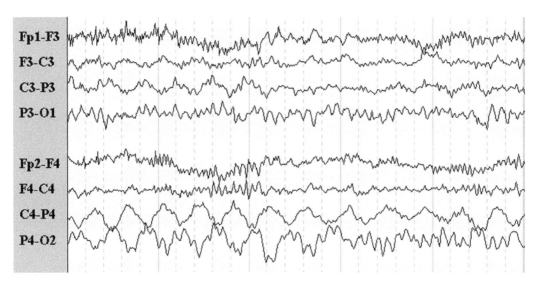

FIGURE 5.3.65 Movement artifact related to hyperventilation. Longitudinal bipolar montage, parasagittal portion.

Movement artifact is also produced by movement of the leads. A small amount of current flows through the electrode leads, and, while this current is miniscule compared to most electrical circuits, there is resistance in the leads and capacitance between the leads. Movement of the leads results in disturbance of the capacitance. The built-up charge can dissipate with loss of the capacitance, and this, too, is recorded on EEG.

How to Avoid Environmental and Machine Artifacts

Electrical artifact, including machine and 60-Hz potentials, can be minimized by the following:

- Recording in an electrically quiet environment, certainly not possible for patients in the ICU;
- Avoidance of ground loops;
- Disconnection of all nonessential electronic equipment from the patient;
- Minimizing the length of the exposed leads;
- Turning off lights and other equipment in proximity to the patient;
- Use of differential amplifiers (which is typical with modern equipment) and equal electrode impedances;
- Use of the 60-Hz filter.

5.4

Abnormal Nonepileptiform EEG

BASSEL ABOU-KHALIL

OVERVIEW

This chapter focuses on nonepileptiform abnormalities, and the following chapter focuses on epileptiform abnormalities. Table 5.4.1 outlines some of the important nonepileptiform abnormalities.

SLOW ABNORMALITIES

Focal Slow Activity

Focal slow activity (Figure 5.4.1) on the electroencephalogram (EEG) usually indicates a focal subcortical structural lesion. The slow activity typically has an irregular appearance. When it consists of persistent nonreactive irregular delta activity, it is often referred to as polymorphic delta activity (PDA). Polymorphic delta activity is most often related to a structural lesion.

The anatomic correlation is often not precise. The area of slow activity is more likely to overlie the structural lesion when the irregular slow activity is very focal. This is more likely when the lesion is close to the surface. The localizing value of focal slow activity is also increased if there is associated attenuation of faster frequencies. Deeper lesions tend to produce more widespread slow activity, without attenuation of faster frequencies (Figure 5.4.2 and 5.4.3).

Slow activity may be laterally displaced with central and parietal lesions; these tend to be associated with temporal slow activity (Figure 5.4.4 and 5.4.5).

Lesions involving one frontal pole or one occipital pole often produce bilateral frontopolar or occipital slow activity.

The slowest delta frequencies tend to be closest to the center of the lesion, with more theta activity in the surround region (see Figure 5.4.6).

If the lesion involves the cortex, there may be voltage attenuation in the center with the slowest frequencies. The slowest irregular delta activity at the center tends to be less reactive, while the faster surround activity tends to be more reactive, attenuating with arousal and stimulation.

Focal irregular slow activity tends to become less prominent in sleep. Focal slow abnormality may be totally missed in sleep (Figure 5.4.7).

Subtle slow activity can be enhanced during EEG review with certain measures including reducing the low-frequency filter cutoff frequency, compressing the time base, and increasing the sensitivity (Figure 5.4.8 and Figure 5.4.9).

The differential diagnosis of focal irregular slow activity is large, with some of the possibilities including

- Tumor;
- Stroke: Ischemic or hemorrhagic;
- Infection: Abscess or encephalitis;
- Trauma: Contusion or hematoma;
- Epileptic focus: Irregular slow activity may be associated with an epileptic focus in the absence of structural lesion;
- Transient focal slow abnormality may be seen in migraine, ischemia, or post-ictal dysfunction after a focal seizure.

Unfortunately, one cannot usually be definitive about the etiology of the slow activity from its appearance. While additional historical information may help the analysis, the diagnosis of focal structural lesions rests largely with imaging studies. However, the time course of slow activity varies depending on the etiology. Focal slow activity after a stroke or head trauma tends to decrease over time, whereas the slow activity associated with a tumor tends to persist. Slow activity as a result of dysfunction such as hemiplegic migraine or post-ictal state usually resolve once symptoms subside.

Focal slow activity may be associated with other types of EEG abnormalities, including

TABLE 5.4.1 ABNORMAL NONEPILEPTIFORM ELECTROENCEPHALOGRAM

Class	Type	Implication
Slow	Focal irregular slow activity	Due to a focal subcortical structural lesion or focal nonspecific dysfunction
	Focal rhythmic delta activity	Association with seizure tendency
	Generalized asynchronous slow activity	Generalized cerebral dysfunction, with a broad differential diagnosis
	Generalized or regional bisynchronous slow activity	Usually due to encephalopathy, with typical manifestation being frontal intermittent rhythmic delta activity (FIRDA) or occipital intermittent rhythmic delta activity (OIRDA)
Attenuation	Focal attenuation	Due to either focal reduction in cortical activity or accumulation of fluid over the cortex (e.g., subdural hematoma)
	Generalized attenuation	Global reduction in amplitude usually due to diffuse loss of cortical activity. Bilateral fluid collection over the cortex is possible.
Increased activity	Focal increase in activity	Most common is skull defect which reduces the attenuation of faster frequencies, a breach rhythm
	Generalized increase in activity	Usually due to encephalopathic disorders, especially excess diffuse beta activity most commonly seen with benzodiazepines
Other abnormal patterns	Periodic discharges	Lateralized periodic discharges (LPDs) are usually associated with an acute structural lesion with associated seizure tendency, but may occasionally be seen with chronic lesions. Bilateral independent periodic discharges (BiPDs) are seen in association with more severe conditions, often in comatose patients. Generalized periodic discharges (GPDs) are seen in various encephalopathies. LPDs and GPDs can be intermediate patterns along the interictal–ictal continuum.
	Alpha-theta coma	Patients with coma from a variety of reasons can have alpha coma, theta coma, or alpha-theta coma. The terms indicate the predominant frequencies. Their prognosis depends on the etiology and is poor if it they are caused by hypoxic encephalopathy.
	Spindle coma	Appearance of spindles in coma, but these are different from sleep spindles. Prognosis depends on etiology but is often less grave than some other patterns.
	Burst suppression	Severe encephalopathy often seen with hypoxic or other encephalopathies or from deep sedation with certain medications

- Widespread asynchronous slow activity in one or both hemispheres. This is more likely to be seen with acute lesions and may mask the focal slow activity.
- Bisynchronous slow activity. This slow activity may have a topographical distribution that is independent from that of the focal slow activity. It may indicate involvement of deep midline structures, as may occur with herniation.
- Focal epileptiform discharges. In some instances, the slow activity may be secondary to epileptiform activity and may be seen in the absence of a structural lesion.
- Asymmetry of physiologic activity including posterior dominant rhythm, mu rhythm, beta activity, and sleep activity, including vertex waves, sleep spindles, and K complexes.

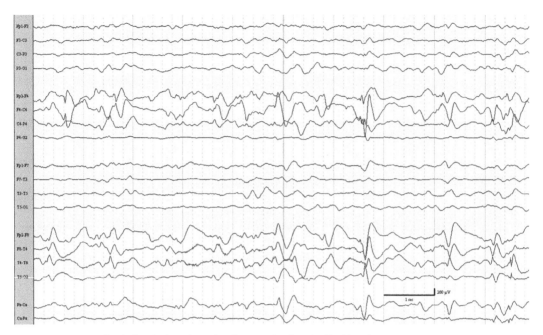

FIGURE 5.4.1 Focal right hemisphere irregular slow activity. Longitudinal bipolar montage.

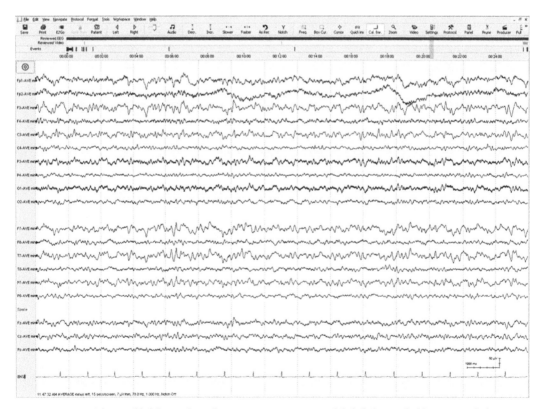

FIGURE 5.4.2 Widespread left hemisphere slow activity in a patient with left thalamic glioblastoma multiforme. Average minus left reference montage.

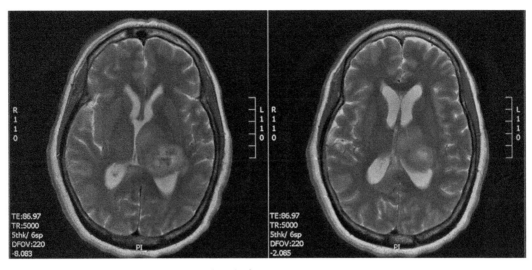

FIGURE 5.4.3 Magnetic resonance imaging (MRI) of patient in Figure 5.4.2.

One form of focal slow activity, temporal intermittent rhythmic delta activity (TIRDA), has a strong association with seizure activity (see Figure 5.4.10).

Intermittent rhythmic theta activity may have a similar association (Figure 5.4.11).

In ICU patients lateralized rhythmic delta activity (LRDA) has been associated with clinical seizures even if not temporal (Figure 5.4.12).

Generalized Asynchronous Slow Activity

Generalized asynchronous slow activity (Figures 5.4.13 through 5.4.15) is the most common EEG abnormality and is extremely nonspecific. It is usually more reactive than focal slow waves, attenuated by eye opening and alerting and increased by relaxation and hyperventilation. A small amount of generalized asynchronous theta

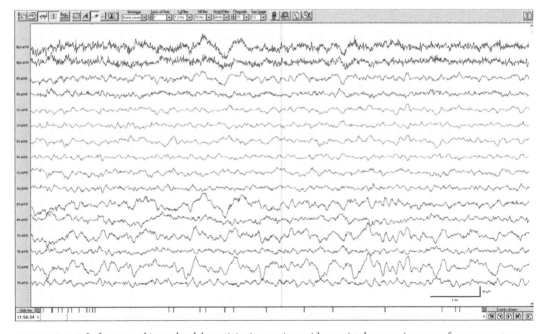

FIGURE 5.4.4 Left temporal irregular delta activity in a patient with a parietal tumor. Average reference montage.

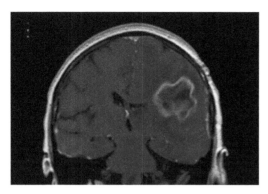

FIGURE 5.4.5 Magnetic resonance imaging (MRI) of patient in Figure 5.4.4.

activity is normal in drowsiness and normal in childhood; it can also be seen in 10–15% of normal adults. When abnormal, it usually indicates widespread subcortical abnormality. Slow activity in the theta range indicates mild dysfunction, whereas slow activity in the delta range means more severe encephalopathy (Figure 5.4.15).

Since generalized asynchronous theta activity is normally present in drowsiness at all ages and in the awake state in children, there should be caution in its interpretation.

Generalized or Regional Bisynchronous Slow Activity

Bisynchronous slow activity may be due to abnormal interaction between the thalamus and the cortex, consistent with overactive thalamocortical circuits. It can be generalized or regional. Even when it is generalized, it usually predominates in one region of the brain, most often frontal. This type of activity is often, but not always, rhythmic and intermittent. In the most recent terminology it is referred to as *generalized rhythmic delta activity* (GRDA). GRDA most often has a frontal predominance or is even restricted to frontal lobe. It was referred to as *frontal intermittent rhythmic delta activity* (FIRDA) (Figures 5.4.16 and 5.4.17). In children it tends to have an occipital predominance and was referred to as *occipital intermittent rhythmic delta activity* (OIRDA) (Figure 5.4.18).

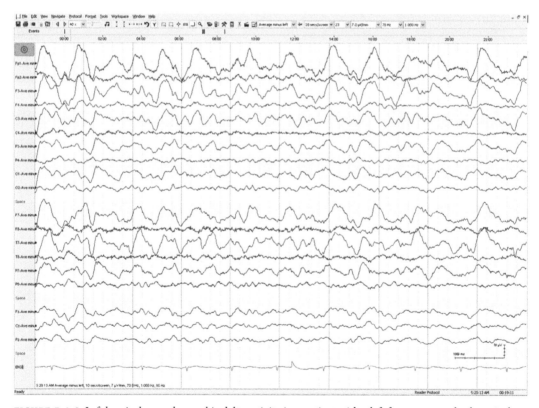

FIGURE 5.4.6 Left hemisphere polymorphic delta activity in a patient with a left frontotemporal subcortical glioblastoma multiforme. Note that the slowest frequencies are over the left frontotemporal region. The left posterior head region has more theta activity. Average reference minus left.

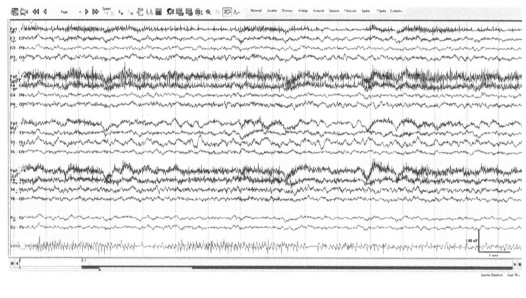

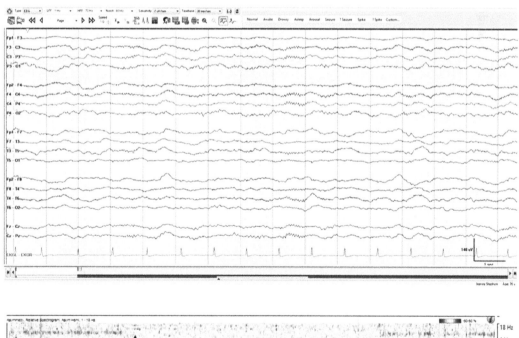

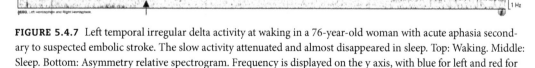

FIGURE 5.4.7 Left temporal irregular delta activity at waking in a 76-year-old woman with acute aphasia secondary to suspected embolic stroke. The slow activity attenuated and almost disappeared in sleep. Top: Waking. Middle: Sleep. Bottom: Asymmetry relative spectrogram. Frequency is displayed on the y axis, with blue for left and red for right predominance. Increased left hemisphere delta activity is demonstrated on waking in the first segment, but fades after the patient falls asleep (*arrow*). Longitudinal bipolar montage.

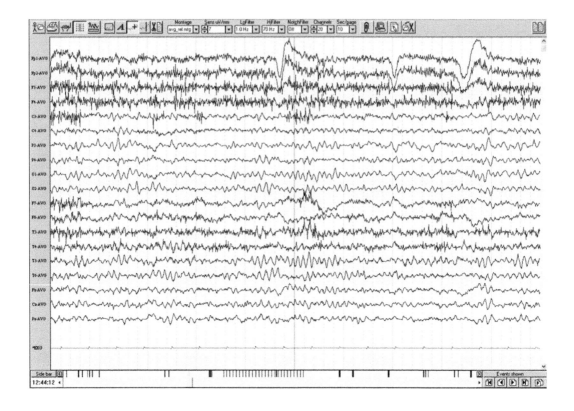

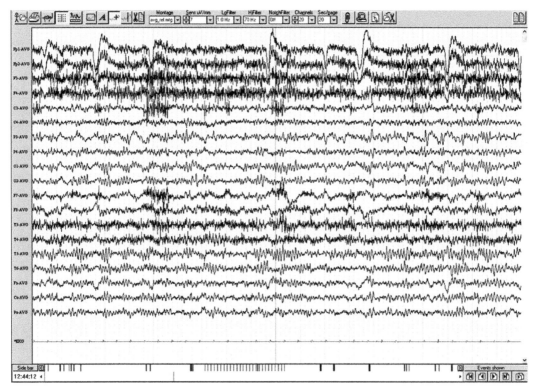

FIGURE 5.4.8 Steps to enhance focal slow activity. Top: Original recording with standard settings. Bottom: Compressing the time base. Next page top: Reducing the low-frequency filter cutoff frequency. Next page bottom: Increasing the sensitivity. Average reference montage.

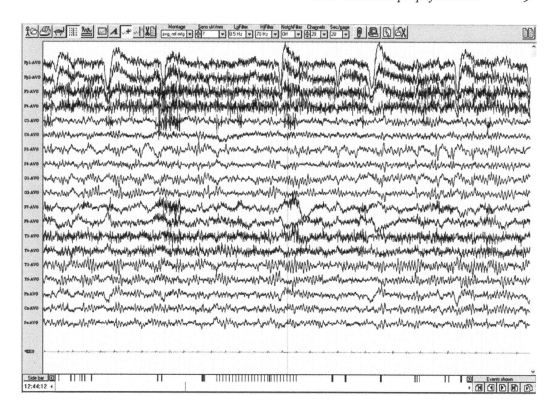

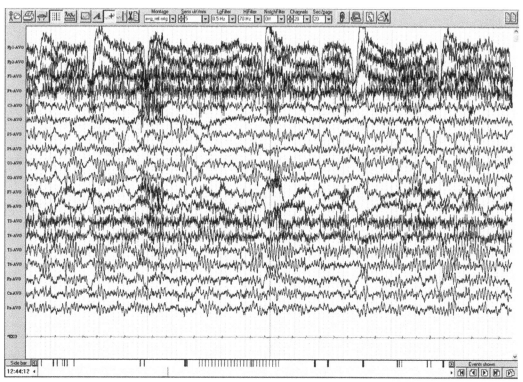

FIGURE 5.4.8 Continued

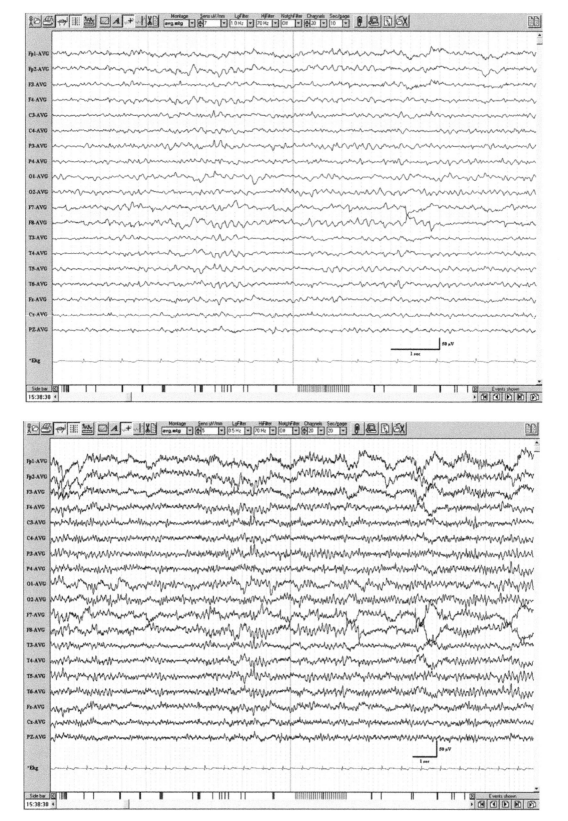

FIGURE 5.4.9 Left occipital focal delta activity brought out by the measures listed in Figure 5.4.8. The patient had a left occipital meningioma. The left occipital region was also involved, as expected with occipital pole source. The electroencephalogram (EEG) also showed right temporal slow activity. Top: Original page (sensitivity 7, low-frequency filter cutoff frequency 1 Hz, 10 sec/page). Bottom: Same page after application of measures used in 5.4.8 (sensitivity 5, low-frequency filter cutoff frequency 0.5 Hz, 20 sec/page). Next page top: Contrasted T1 axial magnetic resonance image showing left occipital meningioma. Average reference montage.

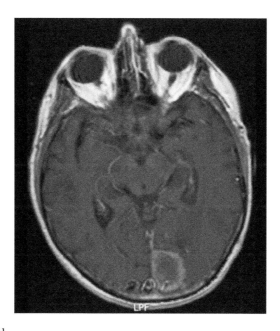

FIGURE 5.4.9 Continued

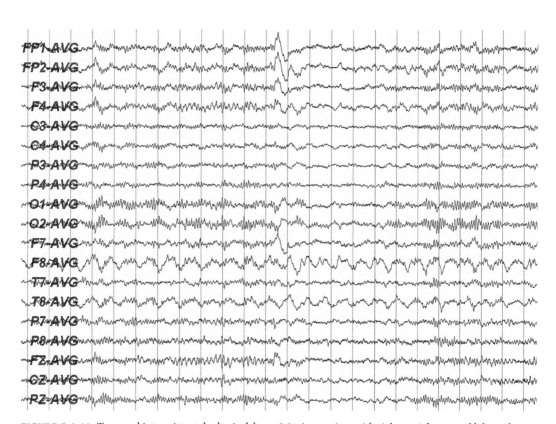

FIGURE 5.4.10 Temporal intermittent rhythmic delta activity in a patient with right mesial temporal lobe epilepsy. Average reference montage.

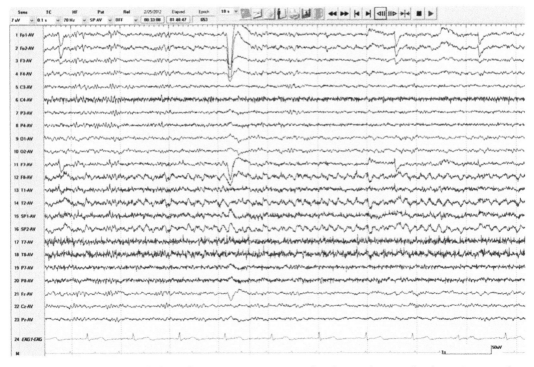

FIGURE 5.4.11 Intermittent rhythmic theta activity in a patient with right mesial temporal epilepsy. Average reference montage.

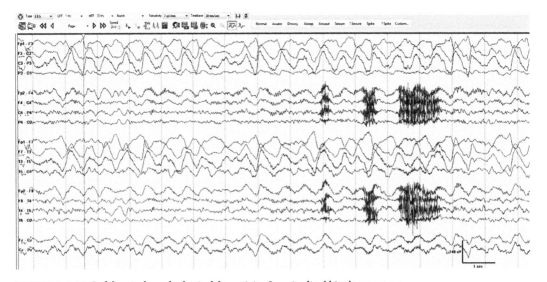

FIGURE 5.4.12 Left hemisphere rhythmic delta activity. Longitudinal bipolar montage.

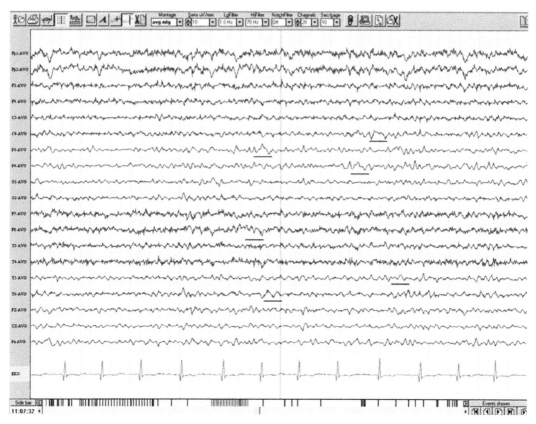

FIGURE 5.4.13 Generalized asynchronous theta activity. Select theta waves are underlined to demonstrate their asynchronous pattern Average reference montage.

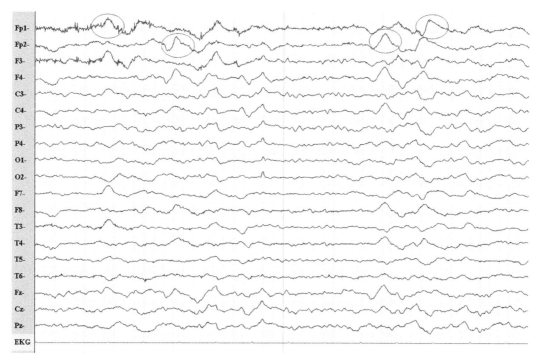

FIGURE 5.4.14 Generalized asynchronous slow activity, predominantly in the delta range. Select waves are circled to demonstrate asynchronous pattern. Linked ear montage.

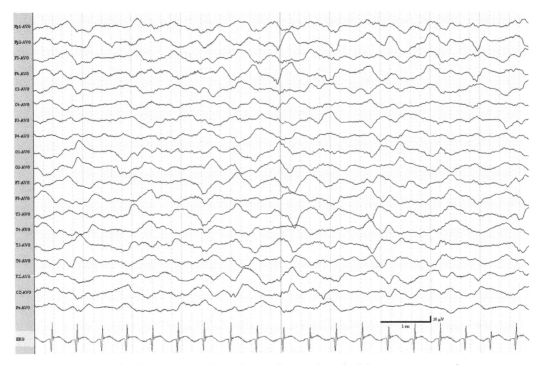

FIGURE 5.4.15 Generalized asynchronous slow activity predominantly in the delta range. Average reference montage.

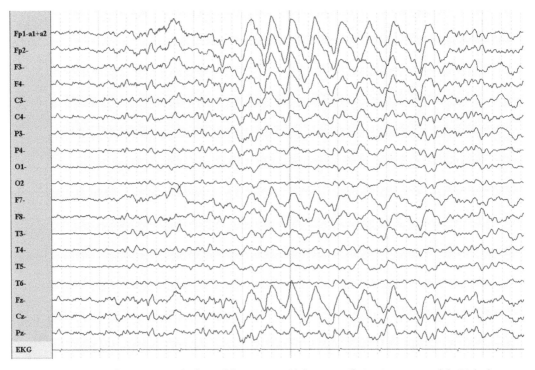

FIGURE 5.4.16 Frontal intermittent rhythmic delta activity with hyperventilation in a young adult. Linked ear reference montage.

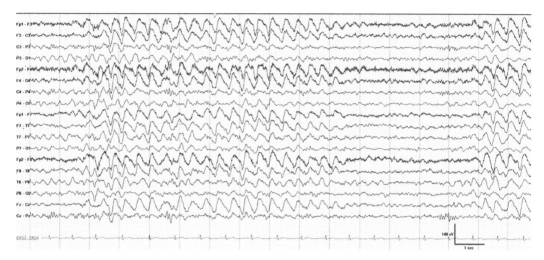

FIGURE 5.4.17 Frontal intermittent rhythmic delta activity (FIRDA) in a 36-year-old man during drowsiness. Longitudinal bipolar montage.

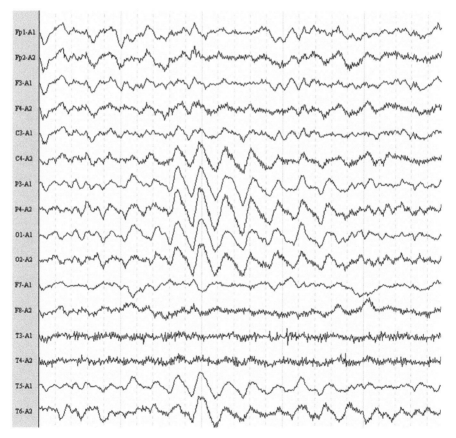

FIGURE 5.4.18 Occipital intermittent rhythmic delta activity (OIRDA) with hyperventilation in a 13-year-old boy. Ipsilateral ear reference montage.

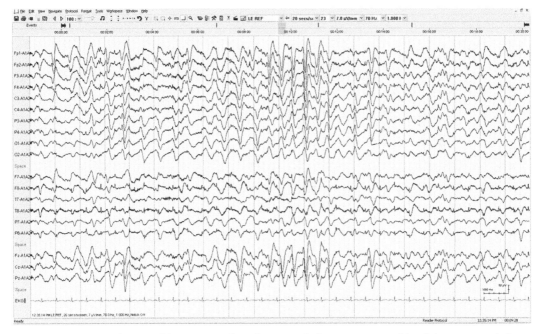

FIGURE 5.4.19 Bisynchronous delta activity with triphasic morphology in a 50-year-old with hepatic encephalopathy and an ammonia level of 168 (normal range 11–35). Linked ear reference montage.

The frequency of GRDA is most often about 2–3 Hz. It is normal in drowsiness and with hyperventilation at any age and normal in waking in children.

When pathological, GRDA can be seen in a wide variety of conditions. The differential diagnosis includes

- Metabolic encephalopathies,
- Degenerative disorders and other conditions affecting cortical and subcortical gray matter,
- Deep midline tumors.

Of these, metabolic encephalopathy may be the most common etiology.

GRDA may have triphasic morphology in patients with metabolic encephalopathy, particularly those with hepatic encephalopathy (Figure 5.4.19).

GRDA may be asymmetrical, but asymmetries may not have lateralizing clinical significance. Lower voltage may correspond to the more abnormal side because of attenuation due to cortical dysfunction, or the side of higher voltage may be more abnormal.

OIRDA in children is uncommonly associated with encephalopathy. OIRDA was reported to be associated with childhood absence epilepsy. There may be subtle spikes embedded in the occipital rhythmic activity in children with childhood absence epilepsy (Figure 5.4.20).

Slowing of the Posterior Dominant Rhythm

Slowing of the waking posterior dominant rhythm (PDR; Figure 5.4.21) is a change in the posterior alpha-range activity to less than 8.5 Hz. Slowing to less than this level is almost always abnormal in adults. The most common degree of slowing is in the theta range, with slowing in the 6.5–8 Hz range. Slowing to less than this is associated with higher levels of disorganization of the background. Interpretation is nonspecific, but this is most commonly seen with encephalopathy or dementia.

It is important to recognize that what may appear as a slow PDR in a longitudinal bipolar montage could be originating anteriorly. It is wise to confirm a slow PDR in an ear reference montage to verify the posterior predominance of the rhythmic activity considered to be a PDR. Figure 5.4.22 is an example of widespread frontally dominant theta activity giving the appearance of a slow PDR.

It is also important not to confuse a normal slow alpha variant with a slow PDR. A slow alpha variant is a subharmonic of the native PDR (Figure 5.4.23).

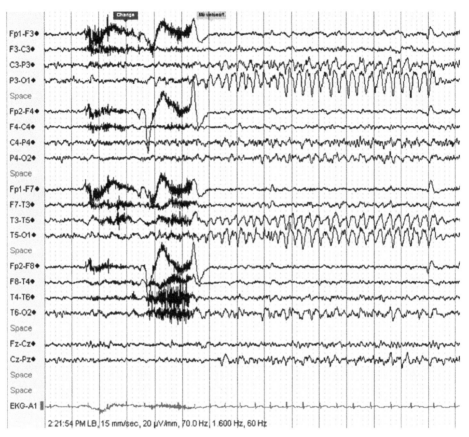

FIGURE 5.4.20 Occipital intermittent rhythmic delta activity (OIRDA) in a 7-year-girl with childhood absence epilepsy. Longitudinal bipolar montage.

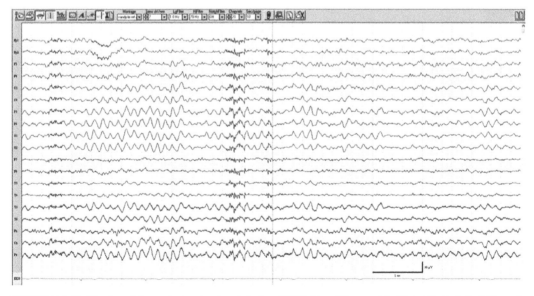

FIGURE 5.4.21 Slowing of the posterior dominant rhythm (6.5 Hz) in a 38-year-old with intellectual disability and generalized epilepsy. Linked ear reference montage.

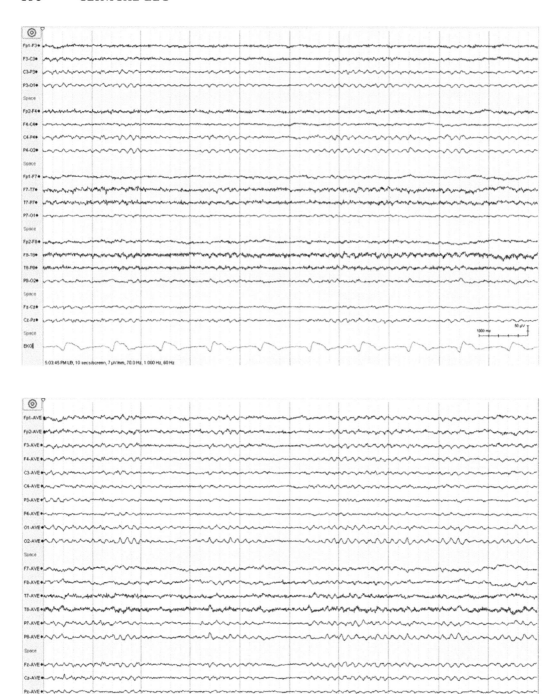

FIGURE 5.4.22 Electroencephalogram (EEG) in a 55-year-old man with 7 Hz rhythmic activity initially misinterpreted as a posterior dominant rhythm (PDR) on longitudinal bipolar (Top) and average reference (Middle) montages. The ear reference montage (Next page top) demonstrated frontally dominant rhythmic activity as the source. It also demonstrated that the patient had a normal 10 Hz PDR after eye closure (Next page bottom).

Top: LB montage. Bottom: Average montage. Next page top and bottom: Linked ear reference montage.

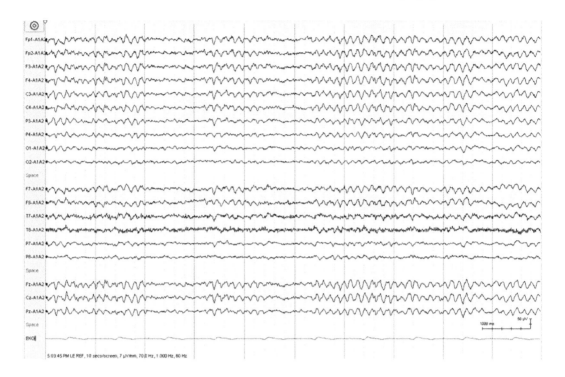

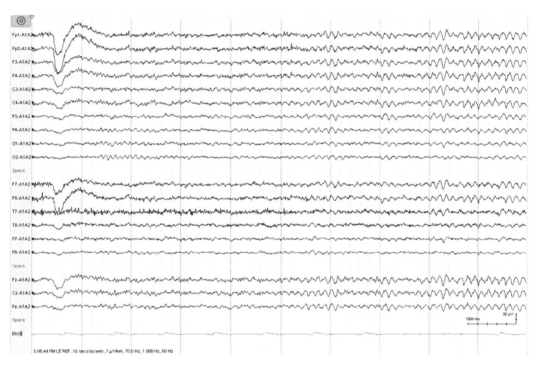

FIGURE 5.4.22 Continued

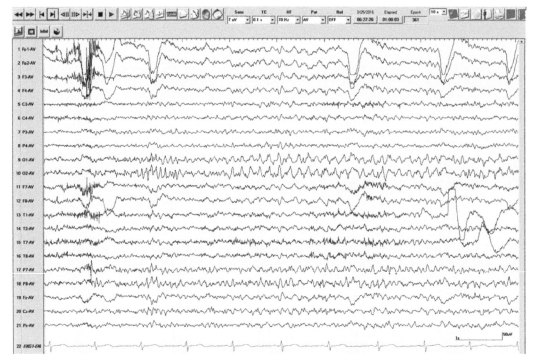

FIGURE 5.4.23 Slow alpha variant alternating with native posterior dominant rhythm (PDR). Average reference montage.

AMPLITUDE ABNORMALITIES

Overview

Amplitude abnormalities can be focal or generalized. Focal amplitude abnormalities include focal attenuation or increase in amplitude. Generalized amplitude abnormalities include global attenuation/suppression or increase in amplitude. The term "attenuation" indicates decreased amplitude of one type of activity (such as activity in a certain frequency) or of all activity. The term "suppression" is a more severe attenuation and is usually used to indicate complete or almost complete disappearance of EEG activity.

Attenuation/Suppression
Focal/Lateralized Attenuation

Focal attenuation (Figure 5.4.24) usually indicates a focal cortical lesion (such as infarct) or focal cortical dysfunction (such as ischemia or post-ictal effect) but may also result from an increased distance between the cortex and the recording electrode, as may be seen from scalp edema, subdural hematoma, and occasionally from dural-based tumors, such as meningiomas.

Since the thalamus has an important role in the cortical generation of rhythmical activity, a thalamic lesion may result in attenuation of the PDR as well as other rhythmic activity on one side. In Figure 5.4.25, attenuation of the left PDR is due to a left thalamic hemorrhage.

Attenuation may affect both normal and abnormal rhythms, as seen in Figure 5.4.26 from a patient with head injury and subsequent left hemisphere infarction. While the right hemisphere is also abnormal, the left hemisphere has greater cortical abnormality resulting in severe attenuation.

Focal attenuation will usually involve multiple electrodes. Focal attenuation that is confined to one channel in a bipolar montage is more likely to be due to an electrical bridge related to a smear of electrode paste (also called a salt bridge), as seen in Figure 5.4.27.

With subdural hematoma, the attenuation is most pronounced with bipolar recordings: there is cortical activity, but the conducting ability of the subdural fluid results in a reduction of potential differences between electrodes and attenuates the recorded potential at the scalp (Figure 5.4.28). The same shunting of potential differences occurs

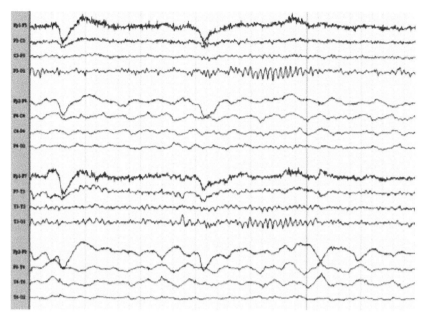

FIGURE 5.4.24 Attenuation of the posterior alpha rhythm on the right after a focal right hemisphere seizure. There is also delta activity in the right hemisphere. Longitudinal bipolar montage.

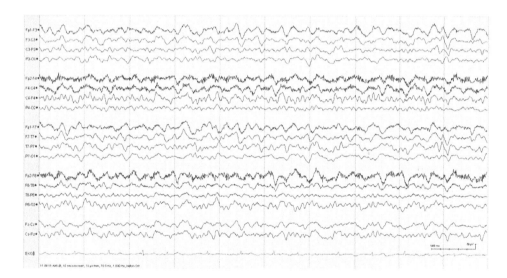

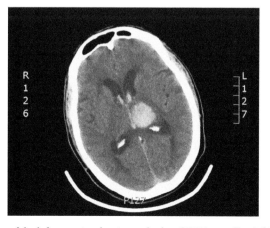

FIGURE 5.4.25 Attenuation of the left posterior dominant rhythm (PDR) as well as left hemisphere predominant irregular delta-theta activity Top: LB montage, in a patient with left thalamic intracerebral hemorrhage. Bottom: Computed tomography (CT) head scan.

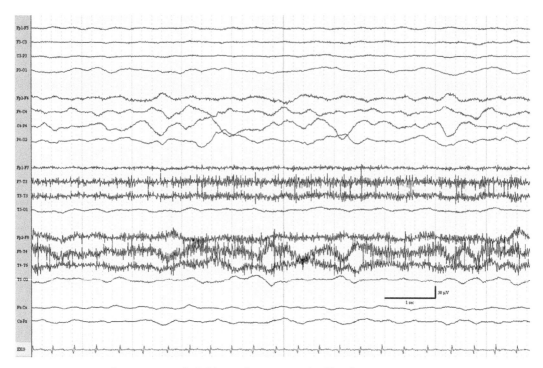

FIGURE 5.4.26 Focal attenuation in the left hemisphere. Longitudinal bipolar montage.

with electrode gel smear on the scalp causing an electrical bridge.

Generalized Attenuation/Suppression

Generalized attenuation or suppression of the background can happen because of three reasons:

- Desynchronization (decreased synchronicity) of cortical activity, as may occur with anxiety;
- Pathological decreased cortical activity due to cortical structural abnormality or dysfunction;
- Increased media between the cortex and recording electrodes (such as fluid collections or tissue).

Decreased synchronicity of cortical activity may occur in an awake, alert state, and is most often seen in anxious individuals. One normal variant seen in a small proportion of adults is a low-voltage background that looks suppressed (Figure 5.4.29). However, a low-voltage EEG would be abnormal in children and adolescents.

Generalized decreased cortical activity can occur with generalized cortical injury or transient dysfunction. Examples of generalized cortical injury include hypoxic-ischemic encephalopathy (HIE), or degenerative conditions such as advanced Huntington's disease; examples of transient dysfunction include drug-induced coma or post-ictal state after a generalized tonic-clonic seizure. Figure 5.4.30 shows EEG suppression from pentobarbital coma.

Excessive fluid or tissue overlying the cortex is more likely an explanation for focal rather than generalized attenuation but may occasionally be bilateral, as in bilateral subdural collections.

Increase in EEG Activity
Focal Increase in EEG Activity

Focal increase in EEG activity is most often the result of a skull defect (Figure 5.4.31). The skull filters fast activity, so the presence of a defect causes increased fast beta activity as well as increased sharpness of less fast activity (sharpness represents a higher frequency component of that activity). Specific rhythms can become more prominent with skull defects in specific regions. For example, if the skull defect is over the central region, mu activity may be exaggerated, and if the skull defect is over the temporal region, a third rhythm could become more prominent. The EEG activity over skull defects in these areas is often referred to as a *breach rhythm*. It is not clear that this should necessarily be considered

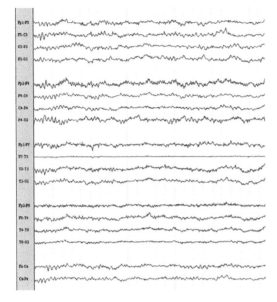

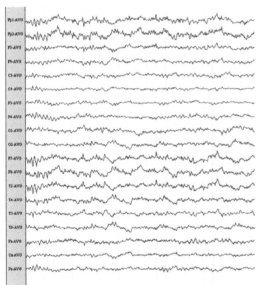

FIGURE 5.4.27 Electrical bridge between F7 and T3 due to smear of electrode paste. Longitudinal bipolar (LB) montage (Top). In the average reference montage (Bottom), F7 and T3 have almost identical activity.

an abnormality. It is rather an expected effect of a skull defect.

Generalized Increase in EEG Activity

Excessive Fast Activity

Excessive fast activity is most commonly seen in patients receiving sedatives such as barbiturates or benzodiazepines. Chloral hydrate usually produces less excessive beta activity. Electromyogram (EMG) activity from scalp muscles can appear as fast activity if its voltage is low and when the high-frequency filter is used. Muscle artifact can be attenuated by asking the patient to relax and open the mouth.

Excessive beta activity beyond what is expected from sedative medication could be interpreted as a minor abnormality.

The patient recorded in Figure 5.4.32 has been treated with clonazepam and has some generalized slow activity as well as excessive beta activity.

Excessive beta activity superimposed on rhythmic delta, termed "extreme delta brush," is an EEG pattern seen in some patients with anti-N-methyl-D-aspartate (NMDA) receptor antibody limbic encephalitis. It is associated with a more protracted course of the disease (Figure 5.4.33).

PERIODIC PATTERNS

Overview

Periodic discharges are repeated discharges with other intervening activity between discharges. They can be classified as *lateralized periodic discharges* (LPDs) or *generalized/bilateral periodic discharges* (GPDs). GPDs can be classified as short-interval and long-interval periodic discharges. *Burst-suppression* could also be considered a periodic pattern.

Lateralized Periodic Discharges

LPDs are periodic discharges that are lateralized to one hemisphere (Figures 5.4.34 and 5.4.35). These were previously termed *periodic lateralized epileptiform discharges* (PLEDs), but this term was abandoned because the descriptor "epileptiform" is often inappropriate. This term encompasses discharges that are focal, as well as others that affect one whole hemisphere. Some involvement of the other hemisphere is acceptable. LPDs are usually high in amplitude, at 100–300 μV.

The appearance of LPDs can vary considerably. They may be sharp or blunt, monophasic, biphasic, or polyphasic. Lower voltage LPDs can be difficult to identify in the background (Figure 5.4.36).

The discharge may be simple or complex, with additional fast or rhythmic components superimposed on the waveform (called LPDs+F and LPDs+R) (Figure 5.4.37).

LPDs are most often the result of acute structural lesion, such as stroke, acute infection, or rapidly growing brain tumor (e.g., glioblastoma

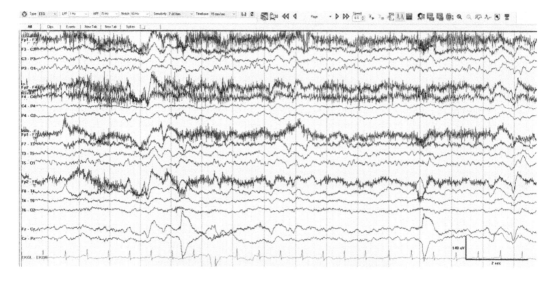

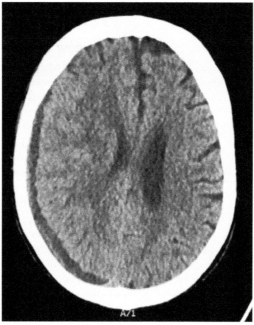

FIGURE 5.4.28 Right hemisphere attenuation Top: Electroencephalogram (EEG) with subdural hematoma. Longitudinal bipolar (LB) montage. Bottom: Computed tomography (CT) head scan.

multiforme). However, LPDs can also occur in patients with acute metabolic disturbance who also have a chronic structural lesion (especially in the setting of alcohol withdrawal). LPDs can also occur in the setting of chronic epilepsy. Therefore, LPDs are not specific for a particular diagnosis. Clinical correlation is required for interpretation. For example, LPDs in the temporal or frontotemporal area can be a sign of herpes encephalitis in a patient with acute onset of fever and seizures (Figure 5.4.38).

The majority of patients with LPDs have clinical seizures. However, there is a controversy over whether LPDs themselves are ictal. The prevailing opinion is that LPDs are not ictal, because more typical rhythmic ictal discharges are sometimes recorded in patients with LPDs (Figure 5.4.39).

However, there are patients with LPDs who have myoclonic jerks synchronous with the discharges, suggesting that they may be ictal in some instances (see Figure 5.4.40).

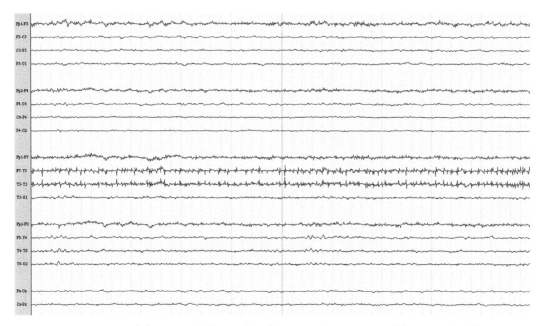

FIGURE 5.4.29 Attenuated electroencephalogram (EEG) as a normal variant in an adult. Longitudinal bipolar montage.

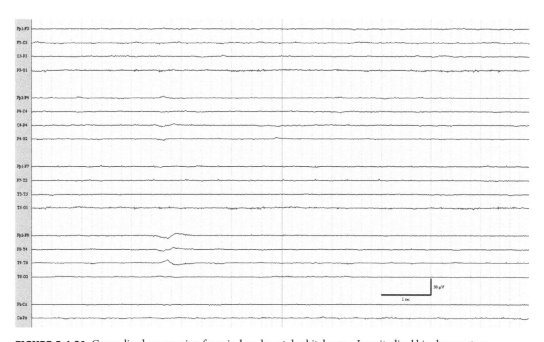

FIGURE 5.4.30 Generalized suppression from induced pentobarbital coma. Longitudinal bipolar montage.

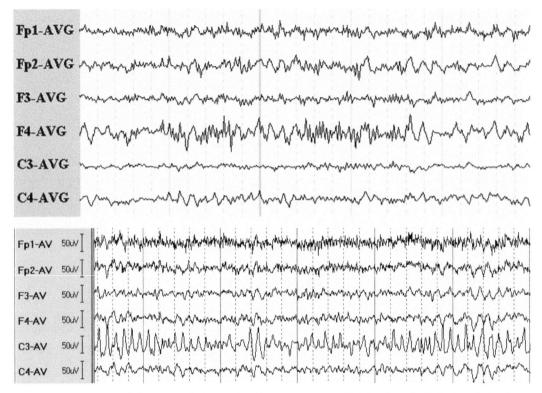

FIGURE 5.4.31 Increased electroencephalogram (EEG) activity over a skull defect (breach rhythm), including beta activity at F4 on top and mu activity at C3 in the bottom. Average reference montage.

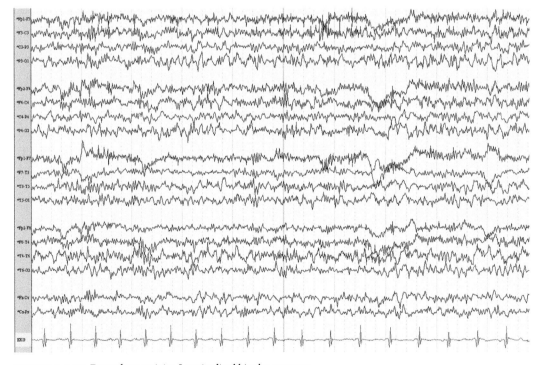

FIGURE 5.4.32 Excess beta activity. Longitudinal bipolar montage.

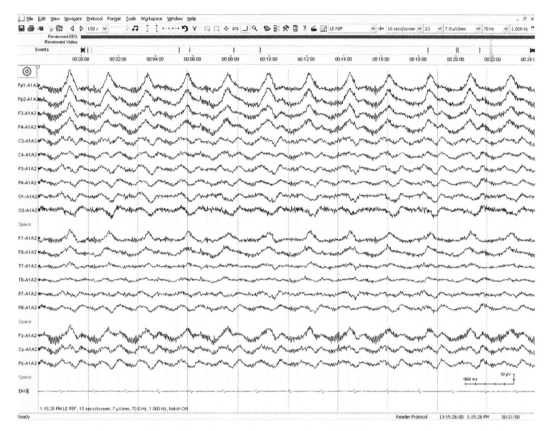

FIGURE 5.4.33 Extreme delta brush in a 38-year-old woman with anti-NMDA receptor antibody encephalitis. Linked ear referential montage.

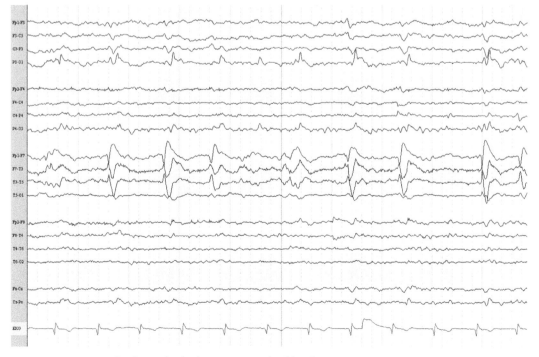

FIGURE 5.4.34 Lateralized periodic discharges. Longitudinal bipolar montage.

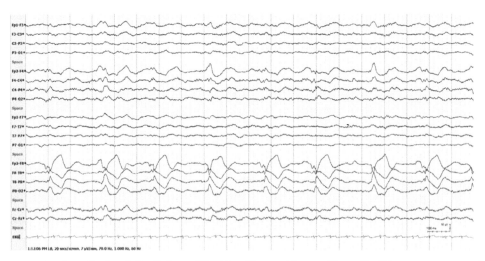

FIGURE 5.4.35 Lateralized periodic discharge (LPD) in a 52-year-old man with small cell lung cancer metastatic to the brain and altered mental status. Longitudinal bipolar montage.

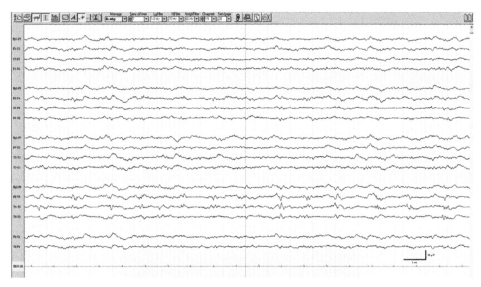

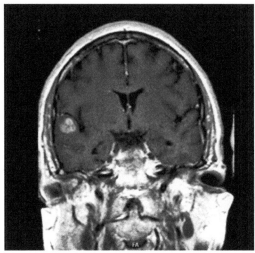

FIGURE 5.4.36 Lower voltage right temporal lateralized periodic discharges (LPDs). Top: Electroencephalogram (EEG) in a patient with a right temporal lesion that was eventually diagnosed as a glioblastoma multiforme. Longitudinal bipolar (LB) montage. Bottom: Magnetic resonance imaging of brain showing the lesion.

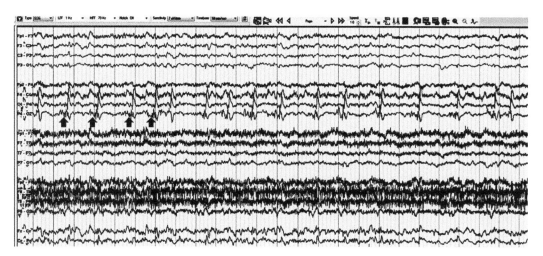

FIGURE 5.4.37 Lateralized periodic discharges (LPDs+ F) in a 67-year-old man admitted for seizures and altered mental status 1 month after a right temporal intracerebral hemorrhage. The arrows point to the fast activity associated with each discharge. Longitudinal bipolar montage.

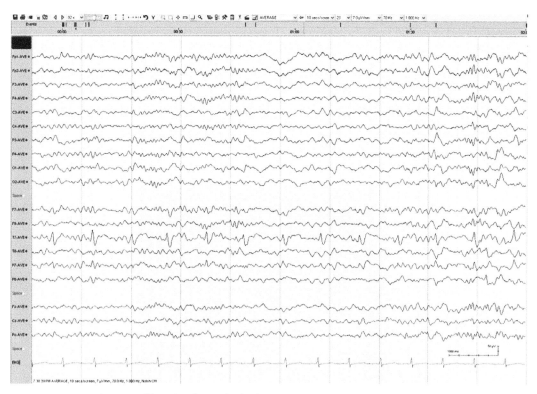

FIGURE 5.4.38 Left temporal lateralized periodic discharge (LPD) in a 59-year-old woman with confirmed herpes encephalitis. Average reference montage.

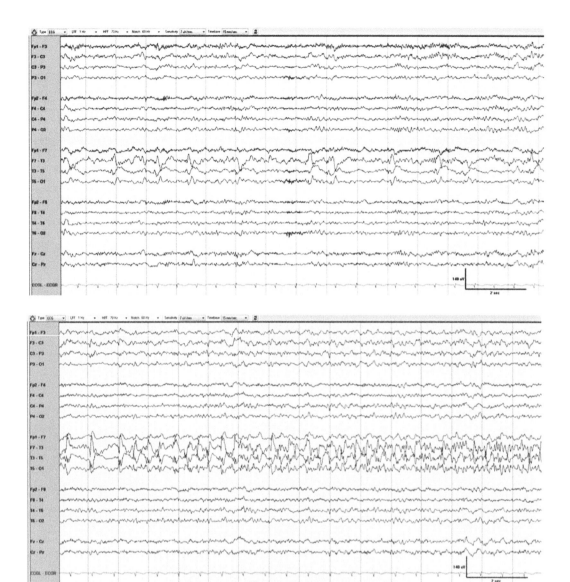

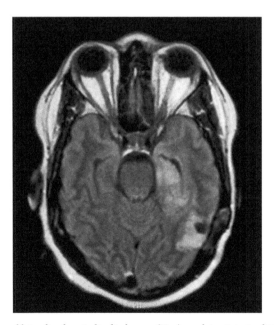

FIGURE 5.4.39 Left temporal lateralized periodic discharges (Top), evolving into traditional ictal discharge (Middle) in a patient with a left temporal glioblastoma multiforme on magnetic resonance imaging (Bottom).

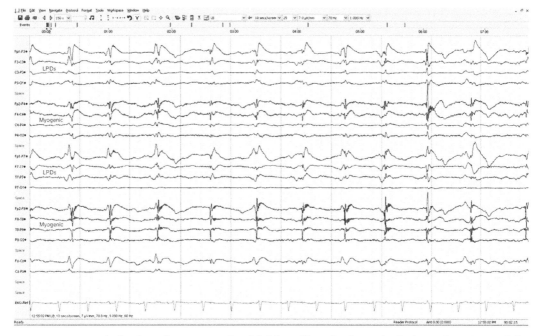

FIGURE 5.4.40 Right facial twitching associated with left frontal lateralized periodic discharges (LPDs). Every left frontal LPD is followed by a muscle twitch artifact on the right. Longitudinal bipolar montage.

LPDs are now considered an intermediate pattern along the interictal-ictal continuum. Certain features can make them closer to the interictal and others closer to the ictal end of the continuum.

Some features have been suggested to increase the odds that LPDs are ictal, including

- Fast or rhythmic activity with the periodic complexes,

- Short interval between discharges, and
- Attenuation of background between discharges.

On the other hand, LPDs with simple monophasic morphology, a focal field, not associated with fast or rhythmic activity, with long interval between discharges, and with background activity in between discharges are more likely interictal (Figures 5.4.41 and 5.4.42).

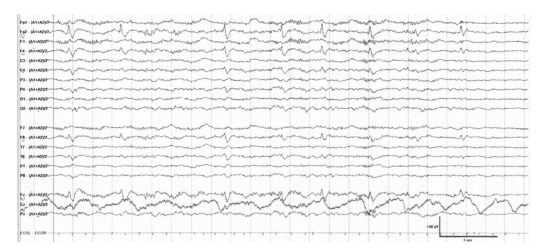

FIGURE 5.4.41 Lateralized periodic discharge (LPDs) that are further apart are closer to the interictal end of the spectrum. Linked ear reference montage.

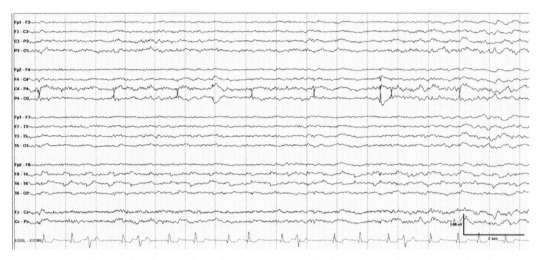

FIGURE 5.4.42 lateralized periodic discharge (LPDs) that are very focal are closer to the interictal end of the spectrum. Longitudinal bipolar montage.

LPDs can occur independently in the two hemispheres, termed *bilateral independent periodic discharges* (BiPDs). BiPDs imply bilateral pathology and patients are usually sicker, often comatose (Figure 5.4.43).

Generalized Periodic Discharges

GPDs are bilateral synchronous discharges that may be prevalent in one part of the brain, usually anteriorly. They are often classified as short-interval or long-interval periodic discharges. Short-interval periodic discharges have a periodicity of 0.5–3 per second. They are more common and less specific than long-interval discharges. The main underlying conditions include metabolic disturbances (e.g., triphasic waves with hepatic encephalopathy), anoxic injury, toxic encephalopathy, Creutzfeldt-Jakob disease (CJD), and

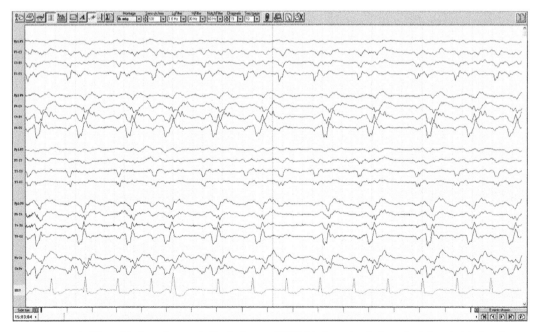

FIGURE 5.4.43 Bilateral independent periodic discharges (BiPDs) independently from the left and right hemispheres with posterior predominance in a 74-year-old woman with bilateral watershed infarcts and unresponsiveness. Longitudinal bipolar montage.

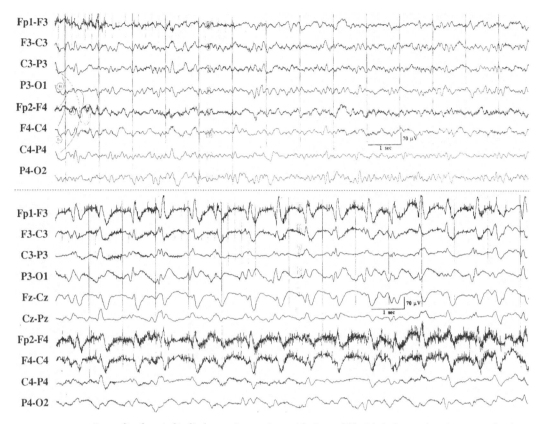

FIGURE 5.4.44 Generalized periodic discharges in a patient with Creutzfeldt-Jakob disease (CJD). Longitudinal bipolar montage.

nonconvulsive status epilepticus. Clinical correlation is always required.

In CJD, the majority of patients will develop periodic discharges in the first 3 months of the disease, as in Figure 5.4.44. Figure 5.4.45 shows a second case of CJD in a 69-year-old with sporadic CJD.

The periodic pattern is not always seen in the patients, as shown for the second CJD case (Figure 5.4.45) in an earlier recording shown in Figure 5.4.46. The periodic discharges evident later in the course are not obvious in this earlier recording. Stimuli can evoke the periodic discharges, as in the recording in Figure 5.4.47 from the same patient. Bursts are evoked by clapping.

In early CJD periodic discharges may be focal, particularly if the pathology is focal (Figure 5.4.48).

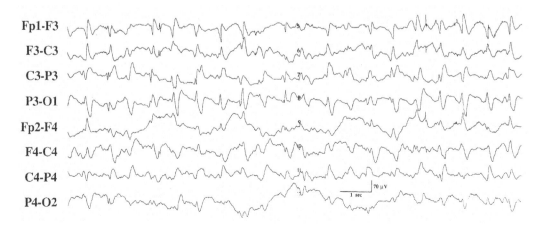

FIGURE 5.4.45 Creutzfeldt-Jakob disease (CJD) case 2. Longitudinal bipolar montage, parasagittal portion.

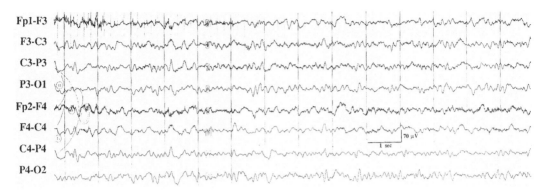

FIGURE 5.4.46 Creutzfeldt-Jakob disease (CJD) case 2. Three weeks prior to the recording in Figure 5.4.45. Longitudinal bipolar montage, parasagittal portion.

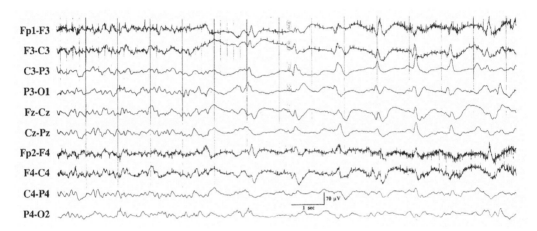

FIGURE 5.4.47 Creutzfeldt-Jakob disease (CJD) case 2. Burst evoked by clapping. Longitudinal bipolar montage, parasagittal portion.

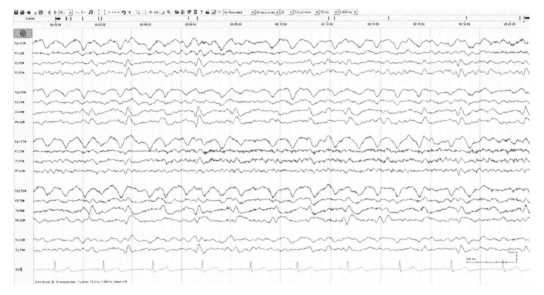

FIGURE 5.4.48 Lateralized periodic discharge (LPD) in a 55-year-old with progressive dementia and documented Creutzfeldt-Jakob disease (CJD) with positive RT-QuiC, positive 14-3-3 protein, and elevated T-tau protein in cerebrospinal fluid (Above). The periodic discharges are right posterior predominant, corresponding to right posterior predominant cortical ribboning on diffusion magnetic resonance imaging (Next page).

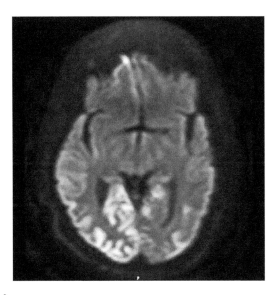

FIGURE 5.4.48 Continued

Short-interval GPDs can be seen in a variety of encephalopathies, including metabolic, toxic, and hypoxic-ischemic etiologies, with examples in the Figures 5.4.49–5.4.51.

GPDs may also be seen transiently after pentobarbital or propofol withdrawal (Figure 5.4.52).[1]

Long-interval periodic discharges have intervals of more than 4 sec between discharges. They are more specific with respect to etiology, particularly when the clinical history is incorporated. Associated conditions include some toxic encephalopathies, as occur with baclofen overdose and

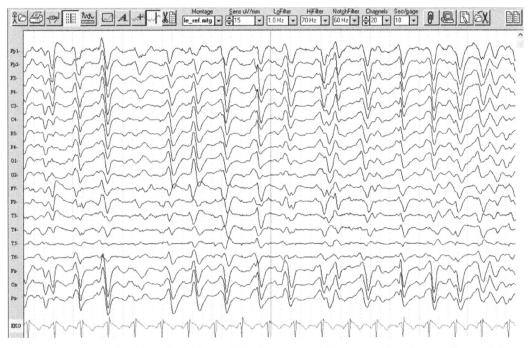

FIGURE 5.4.49 Generalized periodic discharges (GPDs) in a 44 year-old woman with cirrhosis and hepatic failure. Linked ear reference montage.

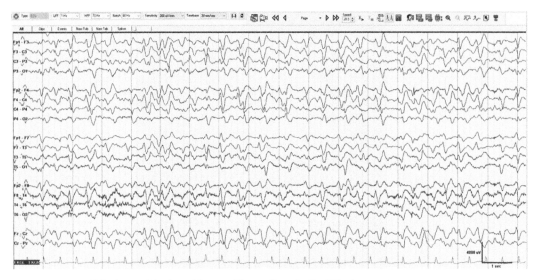

FIGURE 5.4.50 Cefepime toxicity in an 81-year-old man. Longitudinal bipolar montage.

PCP or ketamine effect, anoxic injury, or subacute sclerosing panencephalitis (SSPE). When long-interval periodic discharges are seen in the setting of a dementing illness in a child who also has myoclonic jerks, they are fairly specific for SSPE (Figures 5.4.53). In this condition, the interval between complexes becomes progressively shorter with disease progression.

Anoxia can produce a variety of EEG features; among these are periodic discharges.

Figure 5.4.56 is from a 9-year-old boy who had anoxic encephalopathy due to choking on a ball. The periodic discharges are fairly synchronous between the hemispheres, although the slow activity is markedly asynchronous.

COMA AND ELECTROCEREBRAL SILENCE

Coma

The EEG is often of great value in coma and may help identify the underlying pathophysiology in some cases. Although the EEG is usually nonspecific with respect to etiology, it can distinguish diffuse encephalopathy, focal brain lesions, nonconvulsive status epilepticus, and psychogenic

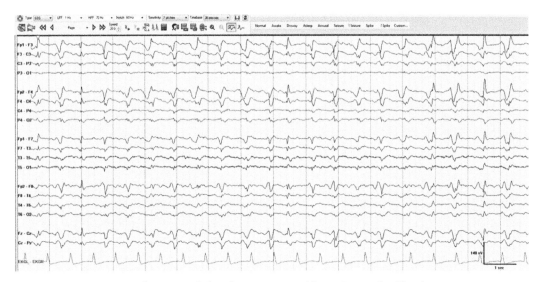

FIGURE 5.4.51 Hypoxic-ischemic encephalopathy in a 57-year-old man. Longitudinal bipolar montage.

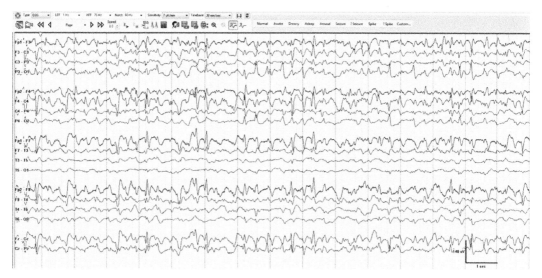

FIGURE 5.4.52 Generalized periodic discharges (GPDs) after withdrawal of pentobarbital used to reduce intracranial pressure after traumatic brain injury in a 25-year-old man. Longitudinal bipolar montage.

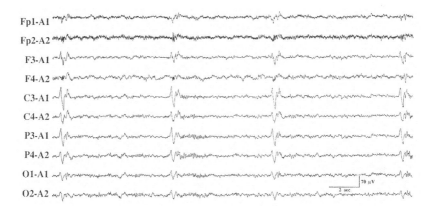

FIGURE 5.4.53 Subacute sclerosing panencephalitis (SSPE). Ipsilateral ear montage.

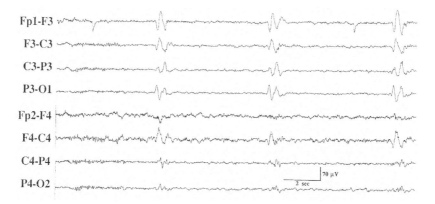

FIGURE 5.4.54 Subacute sclerosing panencephalitis (SSPE) case 2. Longitudinal bipolar montage.

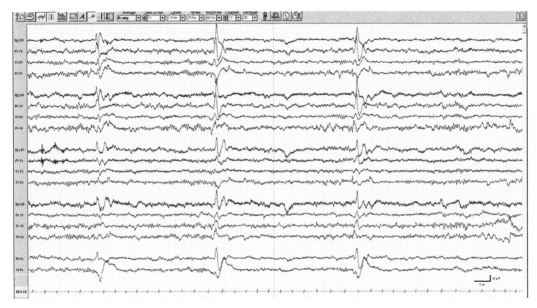

FIGURE 5.4.55 Generalized periodic discharges in a 12-year-old with subacute sclerosing panencephalitis (SSPE). The discharges are 6–10 sec apart, and their periodic nature could be missed on a 10-sec page. Longitudinal bipolar montage with 30-sec page.

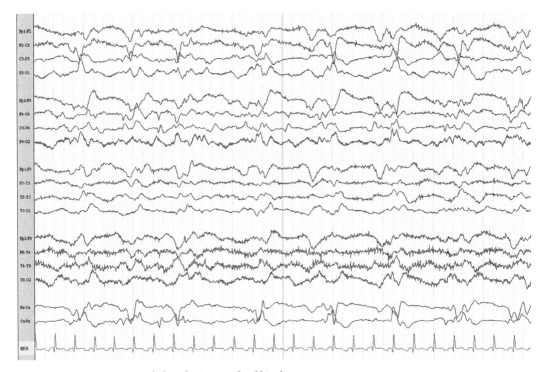

FIGURE 5.4.56 Anoxic encephalopathy. Longitudinal bipolar montage.

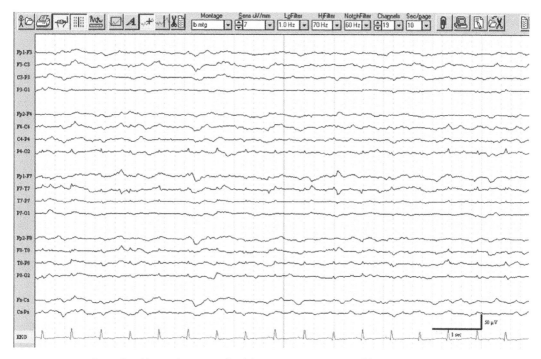

FIGURE 5.4.57 Generalized low-voltage irregular delta activity in a 42-year-old man with severe hepatic encephalopathy secondary to Wilson's disease. Longitudinal bipolar montage.

unresponsiveness (in which case the EEG is expected to be normal). The recordings are usually conducted in the ICU or in the emergency room and therefore are often contaminated with a variety of artifacts. Physiological monitoring with additional electrodes may help identify the source of various artifacts, for example related to respiration, eye movements, or movement or muscle contraction. Intervention, for example with a benzodiazepine challenge, may be necessary during the EEG for diagnostic or therapeutic purposes. The technologist needs to test reactivity after a long segment of recording without stimulation. Testing should include passive eye opening/closure, auditory stimulation, and painful somatosensory stimulation. The EEG can help with prognosis when the etiology is known, particularly with serial recordings. The presence of reactivity is usually a favorable indicator. However, reactivity is not of prognostic value in the case of drug intoxication, when improvement is expected as the drug is cleared.

A metabolic cause is most likely when the etiology is not known. The most common finding is generalized asynchronous irregular delta activity, with or without associated bisynchronous delta activity (Figures 5.4.57 and 5.4.58).

When coma is due to overdose with a sedative medication, generalized low-voltage delta activity may have superimposed beta activity that is slower than the usual beta seen in an awake patient taking sedating medication (Figure 5.4.59).

A deeper level of drug-induced coma leads to a burst suppression pattern as noted in Figure 5.4.60. Baclofen and lithium intoxication tend to be associated with periodic discharges.

Coma due to supratentorial lesions will usually be associated with very abnormal EEG, including focal irregular delta activity and generalized slow activity (Figure 5.4.60).

There may be associated lateralized periodic discharges in one or more location (Figure 5.4.61).

Midbrain lesions are associated with generalized delta activity that is continuous, irregular, or intermittent bisynchronous and rhythmic. When coma is due to a pontine lesion the EEG may be normal or may show a reactive alpha coma (Figure 5.4.62).

Coma due to anoxic brain injury can be associated with many patterns, including generalized slow activity, generalized attenuation, a variety of periodic patterns, burst suppression, alpha/theta coma pattern, and spindle coma pattern.

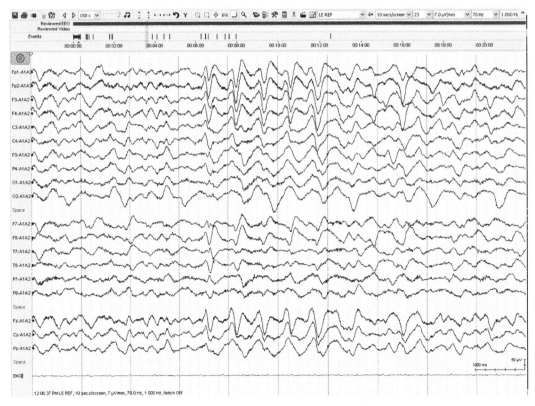

FIGURE 5.4.58 Generalized delta activity with triphasic waves in a 62-year-old man with coma after lung transplant. The coma was secondary to multifactorial metabolic encephalopathy, including renal and hepatic impairment. Ammonia was markedly elevated at 245 (range 18–72). Linked ear reference montage.

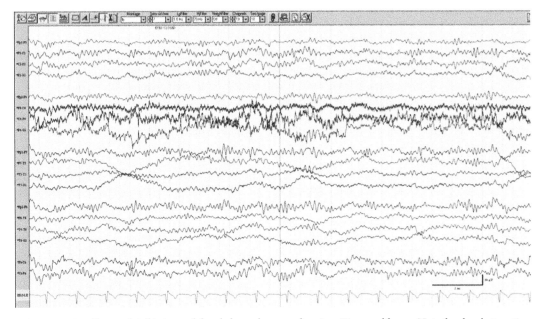

FIGURE 5.4.59 Coma related to tramadol and alprazolam overdose in a 21-year-old man. Note the slow beta activity overriding irregular delta activity. Longitudinal bipolar montage.

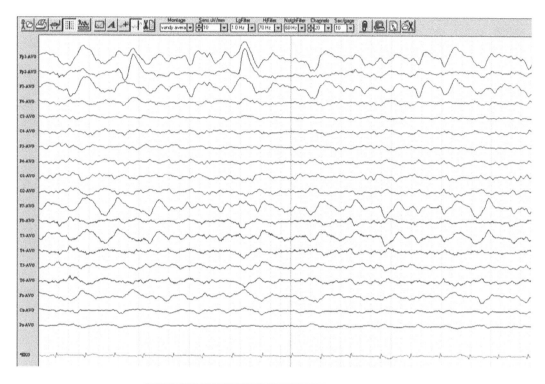

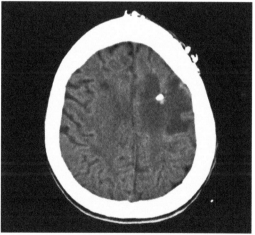

FIGURE 5.4.60 Top: Left frontal focal delta superimposed on generalized low-voltage irregular delta activity in a patient with subarachnoid hemorrhage, hydrocephalus, and edema around left frontal shunt; average reference montage. Bottom: Computed tomography head scan showing hemorrhage and edema.

Burst-Suppression Pattern

The burst-suppression pattern (Figure 5.4.63) consists of epochs of relative flattening of the background (suppression) alternating with epochs of mixed frequency EEG activity (bursts). The bursts usually have a polymorphic appearance, but may contain high-voltage epileptiform activity, especially in some patients who are placed in drug-induced coma because of refractory status epilepticus. The burst-suppression pattern is not specific for any particular etiology. The most common causes are hypoxic-ischemic encephalopathy and medication-induced. With drug-induced coma, the deeper the coma, the shorter the bursts and the longer the periods of suppression. Eventually complete suppression is reached.

When seen in association with hypoxic-ischemic encephalopathy, the burst-suppression

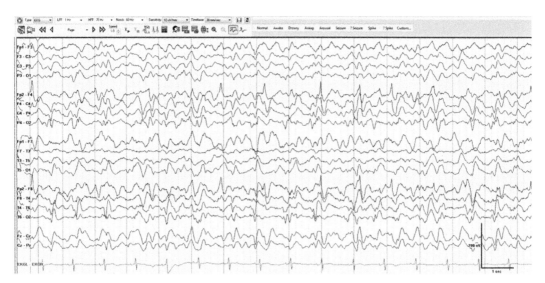

FIGURE 5.4.61 Independent right frontopolar and right occipital periodic discharges superimposed on generalized slow activity in a 62-year-old man with severe traumatic brain injury, right frontal hemorrhage, and multiple contusions. Longitudinal bipolar montage.

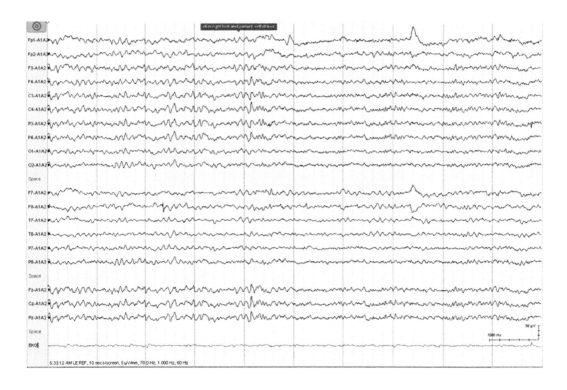

FIGURE 5.4.62 Alpha activity attenuating with stimulation in an 85-year-old woman with central pontine stroke. Above: Reactive alpha in a woman with pontine stroke. Linked ear ref montage. Next page: Diffusion weighted magnetic resonance image showing pontine stroke.

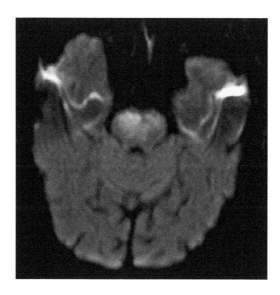

FIGURE 5.4.62 Continued

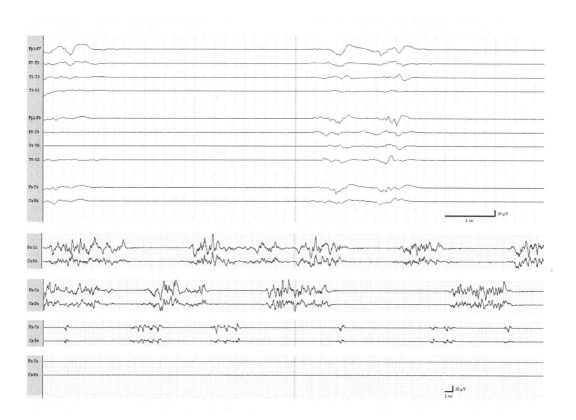

FIGURE 5.4.63 Burst-suppression pattern. The top figure shows 10 sec of electroencephalogram (EEG) with periods of suppression separating two bursts of mixed-frequency activity in the setting of drug-induced coma. The lower segments show compressed EEG demonstrating progressive shortening of the EEG bursts and prolongation of the periods of suppression with deepening coma. *Top panel*: Longitudinal bipolar montage lateral portion and vertex. *Bottom panels*: Longitudinal bipolar vertex channels.

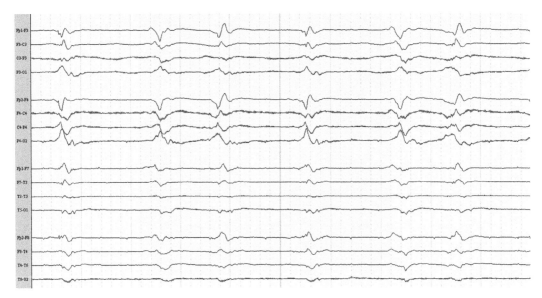

FIGURE 5.4.64 Burst-suppression pattern after anoxic injury in a 76-year-old man. Longitudinal bipolar montage.

pattern is indicative of a poor prognosis for neurological recovery. In fact, any periodic pattern is a poor prognostic indicator in this clinical setting (Figure 5.4.64).

Alpha Coma

The EEG is dominated by alpha activity, which is usually nonreactive in a patient in coma, most commonly due to anoxia. Alpha coma (Figure 5.4.65) prognosis depends on etiology of the coma. Prognosis is poor when due to anoxic brain injury. In this setting the alpha activity is most often generalized or frontally dominant and nonreactive to stimulation.

Spindle Coma

Spindle coma (Figure 5.4.66) may resemble normal sleep, except that the patient is in coma and unresponsive to stimulation. The prognosis depends on the etiology. It is favorable when the etiology is toxic-metabolic, if the derangement can be reversed; less favorable if the etiology is hypoxic-ischemic encephalopathy; and most unfavorable if the etiology is brainstem stroke.

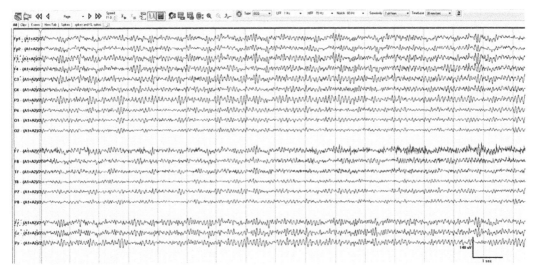

FIGURE 5.4.65 Alpha coma after hypoxic brain injury with asystole in a 42-year-old man. Exam revealed no brainstem reflexes, and the patient died the next day. Linked ear reference montage.

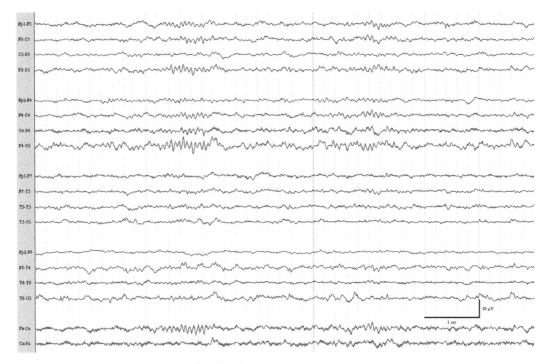

FIGURE 5.4.66 Spindle coma. Longitudinal bipolar montage.

Nonconvulsive Status Epilepticus Presenting as Coma

One of the most important applications of EEG is diagnosis of nonconvulsive status epilepticus (NCSE) in the setting of coma or altered mental status. Since there may be limited clinical signs to make the diagnosis, the EEG and intervention during the EEG are crucial. EEG criteria were proposed in an expert consensus.[2]

- Spikes, poly spikes, sharp-waves, sharp-and-slow-wave complexes recurring at greater than 2.5 Hz

Or

- Spikes, poly spikes, sharp-waves, sharp-and-slow-wave complexes recurring at 2.5 Hz or less or rhythmic delta/theta activity (>0.5 Hz) *and* one of the following:
  - EEG and clinical improvement after IV antiseizure medication, or
  - Subtle clinical ictal phenomena during the EEG patterns mentioned above, or
  - Typical spatiotemporal evolution.

"Spatiotemporal evolution" refers to

- incrementing onset with increase in voltage and change in frequency, or

- evolution in pattern, with change in frequency greater than 1 Hz or change in location, or
- decrementing termination, in voltage or frequency.

If EEG improvement occurs without clinical improvement, or if fluctuation occurs without definite evolution, this should be considered *possible NCSE*.

The preceding criteria apply to patients without known epileptic encephalopathy. For patients with known epileptic encephalopathy who may have alarming patterns in the interictal state, the criteria require an increase in prominence or frequency of the features mentioned, as compared to baseline, with observable change in clinical state and improvement of clinical and EEG features with intravenous anti-seizure medications.

Figures 5.4.67 through 5.4.69 show patients with post-anoxic status epilepticus demonstrating some of the spectrum of EEG findings.

Electrocerebral Inactivity

Electrocerebral inactivity (ECI) or *isoelectric EEG* represents absence of electrocerebral activity. The definition of ECI is no cerebral activity greater than 2 μV. This is often called *electrocerebral silence* (ECS). "Isoelectric EEG" is another term that has been widely used but brain death recordings are

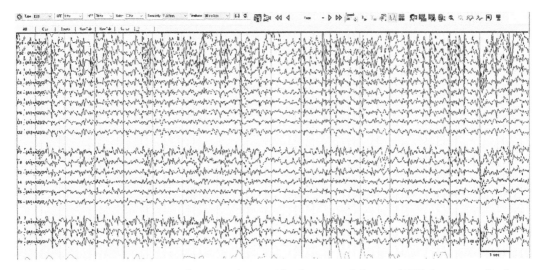

FIGURE 5.4.67 Post-anoxic status epilepticus with coma. The electroencephalogram (EEG) shows generalized frontally dominant spikes at ≥4 Hz. Linked ear reference montage.

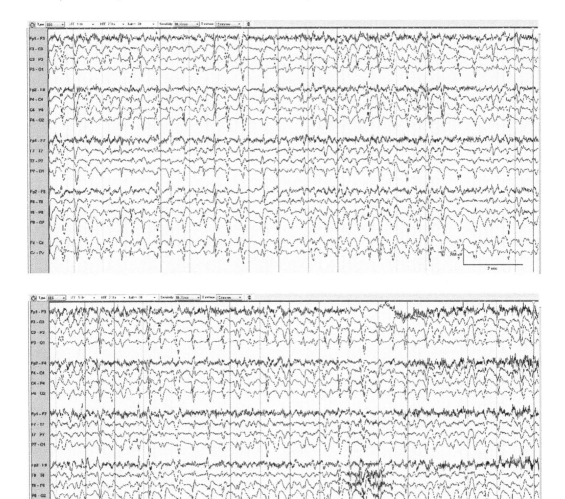

FIGURE 5.4.68 Nonconvulsive status epilepticus (NCSE) with 3/sec fluctuating periodic activity. The patient was noted to have intermittent twitching of the extremities. Three frames, Middle, Bottom, Next page. Longitudinal bipolar montage.

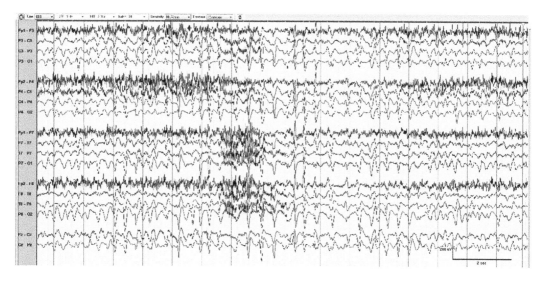

FIGURE 5.4.68 Continued

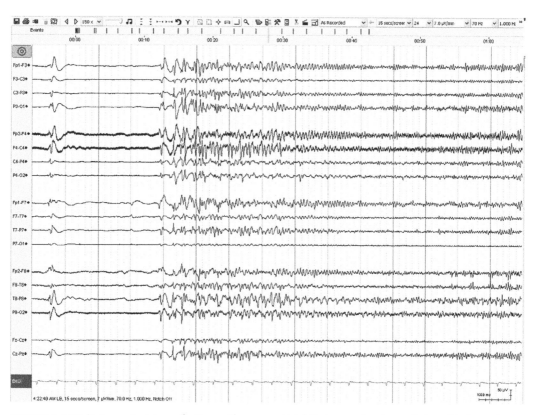

FIGURE 5.4.69 Post-anoxic status epilepticus with recurrent ictal discharges, showing evolution with decreasing frequency. Five frames. Longitudinal bipolar montage.

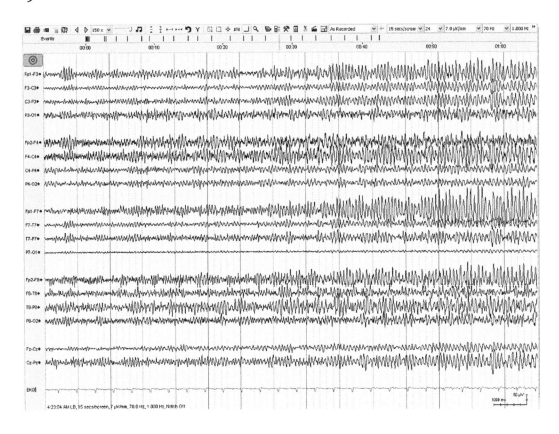

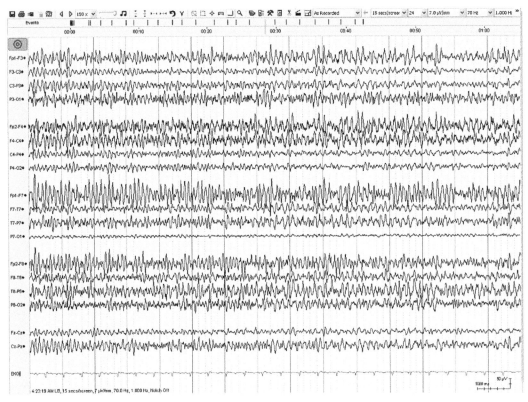

FIGURE 5.4.69 Continued

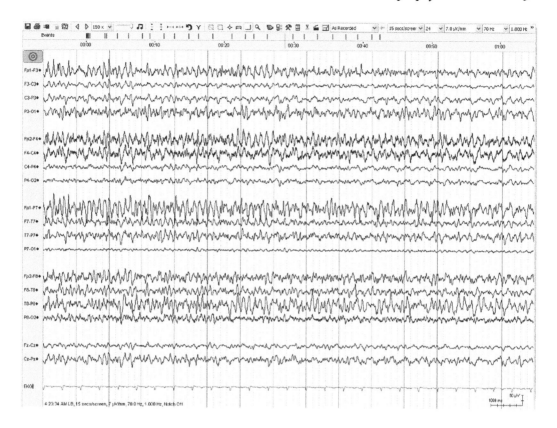

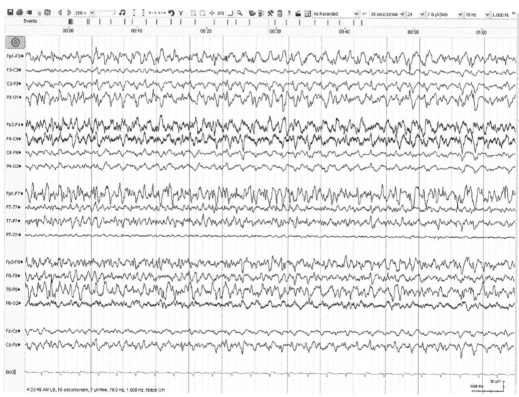

FIGURE 5.4.69 Continued

never isoelectric (having no electrical charge or potential difference), and if they appear that way then there is something wrong with the recording system.

The technical requirements of an ECI EEG are

- Minimum of 8 scalp electrodes; electrodes greater than 10 cm apart;
- Electrode impedance between 100–10,000 ohm;
- High-frequency filter 30 or greater; low -frequency filter 1 or less;
- Hypothermia, drug intoxication, shock must be excluded;
- Record should be more than 30 min long at a sensitivity of 2μV/mm;
- Physiological monitoring must include electrocardiogram (EKG). Other physiological monitoring, such as respiration and EMG, is very helpful.

The background will look totally flat at a sensitivity of 7 μV/mm, except for artifact. However, at a sensitivity of 2 μV/mm, the recording is never perfectly flat. The residual activity of more than 2 μV in the EEG should be proved to be of artifactual origin. In fact, artifacts are a major problem in interpretation. The artifact most commonly encountered is EKG artifact, which may take on a variable appearance at the scalp. Demonstrating perfect correlation with the EKG channel is usually sufficient to prove the activity is not cerebral. The same is true for artifact due to respiration.

However, a variety of rhythmic activities can be due to machine artifact, movement artifact, or muscle artifact. The EEG technologist may need to disconnect nonessential equipment, reposition the patient, pad respirator tubes with towels, or move electrodes. Occasionally neuromuscular-blocking agents can help demonstrate the artifactual origin of some activity.

ECI not necessarily equivalent to brain death. The criteria for determination of brain death include EEG as a confirmatory test if the other criteria are met (see Figure 5.4.70). An ECI EEG indicates neocortical death and is supportive of the diagnosis of brain death in conjunction with the appropriate exam findings, if performed in

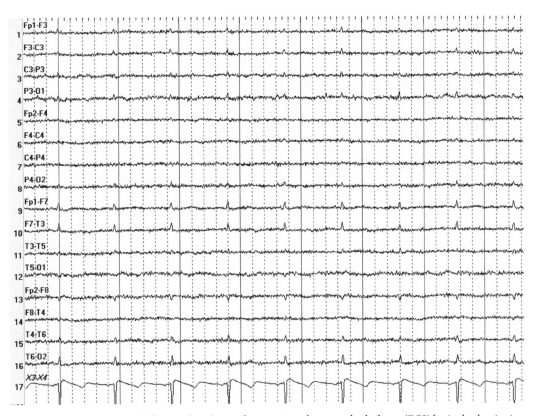

FIGURE 5.4.70 Electroencephalogram (EEG) recording meeting electrocerebral silence (ECS) brain death criteria. Longitudinal bipolar montage.

accordance with accepted technical guidelines in the appropriate clinical situation.

CRITICAL CARE TERMINOLOGY

The American Clinical Neurophysiology Society (ACNS) released guidelines for standardized critical care EEG terminology.[3] The most important guidelines pertain to rhythmic and periodic patterns. In the description of patterns, a main term for distribution should be followed by main term for pattern, then applicable modifier

Table 5.4.2 is a high-level synopsis of this scheme, but the source document has extensive details which should be consulted.

Main Term 1 includes Generalized (G), Lateralized (L), Bilateral Independent (BI), and Multifocal (MF). Generalized refers to a bilateral

synchronous pattern, even if it is restricted to one bilateral region, such as bifrontal. Lateralized includes not only strictly unilateral but also bilateral synchronous but asymmetric patterns. Bilateral Independent designates independent lateralized patterns without synchrony between the hemispheres. Multifocal designates three or more independent lateralized patterns with at least one in each hemisphere.

Main Term 2 includes: Periodic discharges (PD), Rhythmic delta activity (RDA), Spike-and-wave or sharp-and-wave (SW). Periodic discharges are relatively uniform recurrent waveforms separated by relatively constant interval. Discharges are defined as waves of maximum three phases (two baseline crossings) or a wave of any number of phases which lasts 0.5 sec or

---

TABLE 5.4.2 AMERICAN CLINICAL NEUROPHYSIOLOGY SOCIETY (ACNS) GUIDELINES FOR NOMENCLATURE OF RHYTHMIC OR PERIODIC PATTERNS

A

Main term 1: Distribution

Main term	Stands for	Optional qualification	Requirement
G	Generalized	Predominance (frontal, midline, or occipital)	Bilateral, bisynchronous, and symmetric pattern; may have restricted field
L	Lateralized	Unilateral or bilateral asymmetric; hemisphere and lobe	Includes unilateral and bilateral synchronous but asymmetric Can be focal, regional, or hemispheric
BI	Bilateral Independent	Lobe/hemisphere most involved	Independent lateralized patterns in each hemisphere
MF	Multifocal	Lobe/hemisphere most involved	At least three independent patterns, with at least one in each hemisphere

B

Main term 2: Pattern

Main term	Stands for	Requirement
PD	Periodic Discharges	Relatively uniform waveforms recurring with relatively regular intervals (<50% variability for majority of intervals); at least six cycles are required
RDA	Rhythmic Delta activity	Relatively uniform waveforms repeating without an interval at <4Hz, with less than 50% variability in cycle duration for majority of cycles; at least six cycles are required
SW	Rhythmic Spike-and-Wave, Sharp-and-Wave or Polyspike-and-Wave	Recurring complexes with consistent relationship between the spike (or polyspike or sharp wave) component and the slow wave, with no interval between one complex and the next; at least six cycles are required

TABLE 5.4.2 CONTINUED

C

Plus (+) modifiers

Modifier	Stands for	Definition	Where applicable
+F	Superimposed fast activity	Theta or faster, rhythmic or not	Applies to PD or RDA only
+R	Superimposed rhythmic activity	Rhythmic or quasi-rhythmic delta activity	Applies to PD only
+S	Superimposed sharp waves or spikes, or sharply contoured	>1 sharp wave or spike every 10 sec (not periodic and not SW) or RDA that is sharply contoured	Applies to RDA only
+FR	Superimposed fast as well as rhythmic activity		Applies to PD only
+FS	Superimposed fast activity as well as sharp waves/spikes/sharply contoured		Applies to RDA only
No+	None of the above		

less. When there are more than three phases with a duration of more than 0.5 sec, the term "burst" is more appropriate than "discharge." Rhythmic delta activity refers to recurrent waveform without an interwave interval, with a frequency of 4 Hz or less. Spike-and-wave or sharp-and-wave are defined as spike, polyspike, or sharp wave, as classically defined, followed by a slow wave, with no interval between the complexes.

TABLE 5.4.3 SPORADIC EPILEPTIFORM DISCHARGE PREVALENCE

Descriptor	Definition
Abundant	≥1/10 sec
Frequent	1/min–1/10 sec
Occasional	1/h–1/min
Rare	<1/h

The Plus (+) modifiers can make intermediate patterns that are on the interictal–ictal continuum closer to the ictal end of the spectrum. The modifier "+F" is applicable to both PD and RDA; the modifier "+R" applies only to PD; and the modifier "+S" applies only to RDA.

Additional major modifiers characterize prevalence, duration, frequency, sharpness, amplitude, polarity, evolution, and stimulus induction. Minor modifiers describe onset, presence or absence of triphasic morphology, and presence or absence of lag.

The guidelines also address the prevalence of sporadic epileptiform discharges (Table 5.4.3).

The background activity is described by symmetry, presence or absence of PDR, background EEG frequency, a peak gradient, variability, reactivity, voltage, stage II sleep transients, continuity, and presence or absence of a breach effect.

5.5

Abnormal EEG in Epilepsy

Interictal Epileptiform and Ictal Discharges

BASSEL ABOU-KHALIL

EEG ROLE IN THE DIAGNOSIS AND MANAGEMENT OF EPILEPSY

The electroencephalogram (EEG) helps to provide support for the clinical diagnosis of epilepsy but should generally not be the basis for that diagnosis in the absence of clinical information.

The EEG has a role in all of the following:

- Diagnosis of epilepsy;
- Diagnosis of status epilepticus;
- Classification of the epilepsy and epileptic syndrome;
- Localization of the epileptogenic zone;
- Prediction of seizure recurrence after a first unprovoked seizure or after anti-epileptic drug withdrawal;
- Assessment of response to therapy in one specific form of epilepsy: idiopathic generalized epilepsy with absence seizures. In this situation, improvement in seizure control is reflected with decreased epileptiform discharges on EEG;
- Infrequently, to provide evidence for the etiology of epilepsy.

When potentials are found that are suspicious for interictal or ictal activity, there is a sequence of questions to be considered in analysis.

- Is the discharge cerebral or artifactual?
- If the discharge is cerebral, is the discharge normal or abnormal?
- If the discharge is abnormal, is the discharge specific for epilepsy (i.e., epileptiform)?
- If the discharge is epileptiform, is the discharge focal or generalized?
- If the discharge is focal, what is the field of the discharge?

This sequence of steps can seem simple, but when faced especially with a difficult interpretation, a consideration of basic analysis can be helpful. For example, multifocal sharp transients in a premature infant may look epileptiform but be normal for the conceptional age. Or, an apparent generalized seizure in an older adult may be associated with focal sharp waves, suggesting secondary generalization of a focal epilepsy due to a structural lesion.

In the routine 20- to 30-min EEG, it is most likely that only interictal abnormalities will be seen. These are the abnormalities most often sought in routine EEGs for epilepsy. Interictal abnormalities that are specific for epilepsy are termed *epileptiform*. It is generally suggested that the term "epileptiform" be reserved for interictal discharges associated with epilepsy, while ictal EEG findings are termed *seizure patterns* or *ictal patterns*. The first routine EEG may be normal in about 50% of instances. With repeated recordings, approximately 90% of patients will demonstrate epileptiform abnormalities. There will be approximately 10% of patients who will always have a normal EEG between seizures.

Seizure patterns are only infrequently seen in the routine EEG. One notable exception to this are those ictal discharges associated with absence seizures. Absence seizures are almost reliably precipitated with hyperventilation in the untreated child with childhood absence epilepsy.

Epileptiform Discharges

These include spikes and sharp waves and combinations of these with slow waves. By definition, spikes are shorter than 70 msec, whereas sharp waves are 70–200 msec in duration. Other epileptiform discharges include spike-and-wave complexes, slow spike-and-wave complexes, sharp-and-wave complexes, multiple-spike complexes (or polyspike complexes), multiple-spike-and-slow-wave complexes (or polyspike-and-slow-wave complexes), multiple-sharp-wave complexes, and multiple-sharp-and-slow-wave complexes.

Many EEG waves have a sharp appearance, but they are only called spikes or sharp waves if they satisfy a number of features, including a relatively high voltage compared to the background; an asymmetric temporal appearance of the wave, typically with a shorter first half and a longer and higher voltage second half; a biphasic or polyphasic morphology; and an after-going slow wave. Spikes and sharp waves should be different from background activity and not just of higher voltage or sharper. The great majority of sharp waves and spikes are surface-negative. They generally have a field that includes more than one electrode. They should be different from what is expected of physiologic activity in the particular field and state of alertness.

Criteria for epileptiform discharges are as follow:

- Voltage: High
- Morphology: Often asymmetrical
  - Shorter lower voltage ascent or first phase
  - Longer higher voltage descent
  - Polyphasic
  - After-going slow wave
  - Different from background
- Polarity: Great majority are predominantly surface-negative
- Duration: Short (but not too short)
  - Spike: <70 msec
  - Sharp wave: 70–200 msec

- Background: Abnormal
- Must have a physiologic field
- Location and state: Unlike normal physiologic transients

Not all the listed features must be present; however, the more features present, the more confident one can be of their epileptiform nature (see Figure 5.5.1).

Figures 5.5.1–5.5.4 illustrate analysis of sharp transients and give examples of different types of transients.

Truly epileptiform discharges may be seen rarely in the absence of epilepsy. This is most likely in children and is particularly true for occipital and Rolandic spikes, as well as for generalized epileptiform activity. It is important that they should be interpreted in the context of the clinical presentation. However, misinterpretation of normal variants such as wicket spikes is the most common error leading to overdiagnosis of epilepsy.

Ictal Discharges Versus Interictal Epileptiform Discharges

Ictal discharges are usually not merely repetitions of interictal discharges and will generally have an appearance different from repetitive interictal discharges (see Figures 5.5.5 and 5.5.6 for interictal and ictal recordings from the same patient). One exception to this fairly clear differentiation between ictal and interictal discharges is generalized absence seizures. The distinction between interictal and ictal discharges is not always clear-cut. For example, in patients with generalized absence seizures, it has been demonstrated

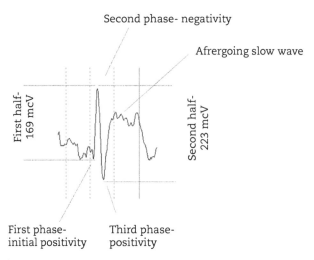

FIGURE 5.5.1 Epileptiform sharp wave demonstrating asymmetrical morphology and an after-going slow wave.

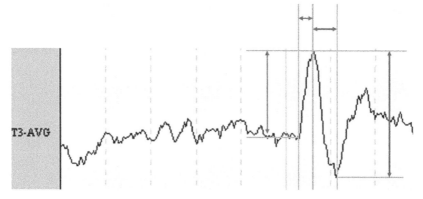

FIGURE 5.5.2 Epileptiform sharp wave demonstrating that the second segment is longer in duration and amplitude than the first segment. Average reference montage.

that a subtle alteration of responsiveness occurs even with a single spike-and-wave discharge if responsiveness is tested with sensitive tools. On the other hand, generalized spike-and-wave discharges that are shorter than 3 sec are generally not appreciated by family members, particularly in the absence of motor accompaniments. Therefore, for practical purposes, one could state that bursts of generalized spike-and-wave discharges are ictal if they last more than 3 sec or if they are associated with clear clinical changes. However, in rare

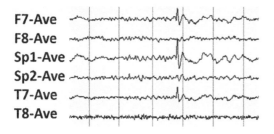

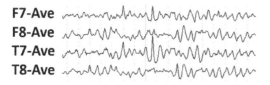

FIGURE 5.5.3 Epileptiform sharp wave (*top*) compared with nonepileptiform sharp transient (*bottom*). Note that the epileptiform transient is asymmetrical, different from the background, with an abnormal background of irregular slow activity on the side of the discharge. The nonepileptiform sharp transient is monophasic and similar to the activity surrounding, except for being of higher voltage and of sharper configuration. Average reference montage.

patients, trains of spike-and-wave discharges lasting longer than 3 sec may not be associated with clinical changes when tested during EEG-video recordings.

Another pattern that can be ictal or "interictal" is that of paroxysmal fast activity noted mainly in patients with Lennox-Gastaut syndrome. In these patients, the paroxysmal fast activity (or generalized polyspike activity) can be associated with generalized tonic seizures or could be totally asymptomatic. Occasionally, such discharges cause arousal as their only clinical manifestation.

Compare the interictal discharge shown in Figure 5.5.5 with the ictal discharge from the same patient in Figure 5.5.6.

FOCAL VERSUS GENERALIZED EEG PATTERNS

Focal Spikes and Sharp Waves

Focal spikes or sharp waves generally suggest focal epilepsy, particularly if there is a single and consistent localization (Figure 5.5.7). For example, consistent right anterior temporal sharp waves suggest right anterior-mesial temporal lobe epilepsy, and consistent left occipital spikes suggest left occipital lobe epilepsy.

Two independent spike- or sharp-wave foci still suggest focal epilepsy in most instances. However, if the discharges are frontal or central, they can be consistent with generalized epilepsy. In generalized epilepsy, "fragments" of generalized epileptiform discharges could be noted, particularly in sleep, in the frontal or central regions (see Figures 5.5.8 and 5.5.9). As a rule, patients with generalized epilepsy will have generalized epileptiform discharges as well as these "fragments."

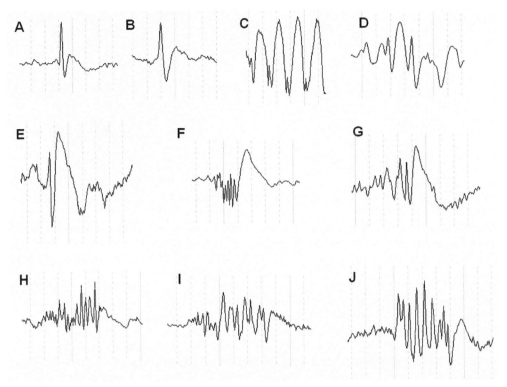

FIGURE 5.5.4 Variety of epileptiform discharges. A: Spike. B: Sharp wave. C: Spike-and-wave complexes. D: Sharp-and-wave complexes. E: Slow-spike-and-wave complex. F: Polyspike-and-wave complex. G: Multiple sharp-and-wave complex. H: Polyspike complex. I,J: Multiple sharp wave complexes. Even though spikes and sharp waves usually have after-going slow waves, the term "spike-and-wave complex" is usually reserved for the situation where the slow wave is very prominent, higher in voltage than the spike.

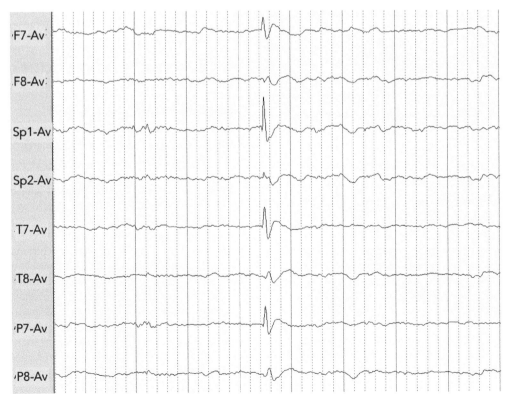

FIGURE 5.5.5 Focal epileptiform discharge a sharp wave.

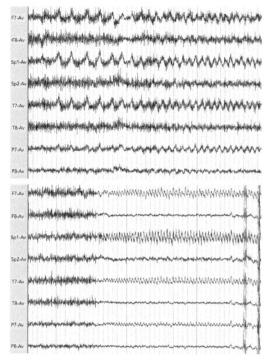

FIGURE 5.5.6 Focal ictal discharge, same patient as in Figure 5.5.5.

When there are two or more independent foci of interictal epileptiform activity, the localization of the epileptogenic focus becomes less certain. Many patients will still have a single ictal focus (i.e., seizures may start in a single location even though interictal epileptiform activity is bilateral or even multifocal; Figure 5.5.10). However, patients with independent foci are more likely to have independent seizure onsets than those with single consistent foci (Figure 5.5.11).

Focal interictal epileptiform discharges may be recorded from regions not involved in the generation of seizures. It is not unusual for temporal sharp waves to be recorded in patients with frontal or parietal epileptogenic zones. While the epileptogenic zone usually generates interictal epileptiform discharges, these may not be visible on scalp EEG if the epileptogenic zone is in a deep location or if the orientation of the dipole is unfavorable. This can lead to a scenario where epileptiform activity recorded on the scalp is unrelated to the epileptogenic zone.

Interictal epileptiform discharges are usually nonspecific with respect to etiology. One exception is focal cortical dysplasia, which can be associated with a pattern of rhythmic epileptiform

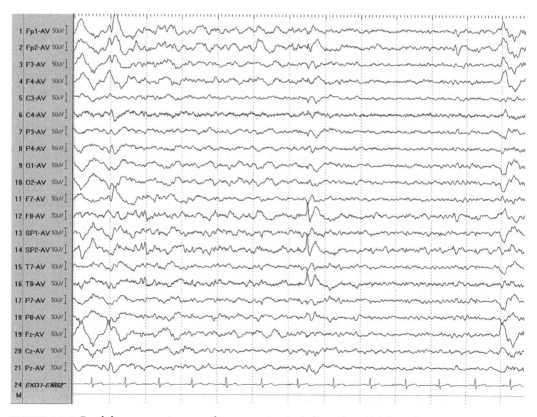

FIGURE 5.5.7 Focal sharp waves. Average reference montage including sphenoidal electrodes.

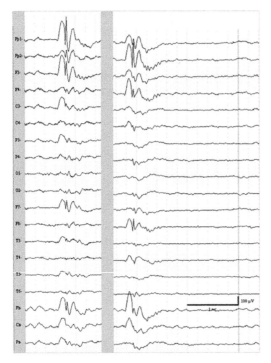

FIGURE 5.5.8 Fragments of generalized discharges. Average reference montage.

discharges (REDs) (Figure 5.5.12). REDs appear to be specific for cortical dysplasia but are not seen in all patients with this pathology. REDs usually coexist with more intermittent interictal epileptiform involving other regions.

Generalized Spike-and-Wave Discharges

Generalized spike-and-wave discharges suggest generalized epilepsy. If they are noted in rhythmic, regular, synchronous, and symmetrical trains, then they are strongly suggestive of the presence of generalized typical absence seizures. Typical absence seizures generally correspond to normal intelligence and normal neurological status. As mentioned earlier, duration of 3 sec or more is usually needed for seizures to be noticed by observers. Occasionally, however, the presence of motor manifestations in these seizures can make shorter discharges associated with clinically detectable seizures. In sleep, generalized spike-and-wave discharges tend to become irregular and longer in duration. In addition, with sleep, there is frequently a change in the morphology to generalized polyspike-and-wave discharges. Therefore, the morphology of these discharges in

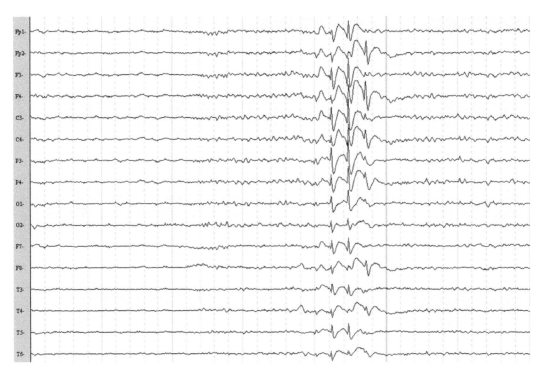

FIGURE 5.5.9 Shifting asymmetries in generalized epilepsy. Average reference montage.

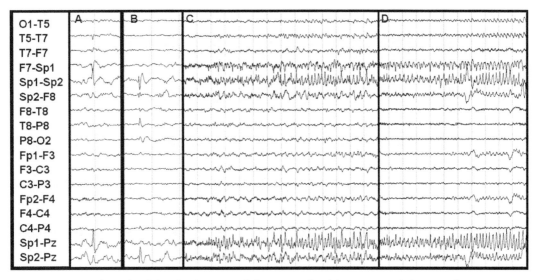

FIGURE 5.5.10 Independent left and right temporal sharp waves (A,B), but consistent left temporal seizure onsets (C,D) in a 46-year-old man with left mesial temporal lobe epilepsy and left hippocampal sclerosis.

sleep cannot predict their morphology in waking (see Figures 5.5.13 and 5.5.14).

Slow Spike-and-Wave Discharges

A frequency of generalized spike-and-wave discharges lower than 2.5 Hz results in the term "slow spike-and-wave" or "atypical spike-and-wave" (Figure 5.5.15). This should be based on the frequency of discharges in waking and not in sleep. Slow spike-and-wave discharges are suggestive of symptomatic generalized epilepsy, such as Lennox-Gastaut syndrome. They are correlated with

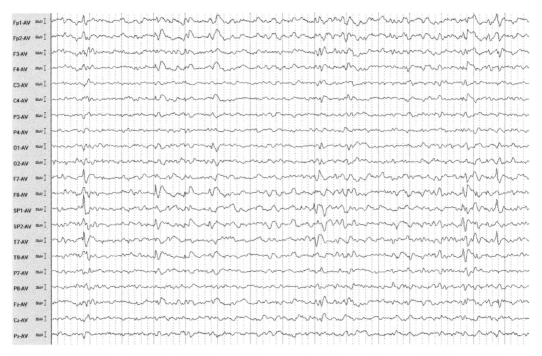

FIGURE 5.5.11 Independent left and right temporal sharp waves in a 34-year-old woman with bitemporal independent seizure onsets. Average reference montage with sphenoidal leads.

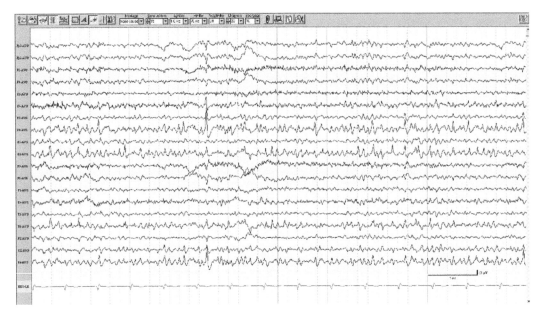

FIGURE 5.5.12 Rhythmic epileptiform discharges involving the right posterior quadrant in a patient with right posterior cortical dysplasia. Average reference montage.

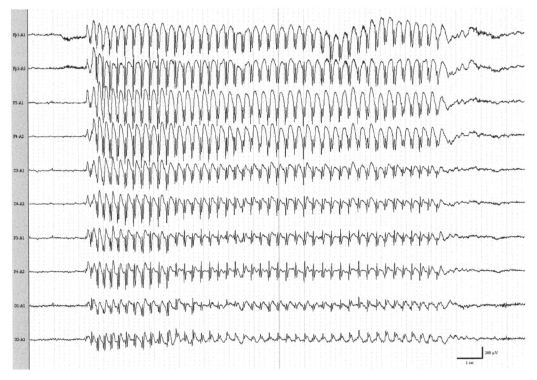

FIGURE 5.5.13 Generalized 3 Hz spike-and-wave. Ipsilateral ear reference montage.

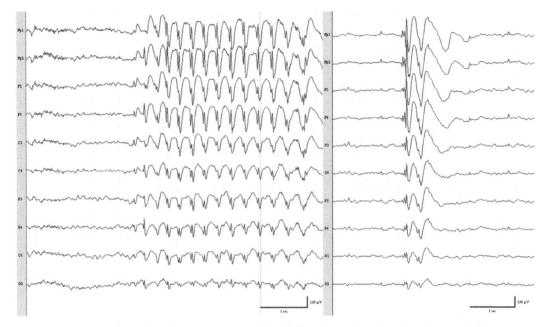

FIGURE 5.5.14 Regular spike-and-wave activity in waking (*left*) and irregular polyspike-and-wave discharges in sleep (*right*) in the same subject. Linked ear reference montage.

atypical absence seizures. Atypical absence seizures are clinically very similar to typical absence seizures except that they may have a lesser alteration of consciousness or responsiveness associated with them and may have a gradual onset and a more gradual termination, as well as more prominent motor features. Slow spike-and-wave discharges are more often asymmetrical and may be associated with focal epileptiform and nonepileptiform abnormalities.

Fast Spike-and-Wave Discharges

Discharges that are faster than 4 Hz are called *fast spike-and-wave discharges* (Figures 5.5.16 and 5.5.17). These typically range from 4 to 7 Hz in frequency. They are seen in association with

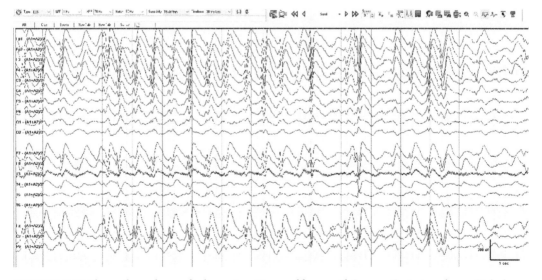

FIGURE 5.5.15 Slow spike-and-wave discharges in a 26-year-old man with Lennox-Gastaut syndrome. Linked ear reference montage.

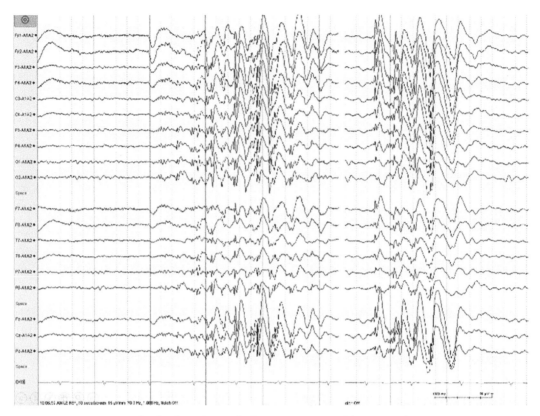

FIGURE 5.5.16 Fast generalized spike-and-wave discharges in a 19-year-old woman with juvenile myoclonic epilepsy. Note the shifting asymmetries. Linked ear montage.

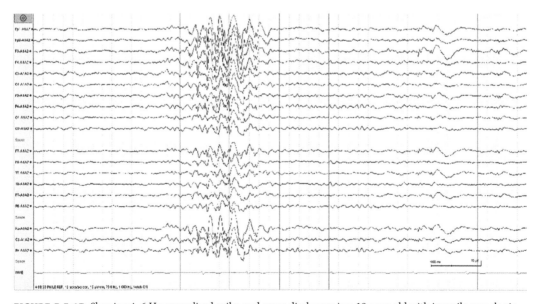

FIGURE 5.5.17 Showing 4–6 Hz generalized spike-and-wave discharges in a 19-year-old with juvenile myoclonic epilepsy. Linked ear reference montage.

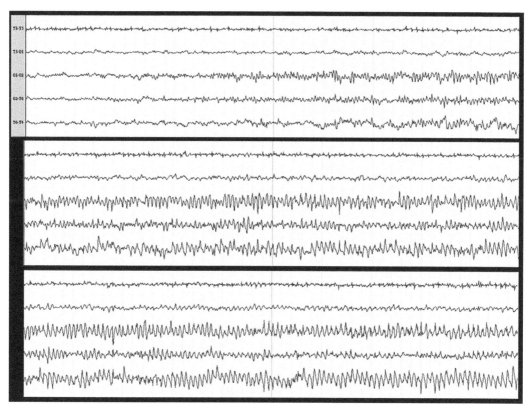

FIGURE 5.5.18 Focal ictal discharge three consecutive 10-sec electroencephalogram (EEG) segments showing onset and initial evolution of a right occipital ictal discharge. The evolution included increase in voltage, decrease in frequency, and widening of field. Posterior circumferential montage.

juvenile myoclonic epilepsy, but also with other idiopathic generalized epilepsies, even in the absence of myoclonic seizures. Fast spike-and-wave discharges tend to be irregular and tend to occur in clusters. These clusters can be associated with myoclonic seizures or could be interictal. In juvenile myoclonic epilepsy, they are most likely to be recorded after arousal, particularly following sleep deprivation.

Focal Interictal Versus Ictal Discharges

Ictal discharges in association with focal epilepsy typically involve rhythmic activity that evolves in frequency, morphology, voltage, and distribution during its course. Although it is most common for discharges to gradually decrease in frequency between their onset and their termination, it is not at all uncommon for frequency to fluctuate, increasing and then decreasing. However, toward the end of the seizure, there is usually a reduction in frequency prior to termination. The end of the seizure is sometimes clear-cut and at other times

not. The post-ictal slow activity can occasionally be difficult to distinguish from the rhythmic ictal activity toward the end of the seizure, which can also be in the delta range.

Focal ictal discharges (Figures 5.5.18 and 5.5.19) may start with voltage attenuation. If this attenuation is focal, it has a localizing value. At other times, the attenuation is diffuse and less useful. The presence of high-frequency beta-range activity at seizure onset suggests neocortical involvement.

Hippocampal seizures will typically start in the theta range and, infrequently, in the alpha range. Seizure onset in the delta range may suggest that the center of seizure activity is at some distance from where the delta activity is recorded. In the case of temporal lobe epilepsy, a theta discharge 5 Hz or higher in the anterior-mesial temporal region should be seen within 30 sec of ictal onset. If not, the temporal localization is less certain.

Focal-onset seizures can evolve to bilateral tonic-clonic activity. The ictal discharge is usually

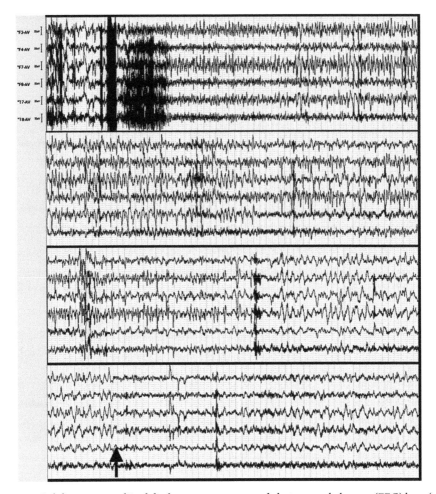

FIGURE 5.5.19 Left frontotemporal ictal discharge on a compressed electroencephalogram (EEG) base (each segment is 60 sec), showing evolution of ictal discharge with increasing amplitude, decreasing frequency, widening field, and an abrupt termination (*arrow*), then postictal slow activity. Each of the frames in this figure represents a continuation of recording from the one above it. Average reference montage.

masked with a confluent muscle artifact in association with the bilateral tonic phase. As the tonic phase evolves to clonic activity, pauses in muscle artifact appear and progressively increase in duration (Figure 5.5.20).

At times, the ictal discharge continues after the muscle artifact stops (Figure 5.5.21).

PATTERNS OF EEG ACTIVITY IN FOCAL EPILEPSY

Temporal Lobe Epilepsy

Mesial Temporal Epilepsy

Irregular delta activity may be the only EEG abnormality in some patients with temporal lobe epilepsy. This is typically recorded from the anterior midtemporal region. Temporal intermittent rhythmic delta activity (TIRDA) is strongly suggestive of temporal potential epileptogenicity. Sharp waves are typically activated in drowsiness and sleep and also increase after the occurrence of seizures, particularly after the occurrence of focal to bilateral tonic-clonic seizures. As a result, in patients whose EEGs are repeatedly normal, one should try to obtain an EEG shortly after a seizure. This can help with the appearance of post-ictal slow activity as well as activation of epileptiform discharges.

In *mesial temporal lobe epilepsy*, sharp waves will typically have a higher voltage anteriorly at F7 or F8. If T1/T2 electrodes are used, they may have equal or higher voltage. If sphenoidal

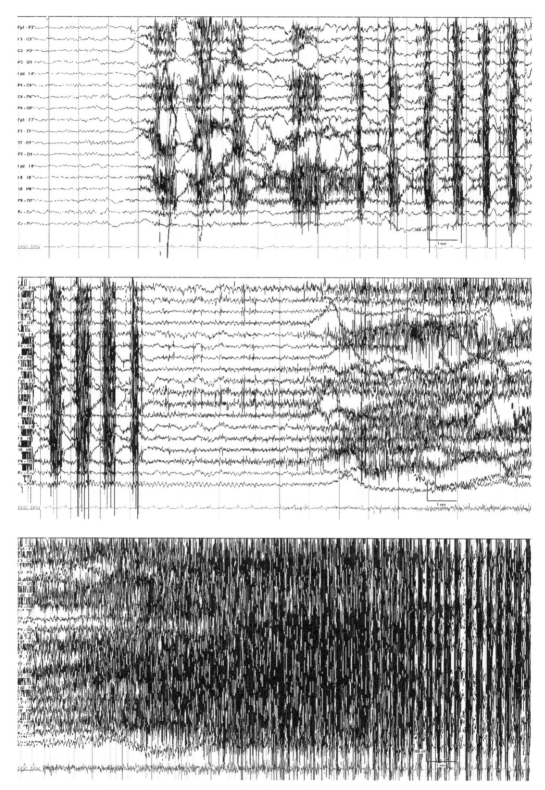

FIGURE 5.5.20 Left hemisphere-onset seizure with evolution to bilateral tonic-clonic seizure. The frames on this and the next page are five frames of a continuous recording. During the tonic phase the electroencephalogram (EEG) is masked with confluent muscle artifact, then clonic activity is associated with characteristic pauses in muscle artifact that progressively increase in duration. Post-ictally, there is generalized suppression of EEG activity. Longitudinal bipolar montage.

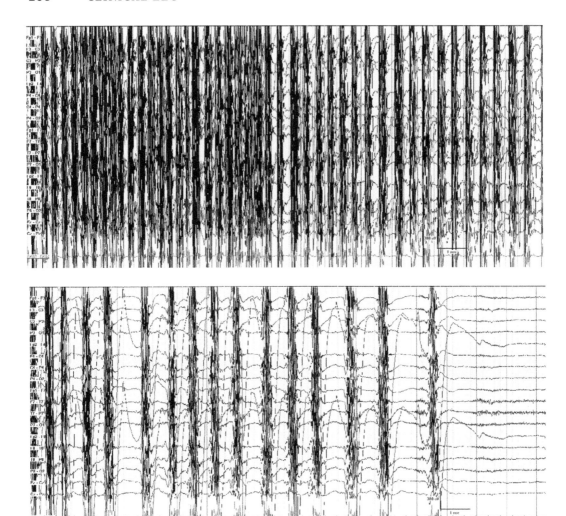

FIGURE 5.5.20 Continued

electrodes are used, they often have the highest voltage (Figure 5.5.22).

There are some patients who have discharges only recorded from the sphenoidal electrodes (Figure 5.5.23).

Ictal discharges associated with hippocampal sclerosis or mesial temporal lesions may have a very focal onset in one sphenoidal electrode (Figure 5.5.24).

Approximately one-third of patients with temporal lobe epilepsy have independent bitemporal epileptiform discharges, particularly in sleep (Figure 5.5.25).

It is very common that, during sleep, the field of epileptiform discharges widens and mirror foci appear. If unilateral focal epileptiform activity is seen in waking and an independent contralateral discharge is noted only in sleep, the waking activity is the most reliable for localization of the epileptogenic zone. In rapid eye movement (REM) sleep, there is also a narrowing of the field and attenuation of mirror foci. Therefore, in patients with bilateral independent epileptiform discharges, those interictal epileptiform discharges recorded in waking or REM sleep are the most reliable for localization. Most patients with bitemporal independent epileptiform discharges will still have unilateral seizure onsets, but they have a higher chance of independent bitemporal seizure onsets than do patients with unilateral epileptiform discharges.

If ictal discharges are unilateral, the side with the highest frequency of epileptiform discharges is typically the side of seizure onset. A small proportion of patients may have generalized spike-and-wave discharges. This is not unexpected, as

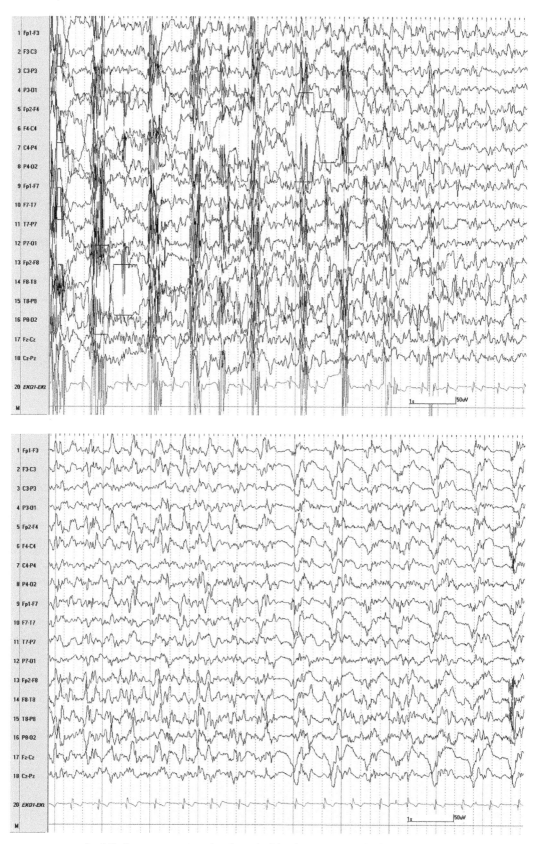

FIGURE 5.5.21 Ictal discharge continuing after the end of the clonic activity. The frames on this and the next page are from the same patient and in order but not continuous. Longitudinal bipolar montage.

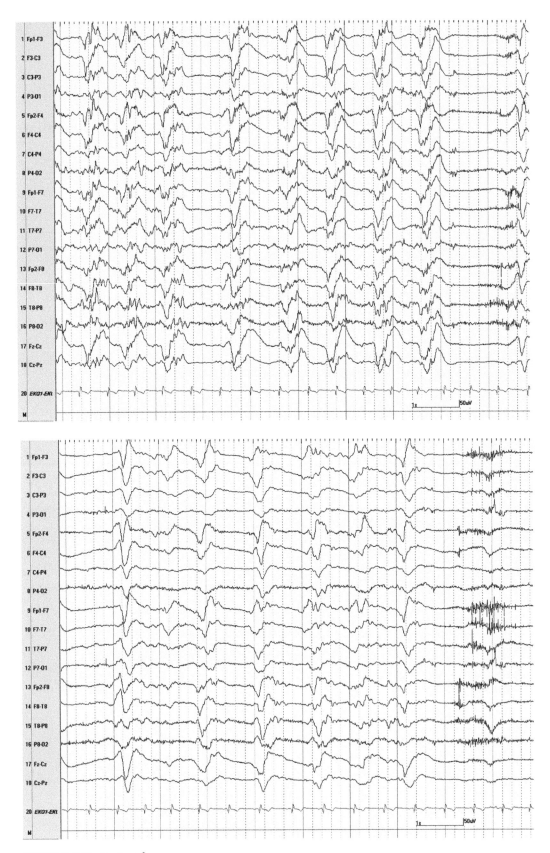

FIGURE 5.5.21 Continued

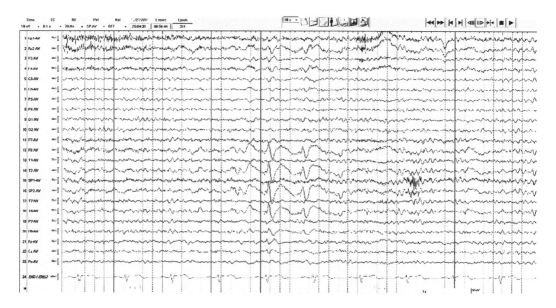

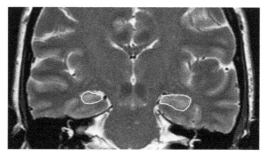

FIGURE 5.5.22 Right temporal sharp waves. (Top) Average reference montage in a patient with right mesial temporal lobe epilepsy and right hippocampal sclerosis. (MRI below EEG from the same patient) The hippocampi are circled to demonstrate the asymmetry. The patient has been seizure-free for more than 2 years after right selective amygdalohippocampectomy.

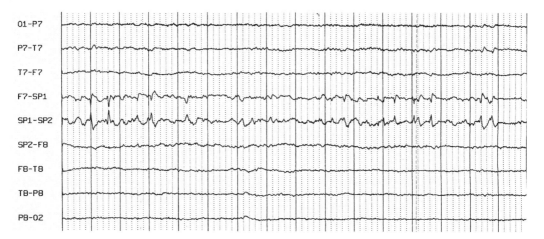

FIGURE 5.5.23 Focal sharp waves and slow activity limited to the left sphenoidal electrode in a patient with mesial temporal lobe epilepsy and hippocampal sclerosis. Sphenoidal bipolar montage.

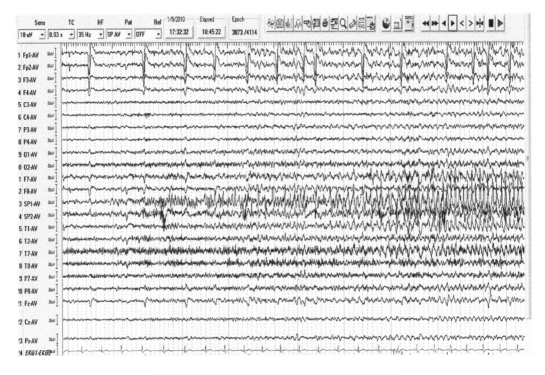

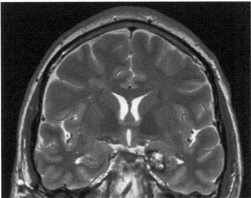

FIGURE 5.5.24 Very focal ictal onset at Sp1 (Top). Average reference montage in a 26-year-old man with a left mesial temporal cavernous malformation (MRI, Bottom).

a high proportion of patients may have a family history of epilepsy as well as a history of febrile convulsions early in life. The generalized spike-and-wave discharges are suspected to be an inherited EEG trait.

Temporal focal aware seizures (Figure 5.5.26) are most often not associated with EEG changes. If they are, the EEG changes tend to be subtle and quite focal.

Focal impaired aware seizures, on the other hand, are almost always associated with a clear-cut ictal discharge. In mesial temporal lobe epilepsy, the ictal discharge is in the theta range at onset or shortly after onset (Figures 5.5.27 and 5.5.28). If sphenoidal electrodes are used, at least 5 Hz rhythmic activity noted in one sphenoidal electrode within 30 sec of seizure onset is strongly supportive of lateralization and localization. In focal to bilateral tonic-clonic seizures of temporal lobe origin, the same EEG changes are seen early on, but the ictal discharge becomes bilateral with extensive diffuse muscle artifact masking the EEG.

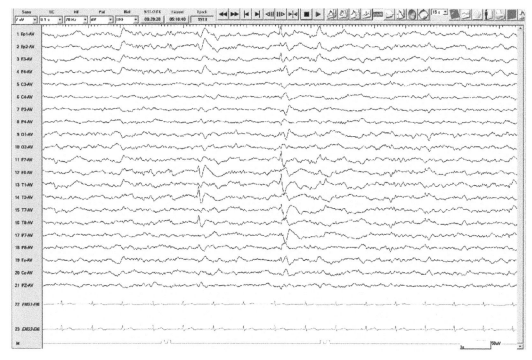

FIGURE 5.5.25 Bitemporal independent sharp waves in sleep. Average reference montage.

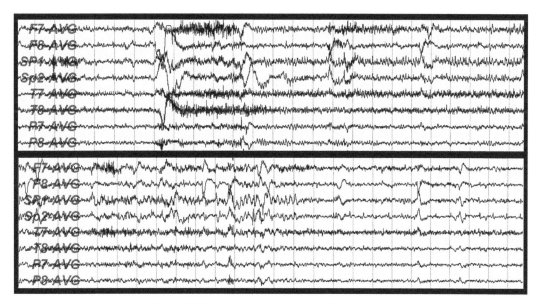

FIGURE 5.5.26 Focal aware seizure of left temporal origin. Average reference montage.

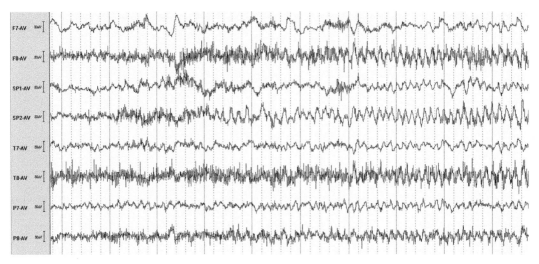

FIGURE 5.5.27 Ictal onset in a patient with right hippocampal sclerosis. The ictal onset is with approximately 6–7 Hz rhythmic activity predominant at Sp2. Average reference montage with sphenoidal leads.

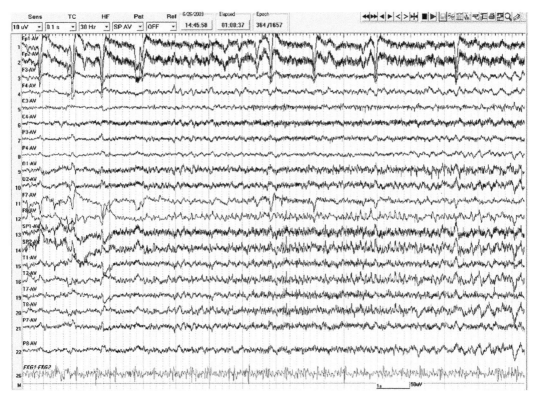

FIGURE 5.5.28 Right temporal ictal discharge in a patient with right mesial temporal lobe epilepsy. The discharge started with 6–7 Hz right temporal rhythmic activity. Average reference montage.

Lateral (Neocortical) Temporal Lobe Epilepsy

It may be difficult to distinguish *neocortical temporal lobe epilepsy* from mesial temporal lobe epilepsy. If sphenoidal electrodes are used, interictal epileptiform activity tends to predominate over a sphenoidal or anterior-inferior temporal electrode in mesial temporal lobe epilepsy, whereas epileptiform activity tends to predominate at T7/T8 or P7/P8 in lateral temporal lobe epilepsy (Figure 5.5.29).

It should be noted, however, that mesial temporal lobe epilepsy and lateral temporal epilepsy groups do not differ in the presence of mesial versus lateral temporal discharges, only in their preponderance. In mesial temporal lobe epilepsy, interictal epileptiform discharges are sharp waves, thought to be propagated from the mesial temporal region. The presence of narrow spikes or spike-and-wave discharges favors a neocortical origin, with locally generated epileptiform activity. TIRDA favors a mesial temporal origin. Lateral temporal ictal onset is more likely to be slower than 5 Hz, often in the delta range. A high-frequency beta-range activity at onset also favors a neocortical localization close to the recording electrode. There is frequent bihemispheric distribution of the ictal discharge at onset, and bilateral spread is more common. A consistent transitional sharp wave (which looks like an interictal epileptiform discharge initiating the seizure) at ictal onset also favors a neocortical origin (see Figure 5.5.30).

Posterior Temporal Lobe Epilepsy

In posterior temporal lobe epilepsy, the interictal epileptiform discharges tend to have predominance in the posterior or midtemporal electrodes and not in the anterior temporal region (see Figures 5.5.31 and 5.5.32). The field may involve the parietal or occipital electrodes.

Ictal discharge onset also tends to predominate in the posterior temporal region and not involve the sphenoidal electrodes (Figure 5.5.33).

Interictal epileptiform activity and ictal onset may be falsely localized in posterior temporal lobe epilepsy. Some patients with posterior temporal lobe epilepsy may have only anterior-inferomesial temporal sharp waves or both posterior temporal and anterior-inferomesial temporal epileptiform activity. In these patients, ictal discharges may also appear to be anterior-mesial temporal. In patients with posterior temporal lesions, such false localization historically resulted in leaving

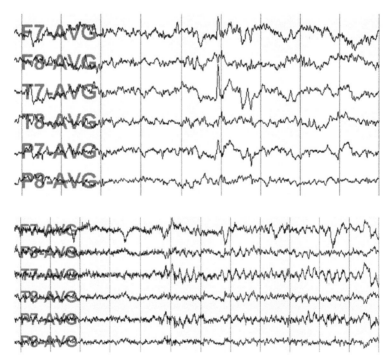

FIGURE 5.5.29 Interictal sharp wave (Top) and ictal discharge (Bottom) in a patient with lateral temporal lobe epilepsy with auditory aura. Both interictal epileptiform activity and ictal discharge predominate at T7. Average reference montage.

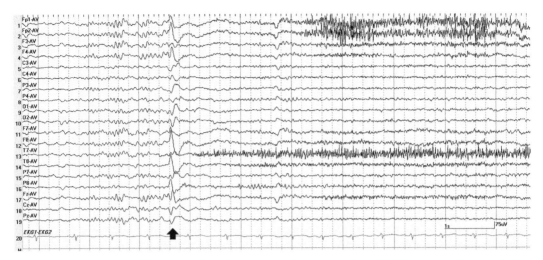

FIGURE 5.5.30 Transitional sharp wave (*arrow*) initiating a seizure in a patient with left neocortical temporal seizure origin. Average reference montage.

the lesion and resecting the anterior temporal and hippocampal regions, with poor surgical results. (Figure 5.5.34).

Frontal Lobe Epilepsy

The frontal lobe is the largest lobe and has surfaces that are invisible or relatively invisible to EEG.

Orbitofrontal onset seizures and mesial frontal onset seizures may have essentially no surface EEG manifestations. In orbitofrontal epilepsy, epileptiform discharges may be recorded from the frontopolar electrodes or from supraorbital electrodes. In mesial frontal lobe epilepsy, the midline electrodes or parasagittal electrodes may record epileptiform discharges. On occasion, these discharges can be confused with vertex waves in sleep (Figures 5.5.35 and 5.5.36). Their occurrence in waking can help resolve this confusion.

Anterior lateral frontal, dorsolateral frontal, and central foci can be associated with focal spike discharges in these regions (Figure 5.5.37).

Secondary bilateral synchrony may occur in frontal lobe epilepsy. This is to be distinguished from the primary bilateral synchrony seen in

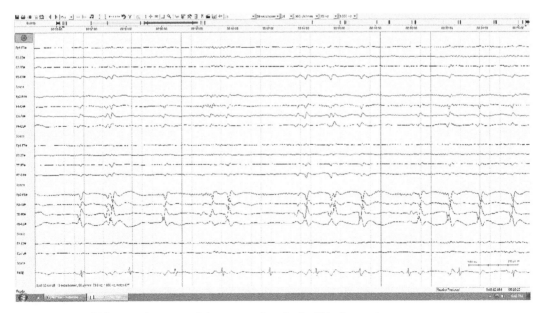

FIGURE 5.5.31 Right posterior temporal sharp waves. Longitudinal bipolar montage.

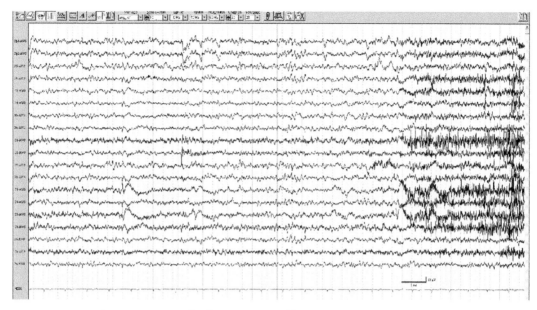

FIGURE 5.5.32 Left posterior temporal spikes in a 46-year-old woman with left posterior temporal seizure onsets. Average reference montage.

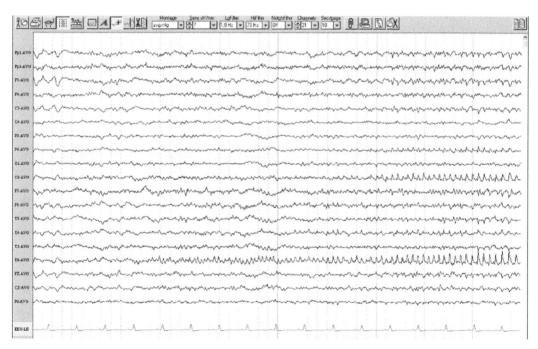

FIGURE 5.5.33 Right posterior temporal ictal onset in a 61-year-old with focal epilepsy and intellectual disability. Average reference montage.

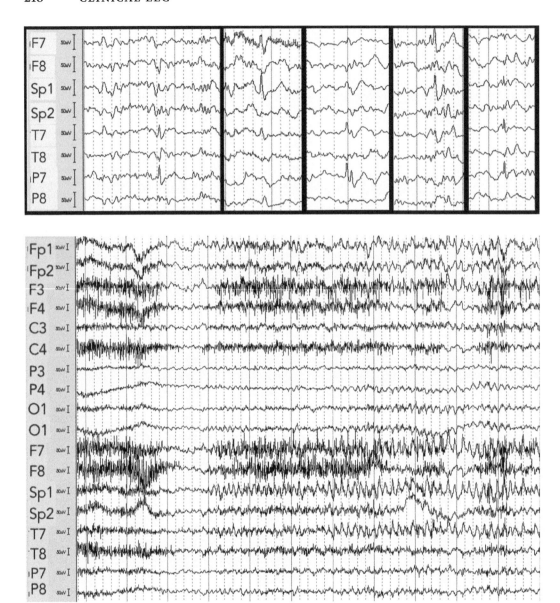

FIGURE 5.5.34 Posterior temporal lobe epilepsy in a patient with a left posterior temporal cavernous malformation. Interictal epileptiform activity (Top) was either anterior-inferomesial temporal (Sp1 and F7) or posterior-mid temporal (P7 and T7). The ictal onset (Bottom) is typical of anterior-inferomesial temporal lobe epilepsy. The patient became seizure-free with lesionectomy, without removal of the anterior and mesial temporal structures. Average reference with sphenoidal leads.

generalized epilepsy. Secondary bilateral synchrony occurs when bilateral synchronous discharges are actually of focal origin. Secondary bilateral synchrony can be suspected when

- Bilateral discharges have a consistent asymmetry,

- There is a consistent lead on one side,
- Some focal discharges are seen only on one side (in addition to bilateral synchronous discharges), and
- A consistent focal slow abnormality or attenuation of normal activity is seen (see Figure 5.5.38).

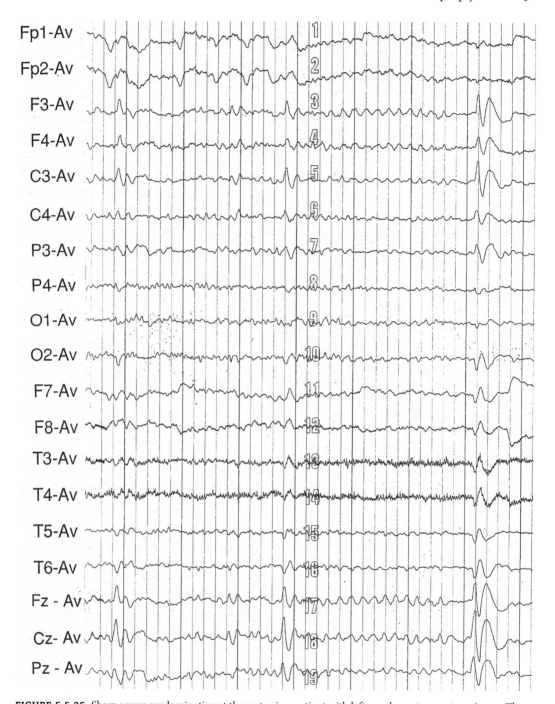

FIGURE 5.5.35 Sharp waves predominating at the vertex in a patient with left supplementary motor seizures. The patient is awake, so these are not vertex waves. Average reference montage.

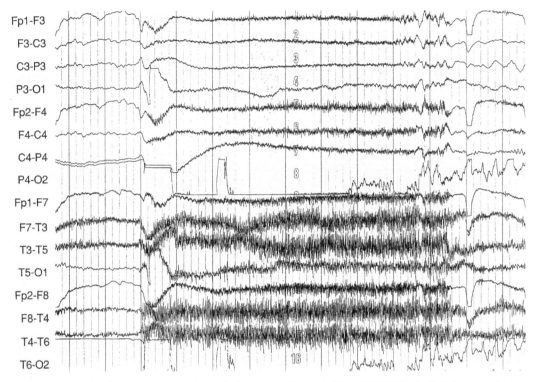

FIGURE 5.5.36 Supplementary motor seizures in the same patient as in Figure 5.5.35. The ictal discharge could be easily missed. Definite electroencephalographic (EEG) changes are noted only toward the end of the discharge at the arrow. Longitudinal bipolar montage.

Frontal lobe seizures have a tendency to become rapidly bilateral/widespread. Seizure spread is at times so fast that a focal onset could be hard to distinguish. The presence of high-frequency focal fast activity at seizure onset suggests good localization of the epileptogenic zone to the region of fast activity (Figure 5.5.39).

Occipital and Parietal Lobe Epilepsies

Occipital lobe epilepsy can be associated with focal spike or spike-and-wave discharges in the occipital region (Figure 5.5.40). It is not uncommon for discharges to be bilateral since volume conduction occurs frequently at the occipital poles (as it does at the frontal poles). Some patients with occipital lobe epilepsy may be photosensitive, with a focal photoparoxysmal response.

Occipital lobe seizures can develop focally or regionally, or can spread to frontal or temporal lobe regions. Seizures starting above the calcarine fissure tend to spread to the frontal lobe, whereas seizures starting below the calcarine fissure tend to spread to the temporal lobe. Occipital lobe seizures that remain regional have a tendency to develop very slowly, starting with beta-range activity that gradually evolves to alpha range and then theta range and then delta range over several minutes. The progression of

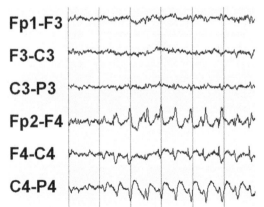

FIGURE 5.5.37 Right frontal lobe spike-and-wave discharges in a patient with a right frontal convexity epileptogenic zone. There is reversal of polarity at F4. Longitudinal bipolar montage.

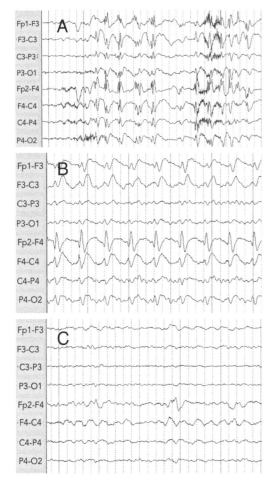

FIGURE 5.5.38 Suspected secondary bilateral synchrony (parts A, B, C). There is a lead on the right (A), a consistent asymmetry with right predominance (A, B), and right frontal slow activity noted intermittently (C). Longitudinal bipolar montage, parasagittal portion.

the ictal discharge can be so slow that the seizure may not be appreciated until the EEG has changed quite drastically.

The EEG is often misleading in parietal lobe epilepsy. Only some patients have focal parietal interictal epileptiform abnormalities and ictal discharges. Many patients have abnormalities in the temporal or frontal regions, resulting in false localization.

Focal Nonconvulsive Status Epilepticus Without Coma

Nonconvulsive status epilepticus without coma can be challenging to diagnose. The pattern that is easiest to recognize may be that of recurrent discrete seizures or merging seizures with waxing and waning amplitude and frequency (Figure 5.5.41).

If waxing and waning ictal activity is not controlled, it may evolve into continuous focal seizure activity, which may be harder to diagnose. The ictal nature of some patterns may be easier to recognize at their termination (Figure 5.5.42).

With continued focal status epilepticus, short periods of attenuation start interrupting the continuous ictal activity (Figure 5.5.43).

PATTERNS OF EEG ACTIVITY IN GENERALIZED EPILEPSY

Idiopathic Generalized Epilepsy

Under the umbrella of idiopathic generalized epilepsy there are several syndromes, including childhood absence epilepsy, juvenile absence epilepsy, juvenile myoclonic epilepsy, and epilepsy with generalized tonic-clonic seizures. These syndromes have in common that the background is expected to be normal. However, children with childhood absence epilepsy may have occipital intermittent rhythmic delta activity (Figure 5.5.44).

Interictal epileptiform discharges are generalized spike-and-wave, usually with bifrontal predominance. When they occur in waking, they usually have a frequency of 2.5 Hz or higher (usually 2.5.4 Hz). In sleep, spike-and-wave discharges can be slower and may have an irregular appearance. In juvenile myoclonic epilepsy, fast, irregular 4–6 Hz spike-and-wave discharge may occur interictally (Figure 5.5.45). They are most likely to be recorded after awakening in the morning. Polyspike-and-wave discharges are also commonly recorded in juvenile myoclonic epilepsy.

Generalized spike-and-wave asymmetries are common, but they typically have shifting predominance. There may also be focal discharges shifting between the left and right frontotemporal region (Figures 5.5.46 and 5.5.47).

Paroxysmal fast activity in sleep is a rare finding in patients with idiopathic generalized epilepsy (Figure 5.5.48). This is more likely to be seen in patients with Lennox-Gastaut syndrome and related structural-metabolic generalized epilepsy.

Photosensitivity with photoparoxysmal response may occur in some patients with idiopathic generalized epilepsy, particularly in women with juvenile myoclonic epilepsy. The

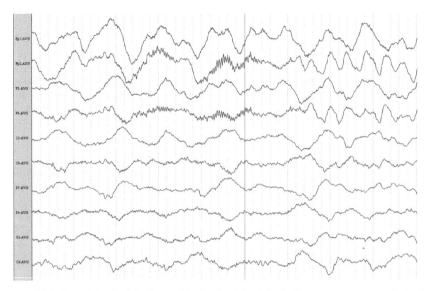

FIGURE 5.5.39 Right frontal fast ictal discharge. The ictal activity is in the beta range at onset. The ictal discharge was associated with left arm twitching. Average reference montage.

photoparoxysmal response usually consists of spikes, spike-and-wave, or polyspike-and-wave activity in association with photic stimulation (Figure 5.5.49). The discharge is usually activated by a range of flash frequencies, most commonly between 10 and 18 flashes/s. In photosensitive patients, the photoparoxysmal response tends to attenuate with age. The photoparoxysmal response is always interpreted as abnormal. It has been suggested that the best correlation with epilepsy occurs if the discharge outlasts the stimulus train; however, this has not been consistently noted.

Eye Closure Sensitivity and Fixation-Off Sensitivity

These two phenomena are more common in idiopathic generalized epilepsy, with both epileptiform discharges appearing within 1–3 sec of eye closure. With *eye closure sensitivity* the duration of the discharge is just a few seconds, whereas with *fixation-off sensitivity* the discharge persists.

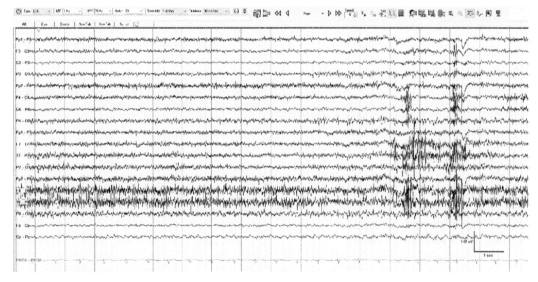

FIGURE 5.5.40 Above and 8 subsequent frames on the next 3 pages. Right occipital lobe seizure discharge with a very gradual evolution in a 32-year-old woman with prior right stroke. Seizures start with flashing lights. Longitudinal bipolar montage.

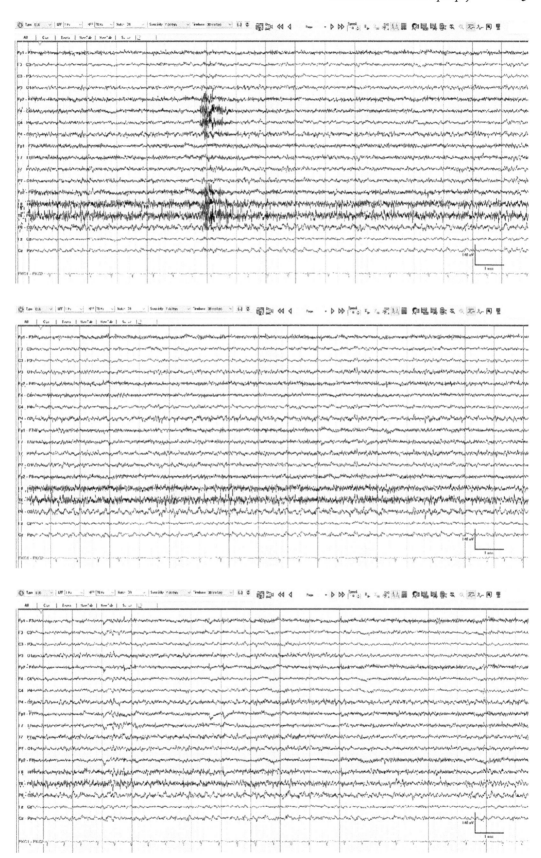

FIGURE 5.5.40 Continued

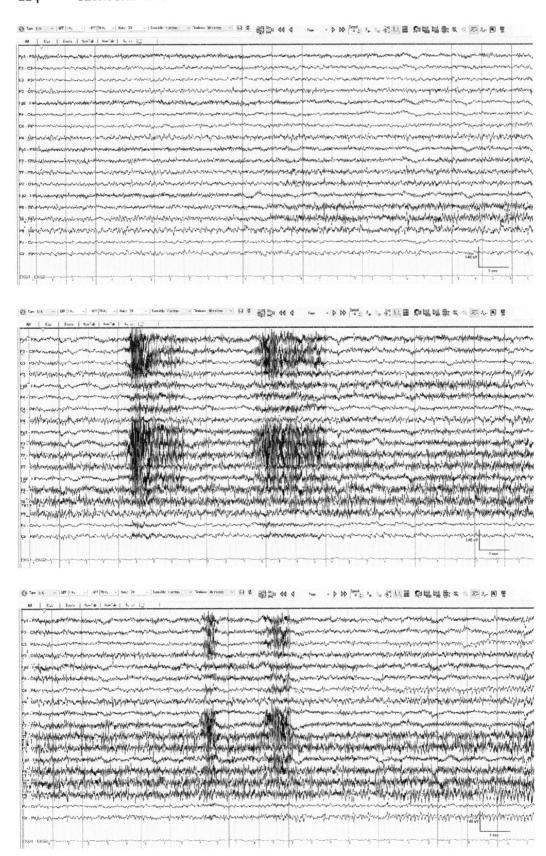

FIGURE 5.5.40 Continued

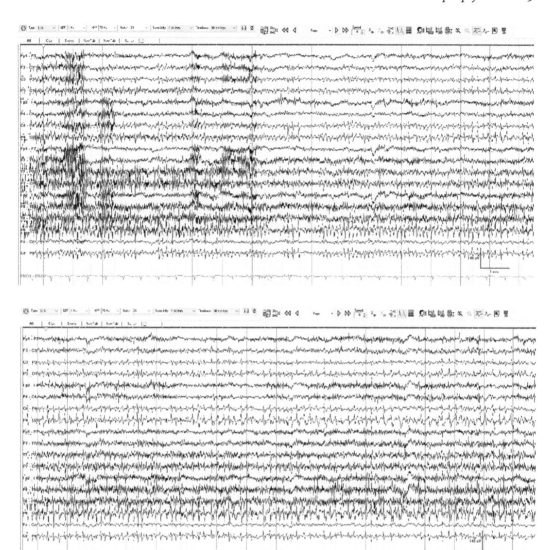

FIGURE 5.5.40 Continued

Figure 5.5.50 shows an example of eye-closure sensitivity.

Figure 5.5.51 shows an example of fixation-off sensitivity.

Fixation-off sensitivity can also be demonstrated with abolition of visual fixation through other means, such as Frenzel glasses.

Ictal Discharges

Ictal discharges in idiopathic generalized epilepsy depend on the seizure type.

Typical absence seizures are usually provoked by hyperventilation in the untreated patient. Hyperventilation should be performed for 5 min rather than the usual 3 min when absence seizures are suspected. A period of hyperventilation can also be repeated for a higher overall yield. Typical absence seizures are associated with generalized synchronous and symmetrical spike-and-wave activity, at a frequency of 2.5.4 Hz, most commonly 3 Hz. The ictal discharge commonly starts at a slightly faster frequency (e.g., 3.5.4 Hz) and ends at a slightly slower frequency (e.g., 2.5.3 Hz). The discharge usually starts abruptly and ends abruptly. The duration is generally shorter than 15 sec. The background returns to normal within a second of termination (Figure 5.5.52).

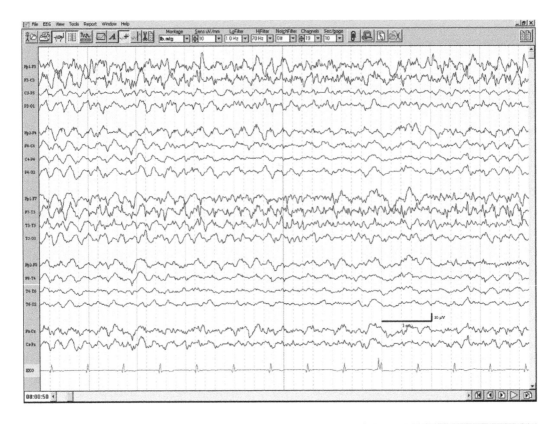

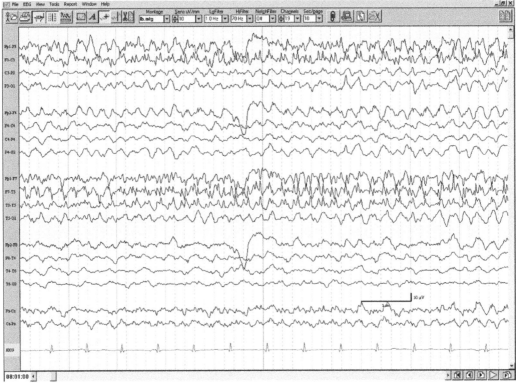

FIGURE 5.5.41 Focal nonconvulsive status epilepticus from the left hemisphere with waxing and waning seizure pattern. The 2 frames on this page and the top frame of the next page are from the same patient and in order but not continuous, and are 10 seconds each. The bottom frame of the next page is from the same patient and shows 8 min of EEG from the left parasagittal chain, with 1 min of compressed EEG per section. The seizure ended in the last section. Longitudinal bipolar montage.

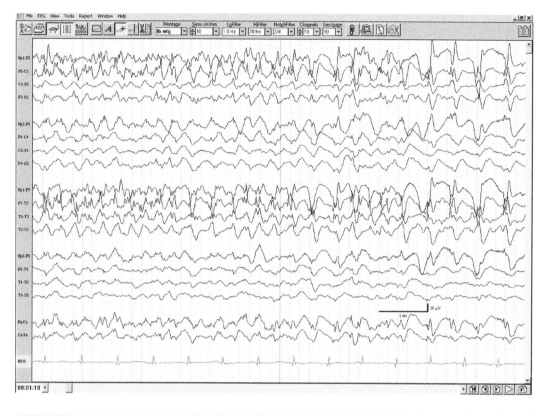

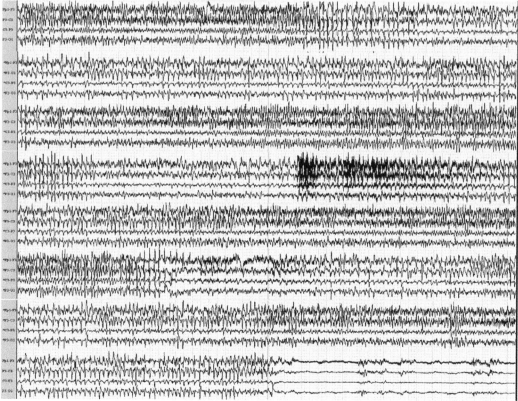

FIGURE 5.5.41 Continued

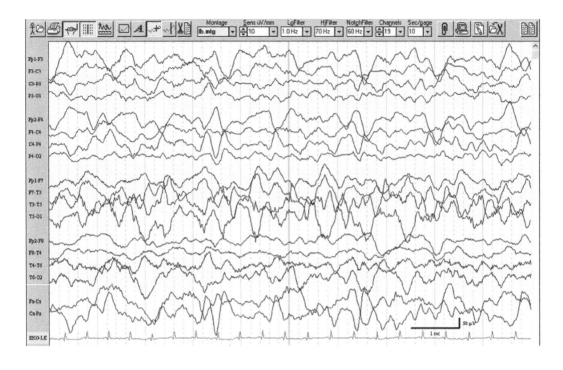

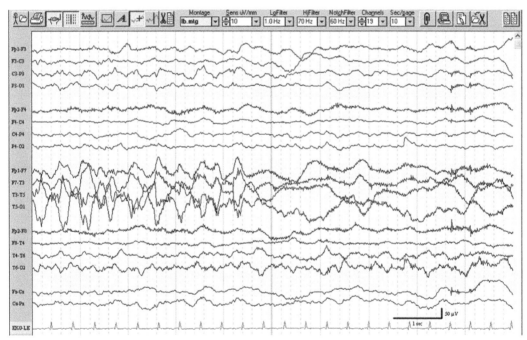

FIGURE 5.5.42 Focal status epilepticus became evident when the ictal discharge terminated. The left temporal slow activity had been present for 8 min from the onset of the recording (Top). The ictal discharge ended after administration of lorazepam (Bottom). The presence of focal high-frequency activity superimposed on slow activity should be a clue to the possible ictal nature of the discharge. Longitudinal bipolar montage.

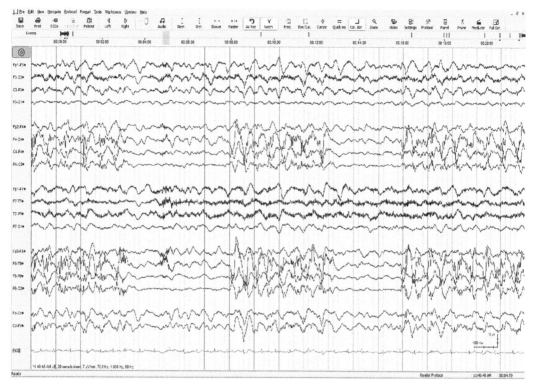

FIGURE 5.5.43 Right hemisphere ictal activity interrupted by short periods of attenuation. Longitudinal bipolar montage.

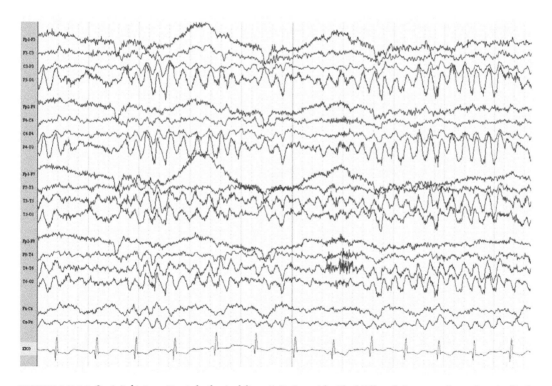

FIGURE 5.5.44 Occipital intermittent rhythmic delta activity in a girl with childhood absence epilepsy. Longitudinal bipolar montage.

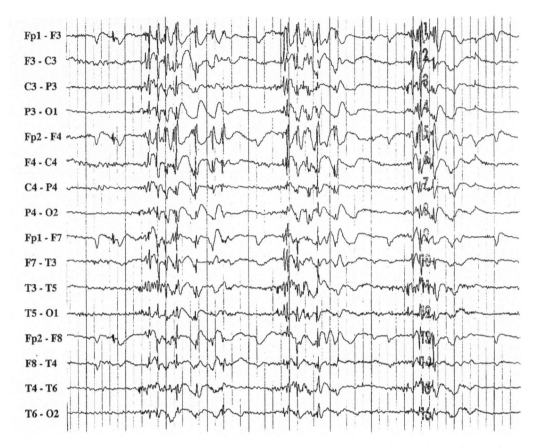

FIGURE 5.5.45 Showing 4–6 Hz irregular spike-and-wave discharges in a patient with juvenile myoclonic epilepsy. Longitudinal bipolar montage.

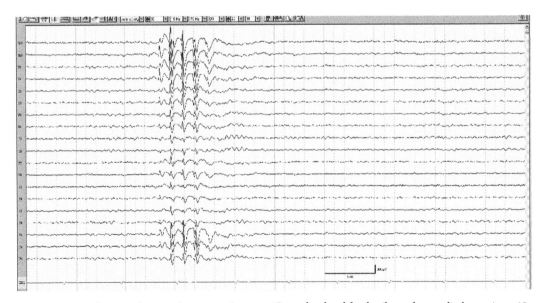

FIGURE 5.5.46 Above and two subsequent frames. Generalized and focal spike-and-wave discharges in an 18-year-old man with idiopathic generalized epilepsy (ear reference montage). Note the shifting asymmetries and shifting focal epileptiform discharges. Average reference montage.

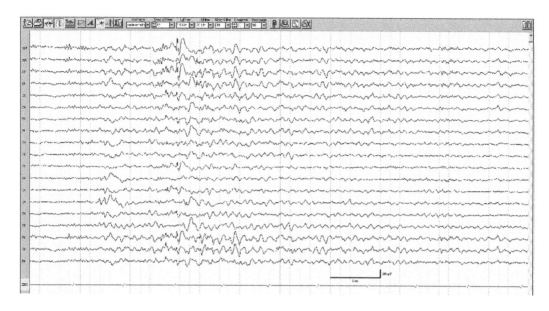

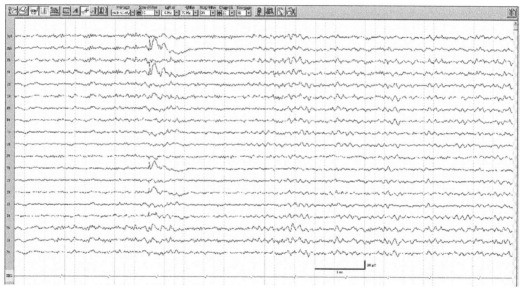

FIGURE 5.5.46 Continued

Generalized spike-and-wave discharges usually have a bifrontocentral predominance, with lowest voltage in the temporal and occipital regions. Rarely, they may appear to have a lead on one side, but with enough seizures recorded the lead will usually shift to the other side with another seizure (Figure 5.5.53).

Figure 5.5.54 shows the slight slowing of the discharge frequency during the seizure.

There may be polyspike-and-wave activity in some patients, particularly with later onset generalized epilepsy (Figure 5.5.55).

The EEG pattern does not clearly correlate with the degree of altered awareness or responsiveness. It had been suggested that a more widespread field of spike-and-wave activity predicts a greater degree of impairment, but this is not necessarily the case, as demonstrated in the example shown in Figure 5.5.56.

Rarely, the spike component is not visible on surface EEG recordings (see Figures 5.5.57 and 5.5.58). It could be that the spike is of low voltage and dwarfed by the slow wave component. It should be noted that some subjects without

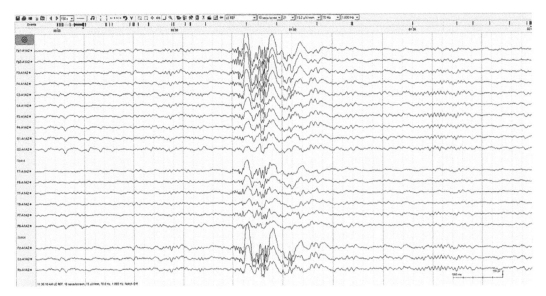

FIGURE 5.5.47 Polyspike-and-wave discharges during sleep in a 27-year-old woman with juvenile myoclonic epilepsy. Linked ear reference montage.

epilepsy may have altered responsiveness during hyperventilation-induced rhythmic delta activity.

The spike-and-wave activity with absence seizures may be intermixed with fast 10–15 Hz rhythms (Figure 5.5.59). The significance of this activity is not known.

Generalized absence status epilepticus may manifest electrographically as very frequent absence seizures (Figure 5.5.60) or more continuous generalized, frontally dominant activity that

tends to be less regular than the brief absence seizure discharges.

Atypical irregular patterns may be seen; the high voltage and frontal predominance may be a tip to consider absence status epilepticus in a patient with altered mental status (Figures 5.5.61 and 5.5.62).

Generalized Myoclonic Seizures

Myoclonic seizures are very brief seizures, and the associated EEG changes are also very brief.

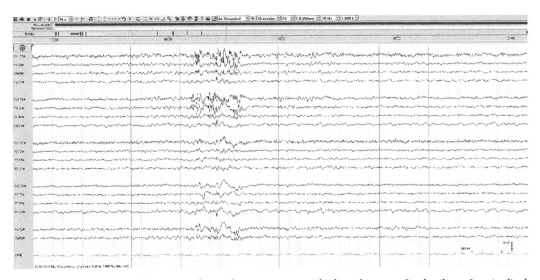

FIGURE 5.5.48 Paroxysmal fast activity during sleep in a patient with idiopathic generalized epilepsy. Longitudinal bipolar montage.

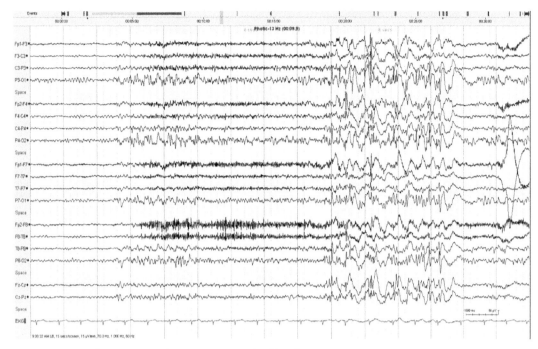

FIGURE 5.5.49 Photoparoxysmal response. Longitudinal bipolar montage.

Typically there will be single or brief serial generalized spike-and-wave discharge or polyspike-and-wave discharge, usually irregular (Figures 5.5.63 and 5.5.64). In juvenile myoclonic epilepsy, myoclonic seizures are accompanied by the 4–6 Hz generalized irregular spike-and-wave discharges seen interictally.

Generalized Tonic-Clonic Seizures

Generalized tonic-clonic seizures occur in many generalized epileptic syndromes. The EEG onset is usually with generalized polyspike-and-wave or spike-and-wave activity. However, this may vary with the specific syndrome. In juvenile myoclonic epilepsy, there may be a cluster of myoclonic

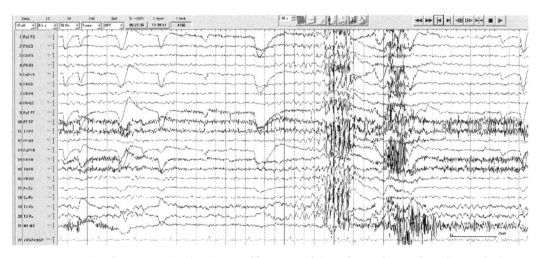

FIGURE 5.5.50 Eye closure sensitivity in a 40-year-old woman with juvenile myoclonic epilepsy. Longitudinal bipolar montage.

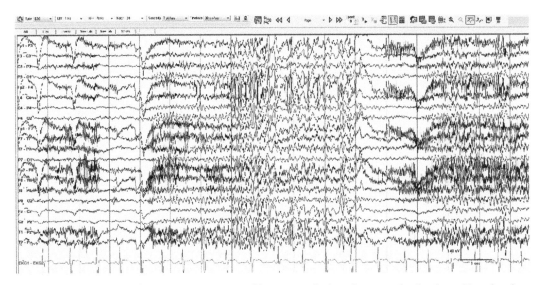

FIGURE 5.5.51 Fixation off sensitivity in a 20-year-old woman with idiopathic generalized epilepsy. Note that the epileptiform activity continues until the eyes open again. Longitudinal bipolar montage.

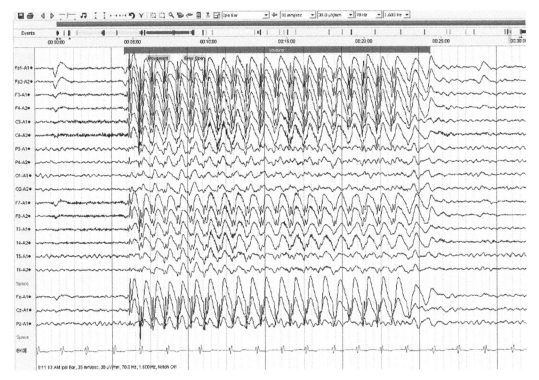

FIGURE 5.5.52 Generalized absence seizure demonstrating typical field, slightly faster frequency at onset than termination, and return to baseline within a second of termination. Ipsilateral ear reference montage.

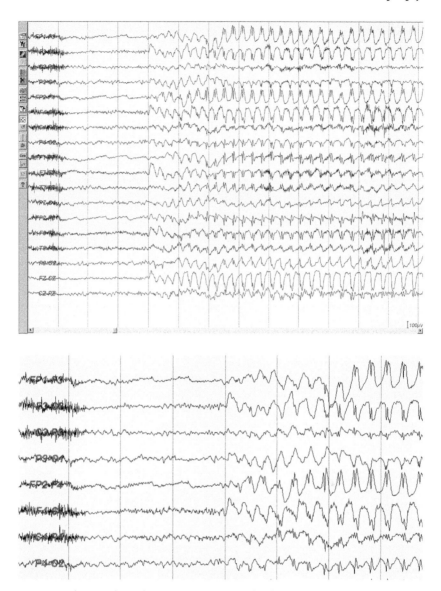

FIGURE 5.5.53 Burst of 3 Hz spike-and-wave activity associated with a generalized absence seizure (Top). There appears to be a slight predominance on the right in the first 2 sec, noted in the zoomed figure (Bottom). Longitudinal bipolar montage.

seizures at onset with the typical fast spike-and-wave or polyspike-and-wave activity, whereas in childhood absence or juvenile absence epilepsy the tonic-clonic seizure may evolve from an absence seizure with the typical 2.5.4 Hz spike-and-wave activity.

For example, Figures 5.5.65 and 5.5.66 show the onsets of a generalized tonic-clonic seizures in patients with juvenile myoclonic epilepsy.

Figure 5.5.67 shows the onset and evolution of a generalized tonic-clonic seizure in a woman with absence epilepsy.

The transition to the tonic phase is with appearance of lower voltage 10–20 Hz activity, at which point the EEG then is usually masked with confluent muscle artifact in association with the tonic phase. As the tonic phase evolves to clonic activity, pauses in muscle artifact

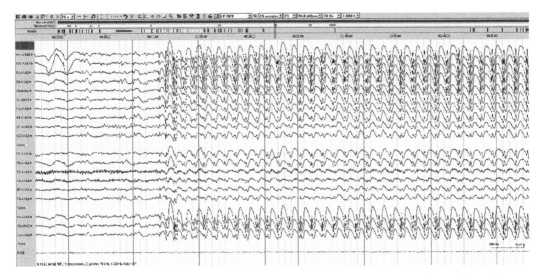

FIGURE 5.5.54 Generalized absence seizure with unresponsiveness in a 16-year-old boy with juvenile myoclonic epilepsy. Note that the generalized spike-and-wave frequency was 3.5 Hz at onset and 3 Hz thereafter. Linked ear reference montage.

appear and progressively increase in duration (see Figure 5.5.67). In paralyzed individuals, the clonic jerks are associated with periodic generalized polyspike-and-wave discharges. The ictal discharge usually ends once the clonic activity stops, after which there is generalized attenuation or suppression for a variable duration. On rare occasions, asymmetries or even focal evolution may occur during the course of the ictal discharge.

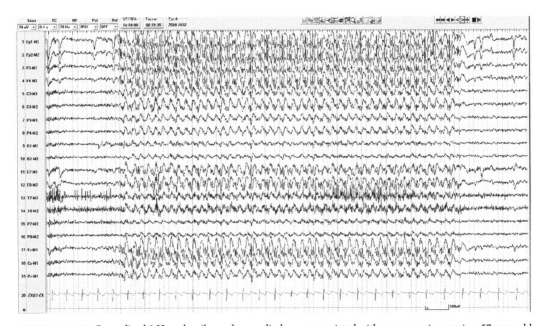

FIGURE 5.5.55 Generalized 3 Hz polyspike-and-wave discharges associated with unresponsiveness in a 57-year-old woman with onset of staring spells and tonic-clonic seizures since age 47. Ipsilateral ear reference montage.

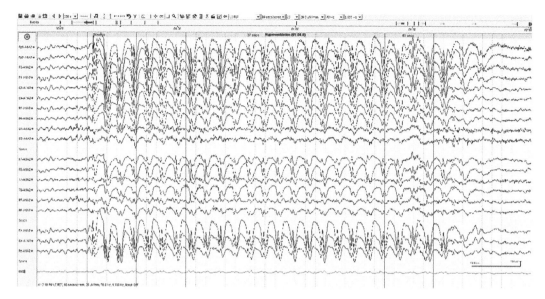

FIGURE 5.5.56 Generalized spike-and-wave burst lasting 8 sec with no associated alteration of responsiveness on testing with commands in a 19-year-old woman with history of absence seizures starting at age 12, but no observed clinical seizures in 5 years. Linked ear reference montage.

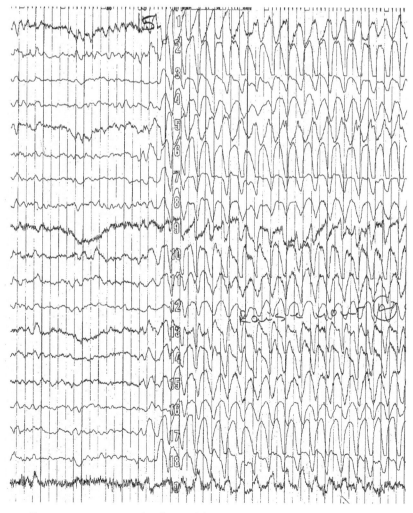

FIGURE 5.5.57 Absence seizure associated with 3 Hz delta activity without visible spike component in a 17-year-old with juvenile myoclonic epilepsy. Longitudinal bipolar montage.

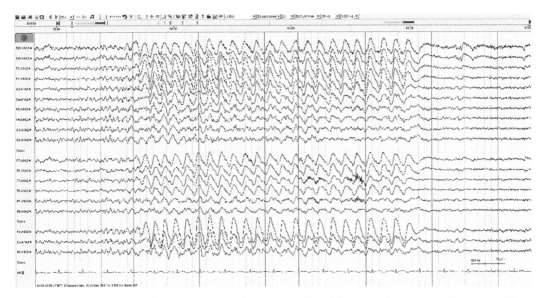

FIGURE 5.5.58 Generalized absence seizure associated with notched delta activity in a 23-year-old woman with juvenile absence epilepsy and pure absence seizures starting at age 18. The notch is the spike component. Linked ear reference montage.

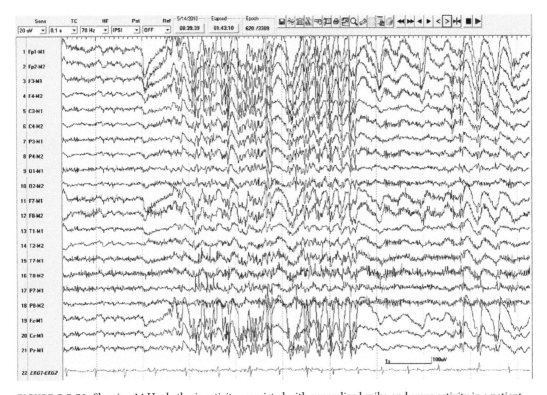

FIGURE 5.5.59 Showing 14 Hz rhythmic activity associated with generalized spike-and-wave activity in a patient with absence seizures. Ipsilateral ear reference montage.

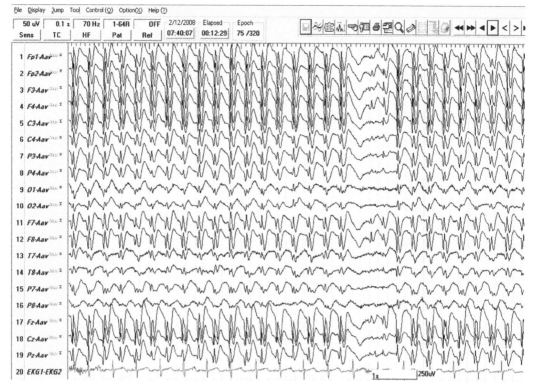

FIGURE 5.5.60 Generalized absence status epilepticus with very frequent, recurrent generalized 2.8 Hz spike-and-wave activity. Linked ear reference montage.

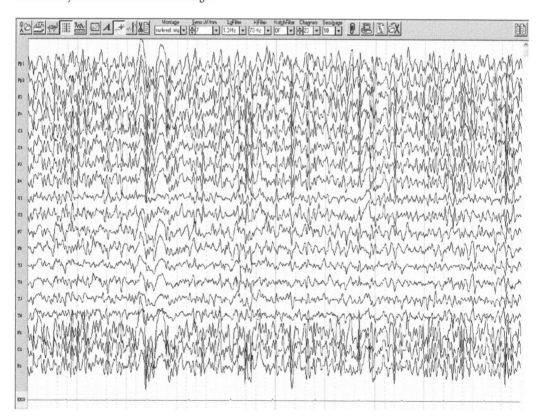

FIGURE 5.5.61 Generalized absence status epilepticus in a 46-year-old man with idiopathic generalized epilepsy who developed mild confusion after starting risperidone. Above: Linked ear reference montage. Note the frontally predominant high-voltage, mixed-frequency sharp activity, including irregular spike-and-wave discharges. Compare with the electroencephalogram (EEG) pattern after the absence status was successfully treated with intravenous lorazepam and valproate. Next page: Ipsilateral ear reference montage.

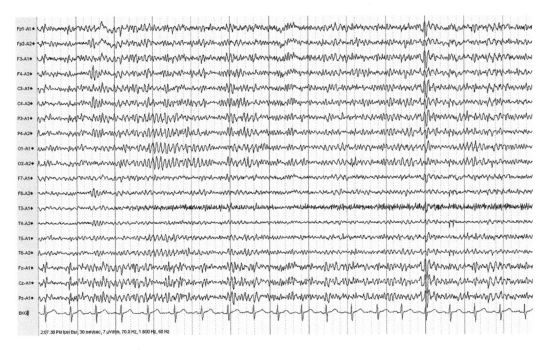

FIGURE 5.5.61 Continued

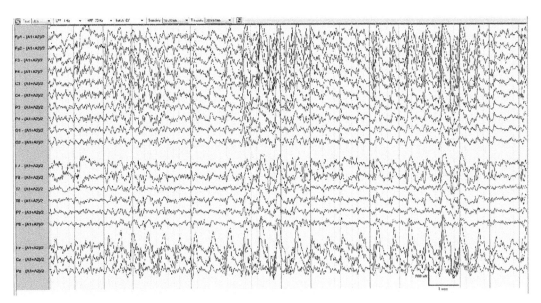

FIGURE 5.5.62 Another example of absence status epilepticus (Above) in a 47-year-old woman with 4 days of confusion. Contrast with the electroencephalogram (EEG) after resolution through appropriate therapy (Next frame). Linked ear reference montage.

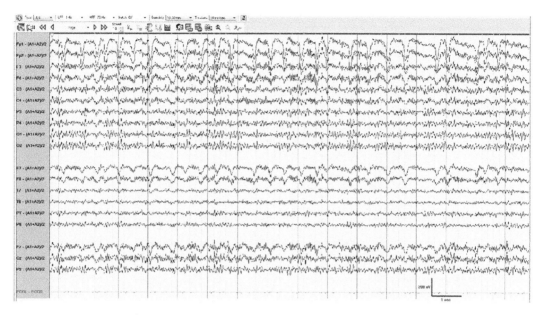

FIGURE 5.5.62 Continued

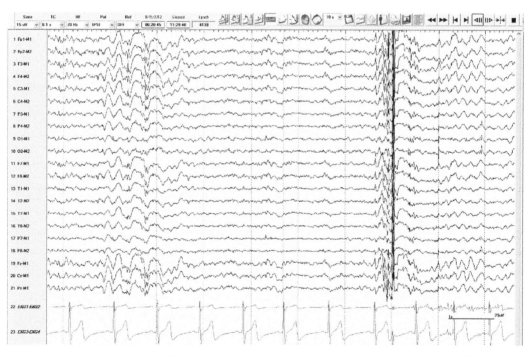

FIGURE 5.5.63 Generalized polyspike-and-wave and spike-and-wave discharges associated with myoclonic seizures in a 22-year-old man with juvenile myoclonic epilepsy. Above: Ipsilateral ear reference montage. Next frame: Longitudinal bipolar montage.

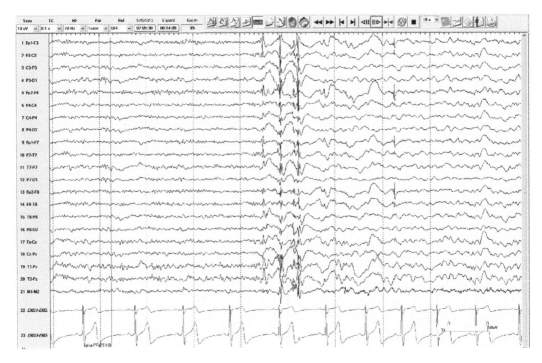

FIGURE 5.5.63 Continued

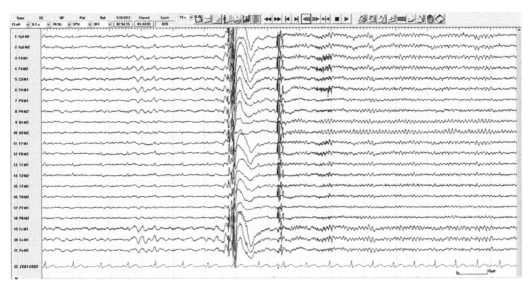

FIGURE 5.5.64 Generalized polyspike-and-wave discharge associated with a myoclonic seizure that caused arousal from sleep in a 25-year-old woman with juvenile myoclonic epilepsy. Ipsilateral ear reference montage.

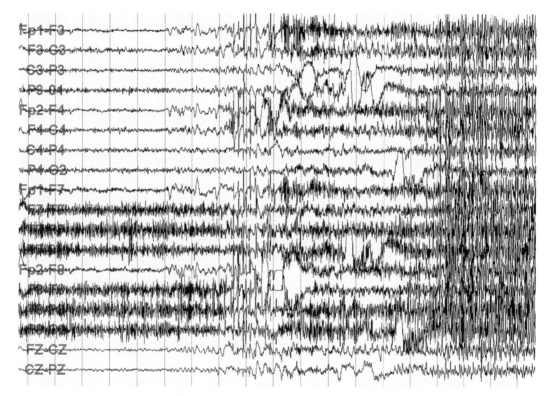

FIGURE 5.5.65 Onset of a generalized tonic-clonic seizure in a patient with juvenile myoclonic epilepsy. Longitudinal bipolar montage.

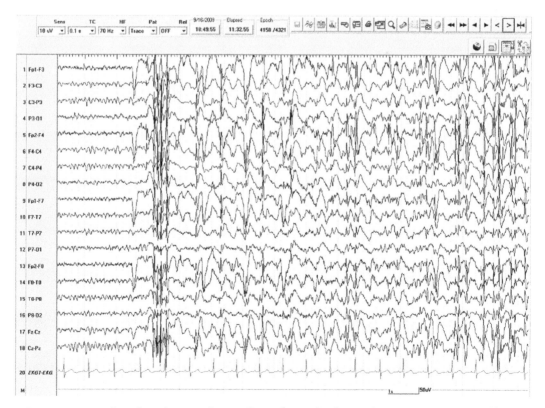

FIGURE 5.5.66 continued on the next frame. Onset of generalized tonic-clonic seizure in a 21-year-old man with juvenile myoclonic epilepsy. Longitudinal bipolar montage.

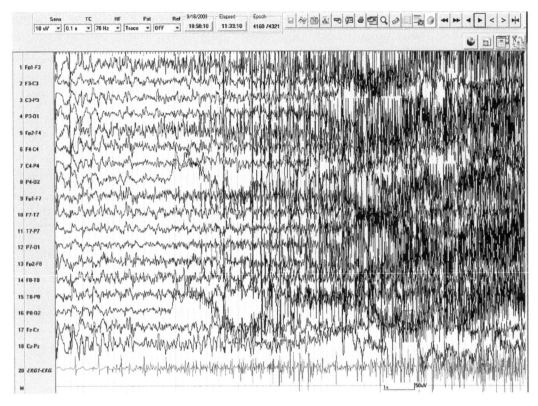

FIGURE 5.5.66 Continued

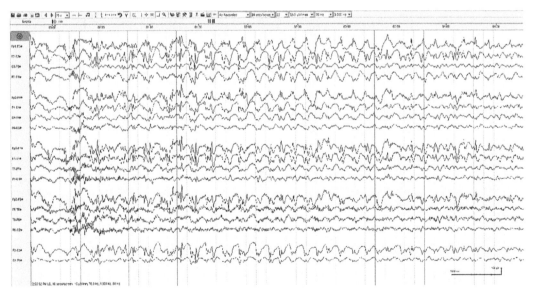

FIGURE 5.5.67 Above and continued on the subsequent 7 frames. Onset of a generalized tonic-clonic seizure in a 27-year-old woman with absence epilepsy. The evolution of the ictal discharge is demonstrated, with postictal suppression. Longitudinal bipolar montage.

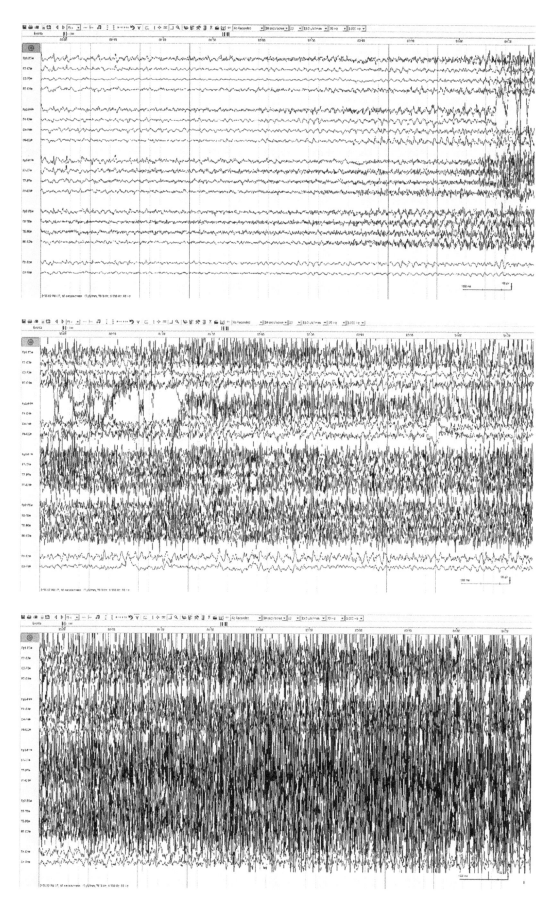

FIGURE 5.5.67 Continued

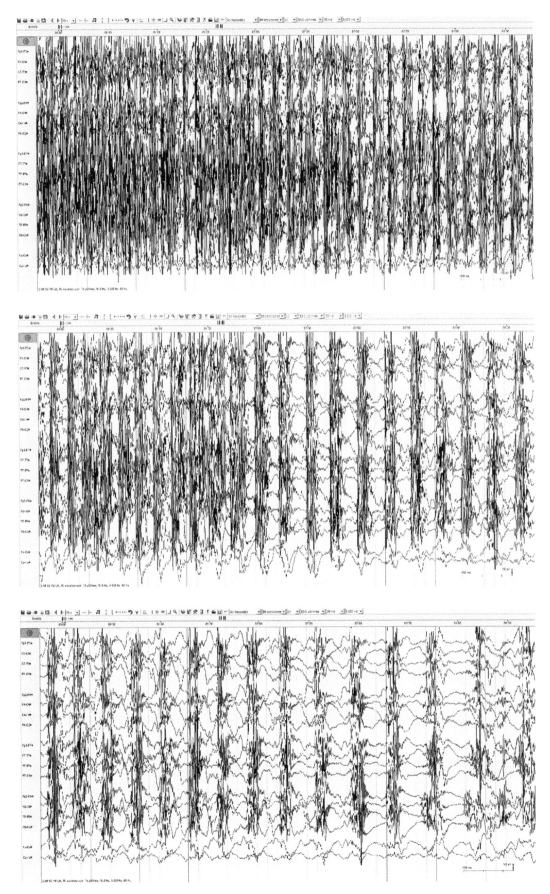

FIGURE 5.5.67 Continued

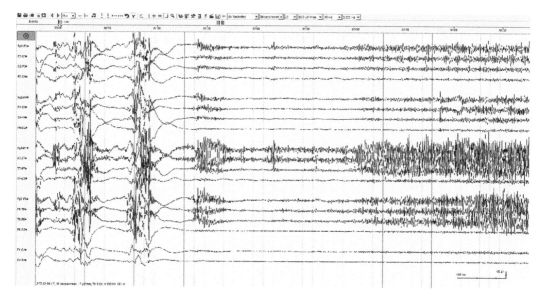

FIGURE 5.5.67 Continued

Lennox-Gastaut Syndrome and Other Structural-Metabolic Generalized Epilepsies

Patients with structural-metabolic generalized epilepsy tend to have an abnormal background, including a slow or absent posterior dominant rhythm and increased slow activity intermingled in the background (Figure 5.5.68).

There may even be focal or multifocal irregular slow activity.

Interictal epileptiform discharges include generalized spike-and-wave or sharp-and- wave discharges that are slower than 2.5 Hz, referred to as "slow spike-and-wave discharges" (Figure 5.5.69).

In sleep, bursts of generalized, high-frequency sharp activity called generalized paroxysmal fast

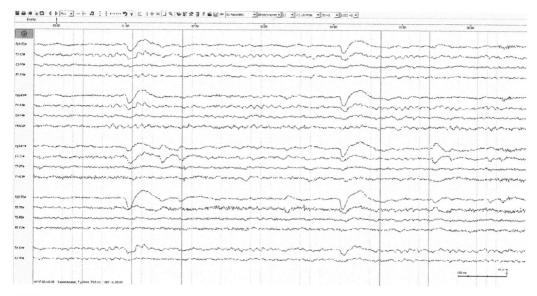

FIGURE 5.5.68 Above and next frame. Slow background in a 37-year-old man with Lennox-Gastaut syndrome. Longitudinal bipolar montage.

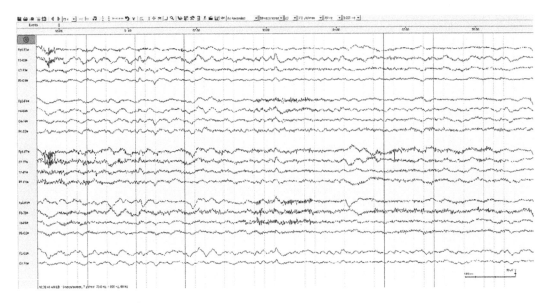

FIGURE 5.5.68 Continued

activity (GPFA) are common and can be seen in almost all patients (Figures 5.5.70–5.5.72). The frequency and voltage can vary considerably. Even though GPFA has the appearance of an ictal discharge, it is only occasionally associated with observable clinical manifestations, namely generalized tonic seizures.

The slow spike-and-wave discharges of Lennox-Gastaut syndrome tend to become less frequent with increasing age, but GPFA tends to persist.

Atypical absence seizures are a common seizure type in structural-metabolic generalized epilepsies, such as Lennox-Gastaut syndrome. The main distinction between typical and atypical absence seizures is electrographic, as the latter have a slower frequency of less than 2.5 Hz (Figure 5.5.73).

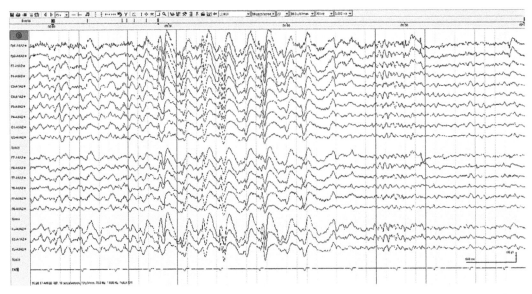

FIGURE 5.5.69 Slow sharp-and-wave discharges in a 27-year-old man with Lennox-Gastaut syndrome. Linked ear reference montage.

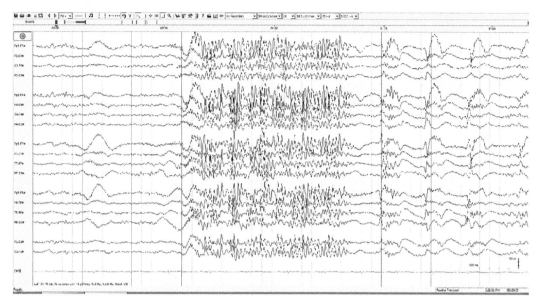

FIGURE 5.5.70 Generalized 11–12 Hz paroxysmal fast activity in sleep in a 56-year-old woman with Lennox-Gastaut syndrome. Longitudinal bipolar montage.

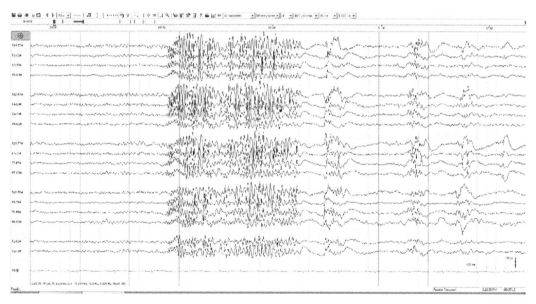

FIGURE 5.5.71 Generalized paroxysmal fast activity in sleep in a 56-year-old woman with Lennox-Gastaut syndrome. The discharge started at 20 Hz and slowed to 13 Hz. Longitudinal bipolar montage.

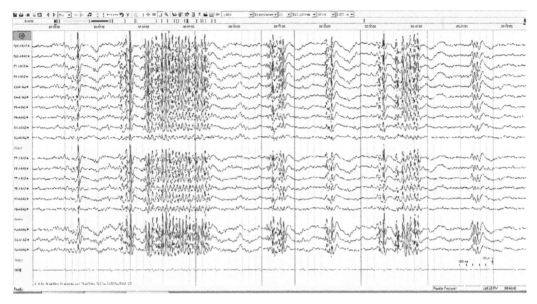

FIGURE 5.5.72 Generalized 10 Hz paroxysmal fast activity in sleep in a 27-year-old man with Lennox-Gastaut syndrome. Linked ear reference montage.

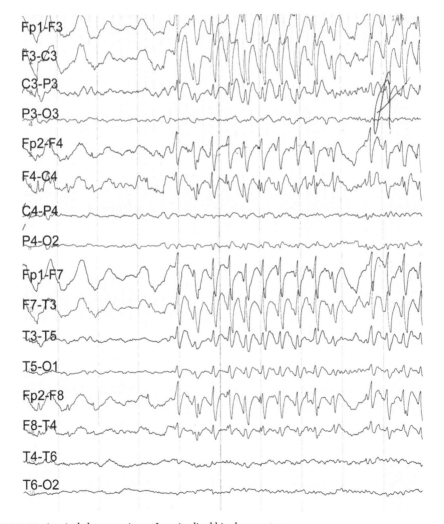

FIGURE 5.5.73 Atypical absence seizure. Longitudinal bipolar montage.

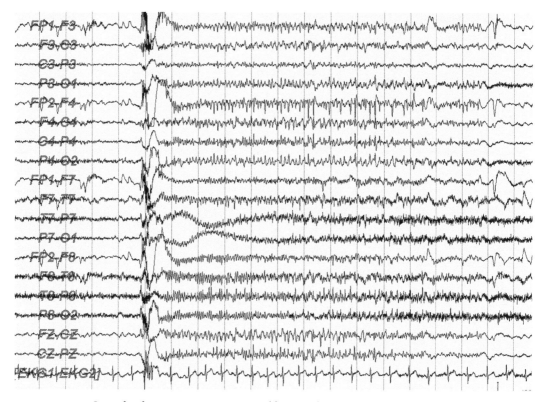

FIGURE 5.5.74 Generalized tonic seizure in a 41-year-old man with Lennox-Gastaut syndrome and seizures since age 5. Longitudinal bipolar montage.

Generalized Tonic Seizures

Generalized tonic seizures are brief episodes of increase in tone, lasting only a few seconds to about 1 min. The clinical manifestation can be mild, with just an increase in neck tone or upward eye deviation, or severe, with marked increase in tone of the axial and appendicular muscles. They usually start in sleep and drowsiness. The corresponding EEG patterns include

- Generalized low-voltage fast activity,
- Generalized voltage attenuation, sometimes preceded by a "transitional" high-voltage sharp wave,
- Generalized 10 Hz activity.

With any of these patterns, the prior background is attenuated at onset. Slower frequencies may become gradually intermixed over the course of the ictal discharge. Figures 5.5.74–5.5.77 show examples.

Generalized Atonic Seizures

Atonic seizures are characterized by loss of tone. They can vary in manifestation from subtle head drops to massive loss of tone with falling. The associated EEG discharge can vary in pattern, including

- Generalized slow spike-and-wave discharge,

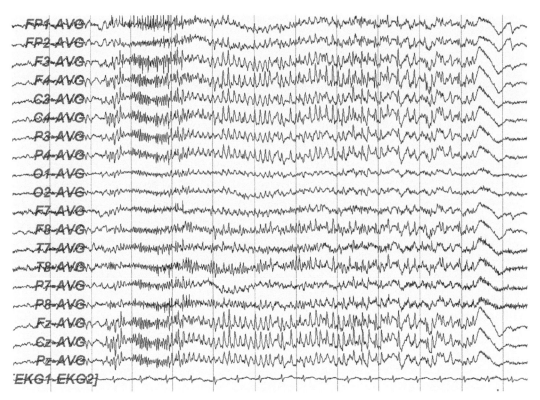

FIGURE 5.5.75 Generalized tonic seizure in a 41-year-old man with Lennox-Gastaut syndrome and seizures since age 5. Note the muscle artifact at Fp1 in association with generalized tonic posturing of extremities. Initial fast activity progressively decreased in frequency. Average reference montage.

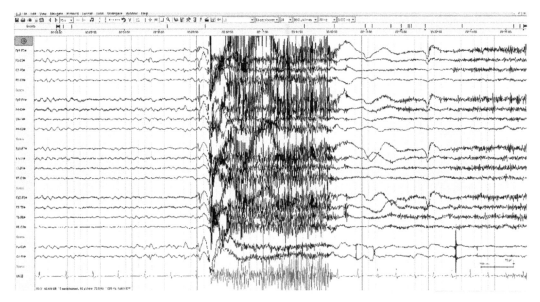

FIGURE 5.5.76 Generalized tonic seizures in a 50-year-old with Lennox-Gastaut syndrome since age 2. The electroencephalogram (EEG) activity is masked with muscle artifact with the first seizure (Above). With the second seizure (Below), initial low-voltage 18 Hz rhythmic activity is noted in the parasagittal regions with central predominance. Clinically there was sustained trunk and neck flexion and bilateral shoulder flexion and abduction, more pronounced in the first seizure. Longitudinal bipolar montage.

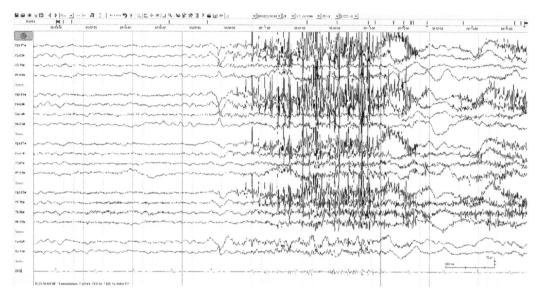

FIGURE 5.5.76 Continued

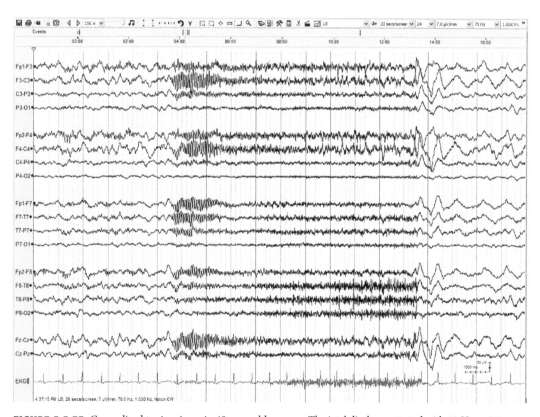

FIGURE 5.5.77 Generalized tonic seizure in 48-year-old woman. The ictal discharge started with 18 Hz activity and evolved with decreasing frequency. Clinically there was associated slight increase in tone resulting in low-amplitude motion of the head and upper extremities. Note the muscle artifact over the electrocardiogram (EKG) channel. Longitudinal bipolar montage.

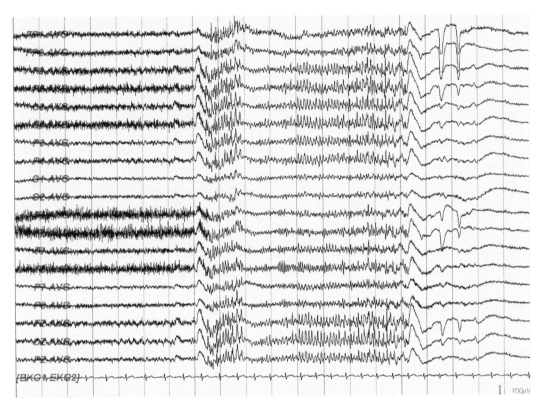

FIGURE 5.5.78 Generalized atonic seizure in a 41-year-old man with Lennox-Gastaut syndrome and seizures since age 5. Note the loss of muscle artifact at seizure onset. Initial fast activity progressively decreased in frequency. Average reference montage.

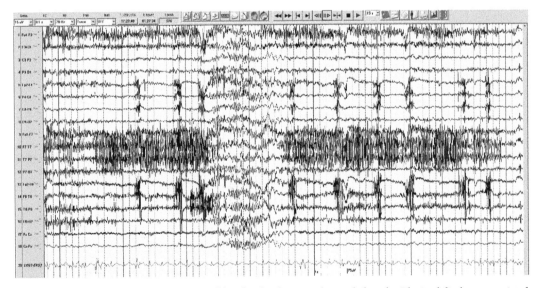

FIGURE 5.5.79 Atonic seizure in a 15-year-old with a developmental encephalopathy. The ictal discharge consisted of 20 Hz low-voltage rhythmic activity. Note the associated loss of muscle artifact during the discharge. Clinically, there was a head drop. Longitudinal bipolar montage.

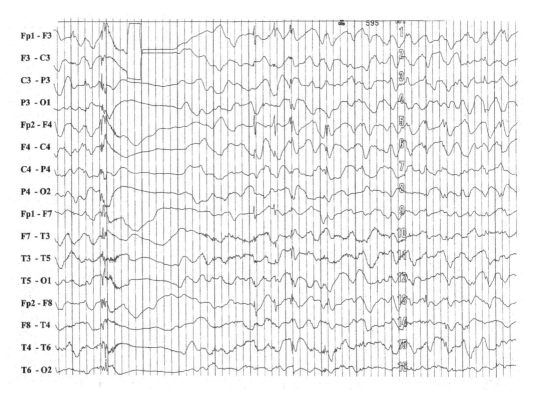

FIGURE 5.5.80 Myoclonic atonic seizure in a 4-year-old with Doose syndrome. The myoclonic jerk is associated with the polyspike discharge, and the atonic phase with the slow wave and attenuation. Longitudinal bipolar montage.

- Generalized voltage attenuation,
- Generalized low-voltage fast activity,
- Combinations of these.

Figures 5.5.78 and 5.5.79 show examples of EEG records with atonic seizures.

In children with Doose syndrome, atonic seizures are preceded by a myoclonic jerk and are called *myoclonic atonic* or *myoclonic astatic* seizures (Figure 5.5.80).

5.6

Status Epilepticus

HASAN H. SONMEZTURK

EPIDEMIOLOGY

The incidence rate of status epilepticus (SE) is estimated to be between 10.3 and 61/100,000 per year. The rate is higher in children younger than 1 year (135–156/100,000) and in individuals older than 65 (15–86/100,000) (Figure 5.6.1). Similar findings were revealed from a recent meta analysis of 43 studies from 2000 to 2016 .[1] The latest population-based epidemiologic study on SE found an incidence of 36.1 per 100,000. The specific incidence rates of nonconvulsive SE (NCSE) and SE with prominent motor phenomena (including convulsive SE) were 12.1 and 24 per 100,000 respectively.[2]

DEFINITION AND CLASSIFICATION

SE has had various definitions: in 2015, the International League Against Epilepsy (ILAE) Task Force on Classification of Status Epilepticus presented the scheme which we use today.[6] The latest definition published by ILAE Task Force states that

> SE is a condition resulting either from the failure of the mechanisms responsible for seizure termination or from the initiation of mechanisms which lead to abnormally prolonged seizures (after time point t1). It is a condition that can have long-term consequences (after time point t2), including neuronal death, neuronal injury, and alteration of neuronal networks, depending on the type and duration of seizures.

T1 is the time after which the seizure is considered to be continuous. T2 is the time after which there is a risk of long-term consequences of the seizure activity. T1 for tonic-clonic SE, focal SE with impaired consciousness, and absence SE

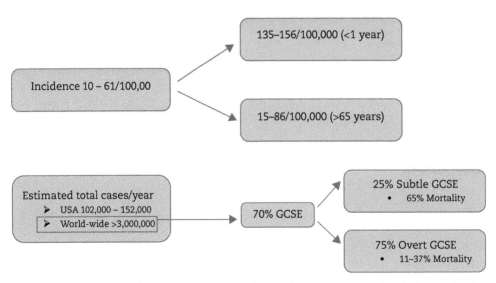

FIGURE 5.6.1 Epidemiology of status epilepticus. Data from multiple sources including DeLorenzo[3] and Treiman[4,5] teams.

TABLE 5.6.1 INTERNATIONAL
LEAGUE AGAINST EPILEPSY (ILAE)
CLASSIFICATION OF STATUS
EPILEPTICUS (SE)

Type of SE	Time (t1)	Time (t2)
Tonic-clonic SE	5 min	30 min
Focal SE impaired awareness	10 min	>60 min
Absence SE	~10–15 min	Unknown

From Trinka et al. 2015.[9]

was 5, 10, and 10–15 min, respectively. T2 for these types of SE was 30 min, greater than 60 min, and unknown, respectively (Table 5.6.1).[7]

Historically, there was no distinction made between these two time points or seizure types. SE was defined as continuous or intermittent seizure activity for 30 min or longer without any recovery to baseline in between the seizures. Later, Lowenstein et al. proposed a practical definition of SE, particularly for convulsive SE, defining the time cut-point as 5 min, at which point aggressive treatment was deemed necessary.[8] The data influencing these earlier definitions were mostly based on animal research and therefore had limitations.

The new classification was built on two semiological pillars with major diagnostic, prognostic, and therapeutic implications. The two semiological axes were presence or absence of predominant motor symptoms and coma and/or impaired awareness (see Box 5.6.1).

BOX 5.6.1   CLASSIFICATION OF STATUS EPILEPTICUS

With prominent motor symptoms
A.1 Convulsive SE (CSE, synonym: tonic–clonic SE)
  A.1.a. Generalized convulsive
  A.1.b. Focal onset evolving into bilateral convulsive SE
  A.1.c. Unknown whether focal or generalized
A.2 Myoclonic SE (prominent epileptic myoclonic jerks)
  A.2.a. With coma
  A.2.b. Without coma
A.3 Focal motor
  A.3.a. Repeated focal motor seizures (Jacksonian)
  A.3.b. Epilepsia partialis continua (EPC)
  A.3.c. Adversive status
  A.3.d. Oculoclonic status
  A.3.e. Ictal paresis (i.e., focal inhibitory SE)
A.4 Tonic status
A.5 Hyperkinetic SE
Without prominent motor symptoms (i.e., nonconvulsive SE, NCSE)
B.1 NCSE with coma (including so-called "subtle" SE)
B.2 NCSE without coma
  B.2.a. Generalized
    B.2.a.a Typical absence status
    B.2.a.b Atypical absence status
    B.2.a.c Myoclonic absence status
  B.2.b. Focal
    B.2.b.a Without impairment of consciousness (aura continua, with autonomic, sensory, visual, olfactory, gustatory, emotional/psychic/experiential, or auditory symptoms)
    B.2.b.b Aphasic status
    B.2.b.c With impaired consciousness
  B.2.c. Unknown whether focal or generalized
    B.2.c.a Autonomic SE

There are also two other treatment response–dependent types of SE which were not included in the latest classification. *Refractory SE* is a term used to describe any SE with failure of first- and second-line agents and requiring third-line anesthetic agents with no seizure control for 60 min or longer, and the term *super refractory SE* is reserved for SE cases with no response to third-line IV anesthetic agents for 24 hours or longer. The latter group most often manifests with coma or severely altered consciousness and minimal or no motor phenomena. *New-onset refractory SE* (NORSE) is by itself a unique entity differing from other SE types and mostly presenting in young adult patients with no prior history of seizures. The etiology of NORSE is unknown but autoimmune processes have been suspected and identified in some patients. Paraneoplastic and infectious etiologies have also been reported. Response to treatment can be poor, and, in one review of four studies (total 23 patients), 61% of the patients either died or became vegetative. Only 22% were reported to have good outcome.

In general, SE patients with prominent motor phenomena have more favorable treatment outcomes compared to SE without prominent motor phenomena. A more striking difference is seen when SE with coma or altered consciousness (poor outcome) is compared to SE without coma or altered awareness (favorable outcome).[10]

Table 5.6.2 summarizes the classification on the semiology axis.[11]

The ILAE task force also defined and grouped the potential etiologies for SE under two major groups, known and unknown. Known etiologies could be acute, remote, progressive, or secondary to a defined electroclinical syndrome. The task force also proposed an "age axis" and grouped SE in selected electroclinical syndromes according to age, from neonatal to elderly.

Attempts were made to structure and organize the electroencephalogram (EEG) correlates of SE, however, due to the heterogeneity of the condition, a specific ictal EEG pattern has not been identified. The EEG findings wildly differ

---

TABLE 5.6.2 SEMIOLOGY OF STATUS EPILEPTICUS

With prominent motor symptoms.	Convulsive SE (TC SE) • Generalized convulsive • Focal onset evolving into bilateral convulsive SE • Unknown whether focal or generalized Myoclonic SE • With coma • Without coma Focal motor SE • Repeated focal motor seizures. (Jacksonian) • Epilepsia partialis continua (EPC) • Adversive status • Oculoclonic status • Ictal paresis (i.e., focal inhibitory SE) Tonic SE Ictal paralysis (focal inhibitory SE)

Without prominent motor symptoms (i.e., nonconvulsive SE [NCSE])	NCSE with coma (including so-called "subtle" SE)
	 NCSE without coma
	 • Generalized
	   • Typical absence status
	   • Atypical absence status
	   • Myoclonic absence status
	 • Focal
	   • Without impairment of consciousness (aura continua, with autonomic, sensory, visual, olfactory, gustatory, emotional/psychic/experiential, or auditory symptoms
	   • Aphasic status
	   • With impaired consciousness
	 • Unknown whether focal or generalized
	   • Autonomic SE

from patient to patient, resembling semiological manifestations. EEG patterns and characteristics are dynamic and destined to change even in the same patient. In general, electrographic findings are described as focal, multifocal, wide-field bihemispheric (bisynchronous/asynchronous), or generalized. EEG patterns often do not show clear onset and offset, evolution in frequency and voltage, or spread. Depending on the point of time that the EEG monitoring is started, the patterns will vary. If the EEG is connected and running at the start of the SE, clear and discrete ictal discharges with associated clinical seizures can be seen. If EEG is initiated hours or days after

onset (i.e., in refractory stage), merged seizures/ictal discharges or patterns like generalized periodic discharges (GPDs) and lateralized periodic discharges (LPDs) can be seen in a continuous, monotonous manner. At the end stage (burnout stage) of SE, GPDs and LPDs can be interrupted or may be seen in a burst suppression pattern.

GPDs or LPDs can have different morphologies with superimposed fast activity, sharp waves or spikes or triphasic waves (Figure 5.6.2). Generalized or lateralized rhythmic delta activity (GRDA or LRDA) can also represent ictal patterns in some SE cases (Figures 5.6.3 and 5.6.4). There also are intermediate patterns that are

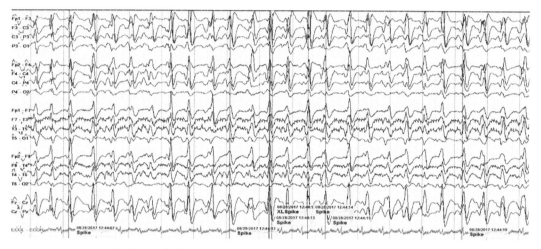

FIGURE 5.6.2 Generalized periodic discharges (GPDs). Longitudinal bipolar montage.

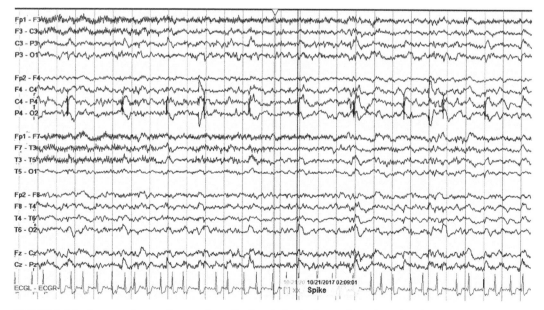

FIGURE 5.6.3 Above and next frame. Lateralized periodic discharges (LPDs). With and without superimposed fast activity. Longitudinal bipolar montage.

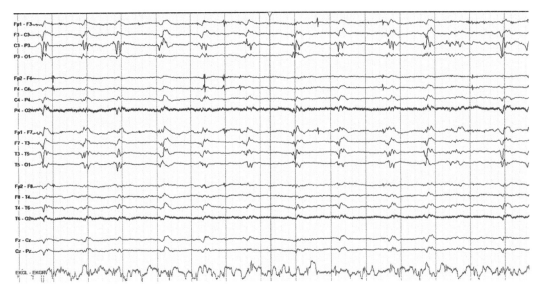

FIGURE 5.6.3 Continued

considered within the spectrum of the interictal-ictal-continuum, and it may not be possible to determine the nature of these patterns by EEG interpretation alone. In patients with altered consciousness or awareness and these intermediate EEG patterns, response to treatment assessment is the key to establishing the diagnosis as definite or possible SE. An anti-seizure medication (ASM) challenge is often required to help determine the nature of these patterns. ASM challenge can be done with a sedating ASM (typically a benzodiazepine, either lorazepam or midazolam) or a nonsedating ASM (typically levetiracetam, fosphenytoin, or lacosamide). The most definitive diagnosis combines clinical pattern, EEG features, and clinical response to therapy. See Table 5.6.3 for unified EEG terminology and criteria for NCSE.[12]

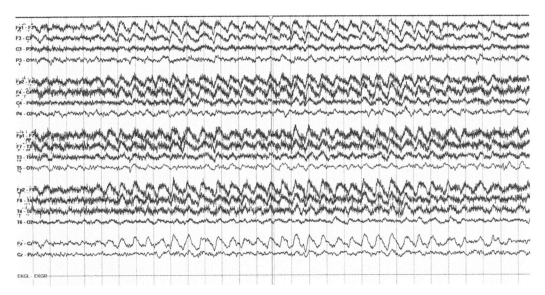

FIGURE 5.6.4 Generalized rhythmic delta activity (Above) versus lateralized rhythmic delta activity (Next frame). Longitudinal bipolar montage.

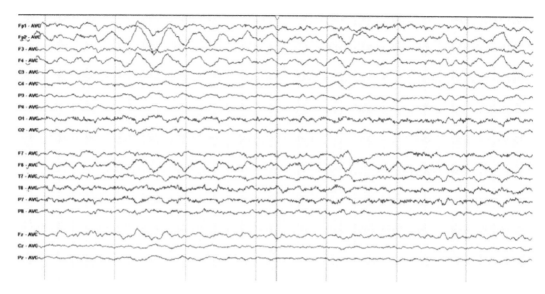

FIGURE 5.6.4 Continued

TABLE 5.6.3 CLASSIFICATION OF NONCONVULSIVE STATUS EPILEPTICUS

Without known epileptic encephalopathy
Epileptiform discharges
>2.5 Hz.

Epileptiform discharges ≤2.5 Hz *and* one:	EEG and clinical improvement after IV ASM, or Sub

With known epileptic encephalopathy
Increased prominence or frequency of the features mentioned above compared to baseline with observable change in clinical state
Improvement of clinical and EEG features with IV ASMs

CONVULSIVE STATUS EPILEPTICUS

Convulsive SE (CSE) is one of the best studied and described form of SE. Even though the term "convulsive SE" generally brings to mind a generalized tonic-clonic SE (GCSE), there are several forms described in the new classification by Trinka et al. These are SE cases with prominent motor phenomena, which can be generalized tonic, clonic, myoclonic, or tonic-clonic seizures either continuous or intermittent without recovery between seizures. Focal rhythmic shaking or twitching SE cases are also classified under CSE (historically called *epilepsia partialis continua*). In recent literature, GCSE was divided into two groups, "overt"

and "subtle." "Subtle" indicated the late nonconvulsive stage of overt GCSE. Both animal and human studies have shown a transition from the convulsive (overt) stage into the (subtle) nonconvulsive stage due to high metabolic and oxygenation demands with progressively decreased supplies as seizures persist. This drop in oxygenation and energy supplies eventually transitions the convulsive stage into the nonconvulsive stage, and that usually corresponds to about the same time a SE becomes refractory and then super-refractory.

The etiologies of GCSE are extensively studied but quite diverse. Some top causes include prior history of epilepsy (approximately two-third of patients), ASM nonadherence or discontinuation, drug (including prescribed and illegal) or alcohol withdrawal, structural brain lesions (acute/chronic), central nervous system infections, and toxic metabolic causes.

EEG findings of GCSE are often masked by intense muscle and motion artifact. However, generalized tonic or clonic muscle artifacts can easily be recognized and differentiated from nonepileptic convulsive events. If EEG is available and connected at the onset of GCSE, it could provide critical information about the classification whether the onset was focal or generalized and assist with better medication selection for therapy. However, most GCSE cases are connected to video-EEG after the onset of convulsions and often after the cessation of convulsions, at which point EEG can identify the presence or absence of after-discharges (NCS or NCSE).

NONCONVULSIVE STATUS EPILEPTICUS

Apart from the new classifications and definitions aiming to describe all forms of SE just detailed, there have also been distinct clinical and historical constellations of SE defining two major groups: convulsive (currently with prominent motor symptoms) and nonconvulsive (currently without prominent motor symptoms) SE. It is critical to know these definitions and nomenclature because a good portion of SE literature has been written using these terms within the past four decades. NCSE became a household name in critical care

units, particularly in neurological ICUs within the past two decades. This is partly because of increased long-term video-EEG monitoring in critical care units. Multiple publications on video-EEG monitoring in critical care units have documented an increasing number of undetected NCSE cases. This opened a new era of critical care EEG monitoring implementing near routine application of long-term video-EEG in neurological ICUs at tertiary care centers all around the United States and in the majority of the developed world. It has been shown that long-term video-EEG monitoring in patients with unexplained

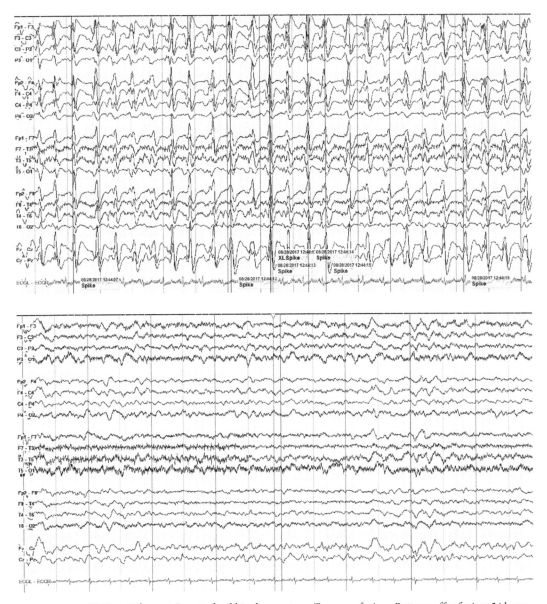

FIGURE 5.6.5 EEG on Cefepime.–Longitudinal bipolar montage, Top: on cefepime, Bottom: off cefepime 24 hours.

altered mental status or coma detects NCSE or nonconvulsive seizures (NCS) in about 15–18% of patients. These SE cases would go undetected and untreated without video-EEG monitoring as they often show minimal to no clinical features or characteristics to help with the diagnosis of ongoing or recurrent seizures. With this new approach, the threshold for obtaining long-term video-EEGs in critically ill patients has dropped dramatically, not only in neurological ICUs but also in medical, cardiac, surgical ICU, and trauma units.

Historically, other terms have been used in place of NCSE in the literature, such as "burnout SE," "subtle SE," or "SE terminans" just to name a few. These were descriptive terms mostly generated because most NCSE cases had a poor prognosis and a good portion of them showed minimal clinical changes, such as very subtle and low-amplitude eyelid myoclonia, hippus, or subtle twitches in face or extremities.

Other historical terms for focal NCSE without loss of awareness are "aura continua" or "simple partial SE." A newly emerging term for this type of status is "focal aware SE." When focal SE occurs with impaired awareness, it was historically called "complex partial SE," and the newly

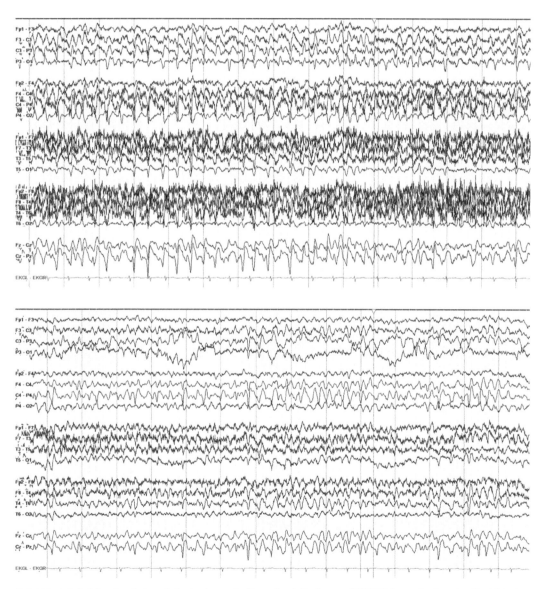

FIGURE 5.6.6 Stimulus-induced rhythmic, periodic, or ictal discharges (SIRPIDs) epoch.–Longitudinal bipolar montage. Top: With stimulation. Bottom: At rest.

emerging term for that is "focal impaired awareness SE."

"Epilepsia partialis continua" has been an established historical name for focal SE with focal motor activity and without loss of awareness. As this type of SE has prominent motor symptoms, it is considered a type of convulsive SE and will be discussed under that topic.

It is important to know there can be electroclinical presentations mimicking NCSE. Particularly certain medications, most importantly cefepime, a fourth-generation cephalosporin, can cause a neurotoxic picture with altered awareness and continuous GPDs on EEG. The majority of these patients will not respond to ASM challenge, and they will not improve clinically or electrographically until cefepime discontinuation (Figure 5.6.5). The case illustrated in Figure 5.6.5 was of a 47-year-old woman with renal failure who was admitted with pneumonia and suspected sepsis treated with cefepime in addition to other antibiotics. On exam she was fully awake but unresponsive and unable to follow commands. Her EEG or clinical picture did not change with lorazepam challenge (total of 6 mg) or levetiracetam (2,000 mg IV load). Patient's cognitive exam normalized and EEG pattern with GPDs disappeared about 36–48 hours after cefepime discontinuation. The patient was moved from the ICU to a regular floor bed 48 hours after cefepime discontinuation. Other implicated medications are ifosfamide, cisplatin, cyclosporin, and other fluoroquinolones.

Stimulus-induced generalized periodic discharges in critically ill patients are commonly seen

TABLE 5.6.4 NEGATIVE AND POSITIVE SYMPTOMS OF NONCONVULSIVE STATUS EPILEPTICUS (NCSE)

Negative symptoms	Positive symptoms
• Anorexia	• Agitation/Aggression
• Aphasia/Mutism	• Automatisms
• Amnesia	• Blinking
• Catatonia	• Delirium/Delusions/Echolalia
• Coma	• Facial twitching
• Confusion	• Laughter/Crying
• Lethargy	• Nausea/Vomiting
	• Nystagmus/tonic eye deviation/hippus
	• Perseveration/Psychosis
	• Tremulousness

as part of severe encephalopathy. Historically, the term "stimulus-induced rhythmic, periodic, or ictal discharges" (SIRPIDs) was used to describe these discharges. These could subside with benzodiazepine challenge, but often lacked associated clinical improvement. Therefore, the true nature of these discharges is not known, and the fact that they subside or disappear with rest and sleep and are exacerbated with stimulation makes an ictal nature of these discharges unlikely (Figure 5.6.6).

Clinical features of NCSE include negative and positive symptoms (Table 5.6.4). Around 75% of critically ill patients with NCSE will have no discernible clinical correlates.

5.7

Advanced Techniques

HASAN H. SONMEZTURK

INTRAOPERATIVE ELECTROCORTICOGRAPHY (ECOG)

Electrocorticography (ECoG) is performed at the time of surgery for electrode placement or resection. When used at the time of electrode placement, ECoG is an aid to determine proper locations for the electrodes. For example, if ECoG shows that discharges are near the margin of a grid, then the coverage area may be revised by moving or adding supplemental electrodes to provide better localization.

When ECoG is used during resection, a recording is usually made before and after the resection. If the patient already had subdural strip electrodes, then these provide the preoperative recording, and the ECoG electrodes are placed for postoperative recording, usually at the margins of the resection. Frequent discharges near the margins are often an indication for further surgery. Discharges that are infrequent or distant from the margin do not necessarily warrant additional surgery.

CRITICAL CARE MONITORING

The American Clinical Neurophysiology Society guidelines for standardized interpretation of critical care EEGs was presented in Chapter 5.4, and neurophysiologists interpreting studies or providing neurologic care in the ICU setting should be familiar with these.

Continuous critical care monitoring is increasingly used for a variety of indications. The most common are post-cardiopulmonary resuscitation (CPR) encephalopathy and seizure monitoring.

Post-CPR Encephalopathy

Encephalopathy after CPR is one of the common reasons for neurologic consultation in the hospital. The widespread use of hypothermia for select patients after cardiac arrest has complicated clinical assessments and prognostication since many

of the previous data regarding clinical findings and prognosis no longer clearly apply to patients who have had hypothermia, whether at the originally used temperature window of 32–34°C or at 36°C, which is often used now. Details of temperature management are outside of the scope of this book, but current guidelines do not favor the higher or lower temperatures.[1] And while initial use was designated for patients with ventricular fibrillation and pulseless ventricular tachycardia who are unconscious after an out-of-hospital arrest, the guidelines current at the time of this writing indicate that it is appropriate to consider hypothermia for patients who are unconscious after recovery from asystole and pulseless electrical activity (PEA), as well as in-hospital arrests; these latter scenarios were previously not recommended for temperature management. Many centers also enforce normothermia after the rewarming period, whether the patient is cooled or not, since hyperthermia may worsen outcome after cardiac arrest.[2]

Recent data suggest that patients with non-shockable rhythm may have better outcomes at 90 days if treated with hypothermia to 33°C rather than controlled normothermia at 37°C.[3]

EEG monitoring is often used to allow for continuous evaluation of brain activity as sedatives are withdrawn, as well as for the identification of seizures or periodic discharges.

Burst suppression immediately after resuscitation, even before temperature management has begun, is an indicator of poor prognosis, whereas patients with just slow activity fare somewhat better.[4] Similarly, burst suppression after rewarming is associated with poor prognosis, while patients with slow activity also fare better.[5]

We hope that our efforts at perfecting post-CPR care, including electrophysiologic monitoring, would result in substantial improvement in outcomes, but data seem to suggest otherwise. Perhaps a larger role is in the identification of patients for whom extensive and expensive efforts are not indicated.[6]

Seizure Monitoring

Patients admitted with status epilepticus benefit from EEG monitoring because discharges can be subclinical after overt clinical seizures are controlled. Also, the location of pathology responsible for the status epilepticus may be evident with long-term monitoring. This should include video recording so that direct behavioral and electrographic correlations can be made. This is discussed in more detail in Chapter 5.6.

ENCEPHALOPATHY IN HOSPITALIZED PATIENTS

An increasing proportion of patients with marked encephalopathy associated with hospitalization, especially sepsis-associated encephalopathy, are found to have seizures.[7,8] The diagnosis of these nonconvulsive seizures in this population is facilitated by longer recordings, and bedside EEG monitoring can be particularly helpful for this. We believe that nonconvulsive seizures in the hospital are significantly underdiagnosed.

EEG findings in some of the common disorders seen with critical care monitoring are discussed in Tables 5.7.1 and 5.7.2. Some specific examples are discussed in more detail later.

EEG in hospitalized patients with encephalopathy can show a wide variety of findings, many of which are actionable. Among them are periodic discharges; suppression, especially if newly developed during the course of the monitoring; unexpected asymmetries; and electrographic seizures.[9] Nonconvulsive status epilepticus in patients with encephalopathy is often identified only after a significant delay.[10]

QUANTITATIVE EEG

Quantitative EEG has a wide variety of applications, some of which include

- Spike detection,
- Seizure detection,
- Mapping,
- Spectral array.

There are many algorithms to accomplish these tasks, but in general terms, mathematical analysis of the digital EEG is performed for these and other purposes.

Spike detection and event detection depend on the frequency components of the signal. For

TABLE 5.7.1 CLINICAL CORRELATES TO ELECTROENCEPHALOGRAM (EEG) FINDINGS WITH CRITICAL ILLNESS

Finding	Clinical correlate
Generalized slowing	Almost any encephalopathy, including renal, hepatic, toxic, sepsis, hypoxic, endocrine
Triphasic waves	Hepatic, renal, some toxicities including lithium and baclofen
Periodic discharges	Symmetric: hypoxic, seizures, Asymmetric or unilateral: Herpes simplex virus (HSV) encephalitis, other focal destructive lesion such as stroke; note that asymmetry does not require visible structural lesion
Beta activity	Coma in patients with prominent beta is most often due to medications, especially benzodiazepines and barbiturates, but this has also been seen with other conditions, especially hypoxic encephalopathy
Normal background	Psychogenic unresponsiveness is the most common cause of coma with normal EEG
	Locked-in syndrome should be considered and repeat neuro exam performed for this possibility

a clinical seizure detection, the combination of movement artifact, plus fast and slow complexes in the EEG, can identify suspected seizures. These seizure detections programs and trendographs have improved dramatically to a sensitivity of nearly 100%. However, specificity (false alarms) are still a major problem. For spike detection, there is often no motor manifestation, so the algorithm may highlight potentials which are of a certain rise-time and amplitude along with a definable field identified from comparison with nearby and distant electrodes of known topography.

Mapping is performed by creating a map on which the positions relate to a surface projection of the brain and the colors and intensities often relate to frequency components and amplitudes. While data are obtained from discrete electrode locations, interpolation is used to estimate the values at points between electrode locations, thereby giving a map with apparent higher spatial resolution than the number of electrodes would actually produce.

TABLE 5.7.2 ELECTROENCEPHALOGRAM (EEG) FINDINGS WITH SELECT CRITICAL ILLNESSES

Disorder	EEG finding
Hepatic encephalopathy	Generalized slowing
	Triphasic waves
Renal encephalopathy	Generalized slowing
	Occasional triphasic waves and seizure activity
Sepsis-associated encephalopathy	Slowing, sometimes seizures
Cefepime neurotoxicity	Nonconvulsive status epilepticus-like electroclinical syndrome (generalized periodic discharges [GPDs] with unresponsiveness)
Herpes encephalitis	Slowing most prominent over the temporal region
	Lateralized periodic discharges are typical but not always seen; repeat study may be needed
Hypoxic encephalopathy	Generalized slowing and suppression
	GPDs, burst suppression, myoclonic status epilepticus (usually indicated grave prognosis)
Psychogenic unresponsiveness	Normal EEG
	Occasional patients with excess beta might have received benzodiazepine for nonepileptic events
Stroke of one hemisphere	Focal polymorphic delta over the region of the stroke
	Occasional periodic discharges
	Occasional seizures

Spectral array displays frequency and power over time and is performed by a frequency analysis of a section of brain, thus giving a principal view of the frequencies. This provides a birds-eye view power analysis of prolonged periods of EEG in a compressed manner. The EEG reader can easily detect high-power regions and jump to the time point of interest to examine the raw data and determine if the reading is ictal or epileptiform in nature. Because spectral array detects anything that has high power, including motion, muscle, chewing, and electrode artifacts, it is quite contaminated and nonspecific. In recent years a new trendograph was developed, the *rhythmic run detection and display* (R2D2). This trendograph detects the power increases only in rhythmic and periodic patterns, thus eliminating most of the muscle, electrode, and motion artifacts. R2D2 is considered one of the most valuable trendographs in the quantitative EEG world.

A host of pathologic and physiologic processes can affect quantitative EEG results. With long-term EEG becoming increasingly common, close inspection of every digital page is becoming increasingly difficult. We are starting to rely more on quantitative EEG to highlight events and seizures. This method may not be perfect but, in some instances, it is better than a naked-eye review when the reader is reviewing multiple 24-hour video-EEG studies.

INTRAOPERATIVE MONITORING

Intraoperative neuromonitoring (IONM) is not a focus of this text but has been widely used by our institution and is an important field of clinical neurophysiology. EEG is just one modality used in IONM. EEG is mostly used to detect sudden ischemic changes as emergent slow activity during carotid endarterectomy (CEA) and aneurysm surgeries in which the surgeon has to clamp the artery while performing surgical work. EEG is most commonly used to determine whether a shunt will be needed during a CEA. If no asymmetry is seen with clamping of the proximal artery, the surgeon proceeds with endarterectomy without shunting, which decreases the risks of embolic strokes.

There are other modalities used for IONM besides EEG. These include somatosensory evoked potentials (SSEPs), transcranial electric motor evoked potentials (TCeMEP), brainstem auditory evoked potentials (BAEPs), and electromyography (EMG). SSEP responses are generated by stimulating the distal nerves, such as the ulnar or median for upper extremity and the tibial nerves for lower extremities. The responses are detected and recorded on the scalp with electrodes roughly located over contralateral sensory cortex, the cervical spine, and Erb's point. The TCeMEP responses are generated by stimulating over the scalp electrodes roughly located over the motor cortex. These are high-intensity stimulations because the signal has to travel through the skull, stimulate the cortex, and generate a motor response in extremities.

BAEP responses are generated with clicks in the ears and recorded over brainstem, midbrain, and thalamic levels with far-field recording. Stimulating and recording electrode nomenclature and positionings is beyond the scope of this chapter and will not be discussed here. EMG is often used to guide the surgeon while doing surgical work around major nerve roots or spinal tracks. EMG electrodes can be attached to cranial nerve muscles or extremity muscles.

With all these modalities, the monitoring neurologist detects the changes from baseline and alerts the surgeon of an issue. For example, if there is unexpected muscle activity, it is possible the surgeon is too close to a nerve root. If there is sudden drop in SSEP amplitudes or a prolongation of SSEP latencies, it is possible the posterior cord is under stress, compressed, or ischemic due to traction or internal pathology (blood, disc etc.). Similarly, motor evoked potentials are used to monitor anterior spinal cord functionality in real time. BAEP monitoring is a very effective modality to monitor the functionality of the eighth nerve during cerebellopontine angle surgeries.

PART 6

Pediatric EEG

6.1

Normal Pediatric EEG

KEVIN C. ESS

OVERVIEW

Interpretation of the electroencephalogram (EEG) of children should be distinct from that for adults as there are complex developmental changes expected with normal rhythms and patterns. Brain function and EEG patterns evolve considerably in predictable patterns as children develop from preterm to term stages, as well as during early and late childhood and into adolescence and young adulthood. Among the many important distinctions seen between pediatric and adult EEG, a few are

- Frequencies comprising the record;
- Organization of the EEG, the "background";
- Evolution of EEG patterns as a function of age;
- Appearance/morphology of epileptiform discharges;
- Unique waveforms seen in childhood.

We will discuss the progression of the normal EEG from the neonatal period forward and discuss important findings that can be seen at individual stages of development.

NEONATAL EEG METHODOLOGY

Neonatal EEG is performed similarly to adult EEG, but the montages are distinct and there is more physiologic monitoring to help determine patient state. Common physiologic monitoring usually includes:

- Respirations,
- Eye movements,
- Electrocardiogram (EKG),
- Electromyogram (EMG) of chin.

Respirations in adults are usually easily differentiated from electrocerebral slow activity, but in neonates and young children, rapid or irregular

respirations can be mistaken for pathologic slow activity. In addition, while apnea is common in preterm and term neonates, clinicians are often concerned about the potential for seizures causing or being related to apneic episodes.

The following data need to be available for interpretation of neonatal studies:

- Age, with well-defined conceptional age based on gestational age plus postnatal age;
- Clinical question being asked;
- Physiological state of the neonate;
- Reactivity of the background.

Conceptional age (CA) is the sum of gestational age at the time of delivery plus postnatal age. This is important as brain development and subsequent EEG patterns usually respect a time-dependent progression whether maturation is intrauterine or post-delivery, as in the case of premature infants. For example, a child delivered at 32 weeks immediately undergoing an EEG would be expected to have similar patterns as another child who was born at 28-week gestation with an EEG performed 4 weeks later.

Physiological state refers to observations regarding level of consciousness and the sleep–wake cycle (e.g., waking, sedated, or asleep). Neonatal EEG as a rule should be long enough to capture natural progression from wakefulness to sleep. Most babies do this frequently enough so that a 1-hour EEG is usually adequate. While physiological monitoring of respirations, eye movements, electrocardiogram (EKG), and chin (electromyogram; EMG) are very helpful to determine the physiological state, in real life, these measurements often do not record well or are prone to artifact. A simple proxy, then, for sleep in neonates is whether, upon video review, eyes are closed (sleep) or open (awake).

For sedated patients, the EEG reader needs to know the agent used. While there are significant limitations to interpreting EEG on sedated patients, many children with, for example, complex cardiac disease are placed on extracorporeal membrane oxygenation (ECMO). They suffer high rates of neurological disease, including strokes and seizures. These patients are always sedated and sometimes paralyzed. EEG is then a critical tool to monitor for seizures while these high-risk patients are on ECMO.

Reactivity of the background refers to response to tactile and auditory stimuli and is important not only for neonates but for most routine and ICU EEGs.

PHYSIOLOGICAL STATE OF NEONATES

Typical sleep–wake patterns evident in children and adults are not seen in premature infants. Normal term infant EEG patterns are not well-developed until 38–40 weeks conceptional age, and further maturation takes many months. At term, there are two sleep stages defined: active sleep (AS) and quiet sleep (QS). These are summarized in Table 6.1.1.

AS is so termed because there are observable small horizontal eye and body movements. Neonates can go directly from wakefulness to AS. Respirations are irregular. AS can be conceived as broadly equivalent as a prelude to rapid eye movement (REM) sleep that appears later in maturation. Theta frequencies predominate in AS, with some delta and beta superimposed. The first AS epoch during sleep is often of higher amplitude than later epochs. Later epochs have not only lower amplitude but also more theta and less delta activity.

QS is so termed because there are minimal to no eye and body movements. Respirations are regular. This is broadly equivalent to non-REM sleep later in maturation. There are two patterns typically associated with QS. One is continuous slow activity predominantly in the delta range. The other is a discontinuous pattern, *Trace Alternant* (TA), with epochs of alternating relatively low-voltage activity punctuated by bursts of theta, which can be sharply contoured. This can occasionally look similar to a pathologic burst suppression pattern, but the interburst activity with TA is typically of higher voltage and comprised of a richer frequency of activities.

NORMAL NEONATAL EEG

The normal neonatal EEG is highly dependent on conceptional age such that patterns need to be described as typical of defined individual periods of brain development. This is a critical point because normal patterns in one period of development can be frankly abnormal in another. The EEG background typical of a term child is usually present by 38 weeks of conceptional age.

EEG findings with different stages of development are presented in Table 6.1.2.

To synopsize, the youngest neonates commonly recorded (about 22 weeks) have a very discontinuous pattern, meaning that there are long periods (up to 2 min) of low-voltage activity punctuated by bursts of high-voltage mixed-frequency activity, which normally includes sharp waves. This *Trace Discontinu* (TD) pattern can look broadly similar to a burst suppression pattern in an adult with severe encephalopathy or sedation but is considered a normal EEG finding for this conceptional age.

With maturation, the periods of low-voltage activity become shorter and have greater activity. That is, the bursts become more frequent and longer, and the differences between the bursts and interburst epochs are much less pronounced as the child approached 38 weeks of conceptional age—the discontinuity is quite modest at that point. As the child approaches 38–40 weeks of conceptional age, sleep–wake cycles become more obvious.

22–29 Weeks Conceptional Age

EEG between 22 and 29 weeks conceptional age consists of TD with mainly low-voltage mixed-frequency activity with interspersed bursts of theta and faster frequencies (see Figure 6.1.1). The interburst intervals can be more than 1 min, especially in very premature infants, although shorter

---

TABLE 6.1.1 NEONATAL SLEEP STAGES

Stage	Description
Active sleep (AS)	Small horizontal rapid eye and body movements with irregular respirations. Theta predominance of the EEG.
Quiet sleep (QS)	Absent to minimal eye movements with regular respirations. One pattern predominating has continuous delta activity with superimposed theta. The other pattern is discontinuous special pattern called trace alternant, with delta and some theta with superimposed bursts of activity.

TABLE 6.1.2 NEONATAL ELECTROENCEPHALOGRAM (EEG) PATTERNS
ACCORDING TO CONCEPTIONAL AGE

Conceptional age	EEG patterns
22–29 weeks	Discontinuous "trace discontinu" pattern with long intervals of low voltage activity up to 2-min duration with brief high-voltage mixed-frequency bursts.
29–31 weeks	Trace discontinu pattern but with shorter interburst intervals. Delta brushes ("delta/beta complex") begin to appear.
32–34 weeks	Discontinuous pattern in quiet and active sleep. Multifocal sharp transients seen.
34–37 weeks	Still a discontinuous pattern in quiet sleep but with progressively shorter interburst intervals. The higher and lower voltage components are more similar in duration, leading to terminology of *trace alternant* as they appear to be alternating with each other. EEG during active sleep (REM-like) is almost continuous. Fewer multifocal sharp transients; more frontal sharp transients. Occasional delta brushes
38–40 weeks	Trace alternant pattern in non-REM sleep with approximately equal burst–interburst duration. May see a continuous slow wave pattern. Fewer frontal sharp transients. Rare delta brushes.

REM, rapid eye movement.

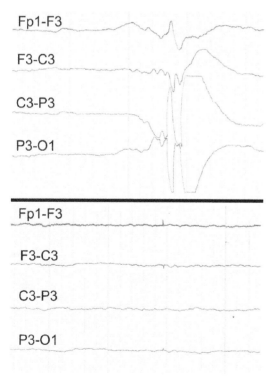

FIGURE 6.1.1 Electroencephalogram (EEG) of a very premature infant.

intervals are typical. The bursts exhibit poor inter-hemispheric synchrony in very young premature infants, but later in this age group there is better synchrony.

The sharp contours of these bursts, along with the quite low voltage of the interburst epochs, can resemble pathological burst suppression. This is differentiated chiefly by knowledge of the age of the patient and clinical condition.

29–31 Weeks Conceptional Age

At 29–31 weeks of conceptional age, while discontinuous patterns persist, there are changes, with the interburst intervals becoming shorter. The interburst intervals also are of higher amplitude still, with a mixed-frequency background. The sleep stages are now present, with the TD pattern mainly seen during QS.

Delta brushes are typical of this conceptional age and are seen in AS. They have the appearance of a delta wave with superimposed fast activity in the beta range, thus leading to an alternative name "delta/beta complexes." They can loosely resemble sleep spindles, but delta brushes are most prominent in the central and occipital regions, whereas the later occurring sleep spindles have a more frontal then central predominance. True sleep spindles are not seen at this age, and wave forms with spindly appearance could in fact represent epileptiform activity.

32–34 Weeks Conceptional Age

Both AS and QS remain discontinuous at 32–34 weeks of conceptional age, but the interburst intervals are of progressively higher amplitude and much shorter.

Delta brushes are seen less often, with the fast component even faster in this conceptional age range. Delta activity is more prominent from the occipital regions.

Multifocal sharp transients are seen in both the waking and sleep states. This can easily be mistaken for pathological sharp waves, but the multifocal nature and the lack of repetitive discharge argues against epileptiform activity (see Figure 6.1.2). This further reinforces a main theme in neonatal EEG: physiological patterns normally seen at one conceptional age (e.g., 33 weeks) would be abnormal at older ages (e.g., 48 weeks). Again, there is a critical need to have an accurate determination of conceptional age to properly interpret a neonatal EEG.

34–37 Weeks Conceptional Age

At 34–37 weeks of conceptional age, AS is now virtually continuous, with irregular delta activity most prominent posteriorly and theta and faster frequencies anteriorly.

QS still shows a discontinuous pattern, but the shorter interburst intervals and higher voltage activity during the interburst intervals suggest more of an alternating pattern of activity and quiescence, with ratios of 1:1 to 1:3. This is the TA pattern.

EMG activity is a reliable indicator of state beginning at this age range, whereas it was not easily seen in younger premature infants; low-amplitude EMG is now seen in REM sleep. Multifocal sharp transients disappear and are replaced with *frontal sharp transients* ("encoches frontales") that are of higher amplitude (see Figure 6.1.3).

Reactivity of the EEG is more prominent than in younger ages, with attenuation of the background with stimulation, and this often represents a change of physiological state.

38–40 Weeks Conceptional Age

These are generally considered term infants, and the EEG pattern that is considered normal features generally continuous patterns while awake with a mixture of theta and delta. Non-REM sleep continues to show evolution of the alternating pattern, with less differentiation of the burst from interburst appearance. The burst–interburst ratio is about 1:1 and represents a mature TA pattern. REM sleep shows a mixed pattern of alpha, theta, and delta with frequent eye movements and irregular respirations (Figure 6.1.4).

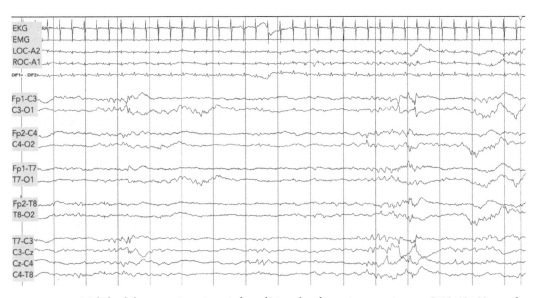

FIGURE 6.1.2 Multifocal sharp transients, in an infant of 37 weeks of gestation, prominent at C3/C4/Cz. Neonatal longitudinal bipolar montage.

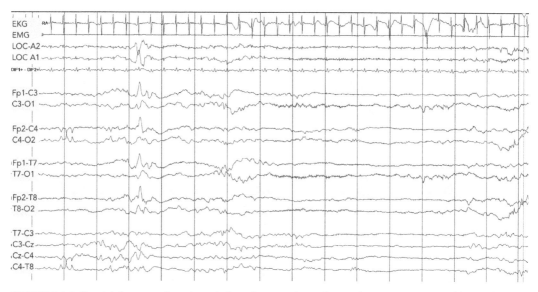

FIGURE 6.1.3 Frontal sharp transients in an infant of corrected age of 37 weeks gestation. Neonatal longitudinal bipolar montage.

Frontal sharp transients are less prominent than in a younger conceptional age range and should abate totally around 2 months post-term. Delta brushes are rare to absent in this age range.

MATURATION OF THE POSTERIOR DOMINANT RHYTHM

The normal waking background of the child depends on age. The posterior dominant rhythm (PDR) is approximately 4 Hz in 4- to 5-month-old infants and becomes faster throughout childhood, reaching 8 Hz by age 3 years, and the average adult frequency of 9–10 Hz by 10 years of age. Figure 6.1.5 shows the maturation of the PDR. The amplitude also tends to be higher than in adults, in the range of 50–100 μV/mm.

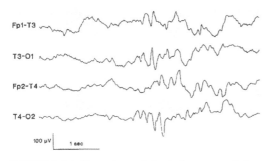

FIGURE 6.1.4 Normal term infant's electroencephalogram (EEG).

POSTERIOR SLOW WAVES OF YOUTH

The slow waves superimposed on and intermixed with the normal posterior waking background are referred to as *slow waves of youth*. These normal findings potentially can be confused with abnormal slow potentials suggesting encephalopathy, especially when seen in young child with a posterior rhythm still in the theta range. Posterior slow waves may have an episodic occurrence or may be seen sequentially. They are usually notched, suggesting that several alpha waves have merged to form them. They are usually not confused with epileptiform activity, although the sequence of an alpha wave followed by a slow wave occasionally suggests a sharp and slow wave complex.

In addition to posterior slow waves, there is more theta anteriorly in young children than in adults, and this, also, should not be interpreted as abnormal.

Neurophysiologists not accustomed to reading pediatric EEGs should be careful to not misinterpret normal slow activity as pathological, or indicative of an encephalopathy. Consideration must always be made to age as well as the state of the patient (Figure 6.1.6).

Posterior slow waves of youth are augmented by hyperventilation, as shown in Figure 6.1.7. This is from the same patient as in Figure 6.1.6.

Posterior slow waves of youth, then, are normal patterns. They are differentiated from pathologic slow waves by the following features:

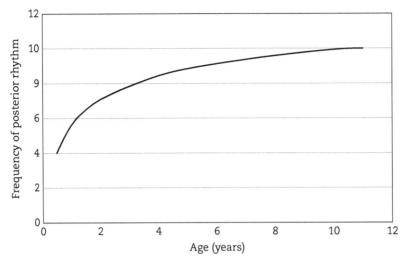

FIGURE 6.1.5 Maturation of the posterior dominant rhythm.

- Otherwise normal background,
- Appearance in wake and light sleep but disappear later in sleep,
- Reactivity to eye opening with attenuation.

They become less evident with growth and are not seen after 30 years of age.

HYPERVENTILATION

Hyperventilation is a key activation technique for children given the higher prevalence of generalized epilepsies seen in this age group. However, hyperventilation in children often produces greater and at times impressive slowing in children compared to adults. This may be due to

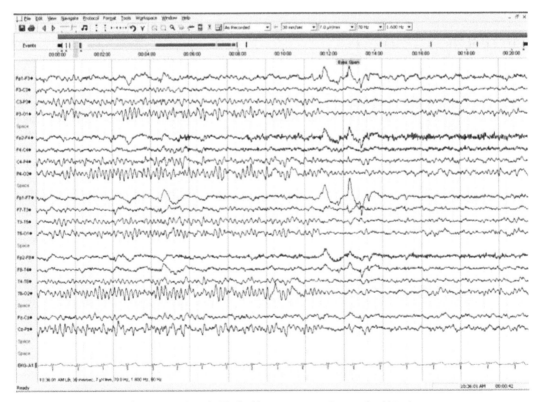

FIGURE 6.1.6 Posterior slow waves of youth, blocked by eye opening. Longitudinal bipolar montage.

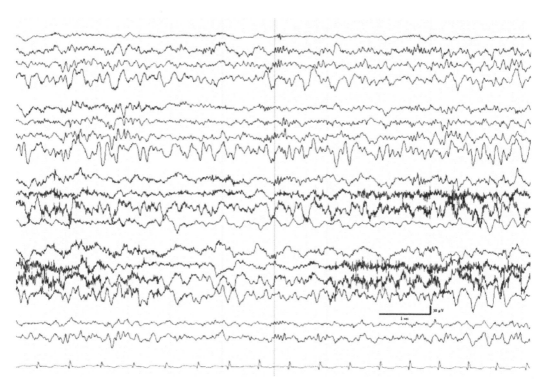

FIGURE 6.1.7 Posterior slow waves of youth, enhanced by hyperventilation. Longitudinal bipolar montage.

physiological responses as a function of age or simply reflect the inclination of children to vigorously hyperventilation when requested. The magnitude and synchronicity of the hyperventilation-related slowing can sometimes be mistaken for generalized seizure activity (see Figure 6.1.8). This is particularly true if there is a notched appearance to the rhythm, a common occurrence when the slow activity is superimposed on faster underlying rhythms. Awareness by a well-trained and experienced EEG technician to this potential pitfall is very important because asking children to follow simple commands during hyperventilation can reliably distinguish normal hyperventilation-induced slowing from generalized epileptiform discharges and actual seizures triggered by hyperventilation. This will help minimize overdiagnoses.

DROWSINESS

One pattern of drowsiness seen in early childhood is that of generalized bisynchronous high-voltage slow waves, often appearing abruptly. This pattern is referred to as *hypnagogic hypersynchrony*. It becomes less frequent with advancing age and is no longer seen by adolescence (see Figure 6.1.9). Similar patterns can also be seen upon awakening and are thus termed *hypnopompic hypersynchrony*.

SLEEP PATTERNS

Sleep should almost always be obtained when the clinical question is seizures since interictal discharges and sometimes ictal discharges are often more common in drowsiness and sleep. For some patients, abnormal electrical activity is only seen in sleep. There is effectively no difference between sedated sleep and natural sleep in terms of patterns. Chloral hydrate is sometimes used as a sedative since it has a wide safety margin, and this agent does not produce the prominent drug-induced beta activity that is typical of benzodiazepines and barbiturates. However, this is considered conscious sedation and requires special documentation and monitoring and can also occasionally alter the EEG patterns.[1]

The sleep records of children and adults are more alike than are the waking records. However, there are maturational changes in children. In addition, sleep activity of children can be particularly sharp and high in voltage, possibly leading to misdiagnoses.

Vertex Waves

Vertex waves (Figure 6.1.10) are not present at birth but begin to appear at about 5 months of age. By 2 years of age they are prominent in Stage 2 sleep, sharp in configuration, and of high

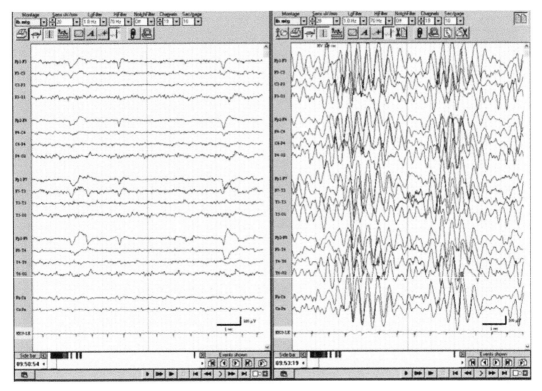

FIGURE 6.1.8 Hyperventilation in a child. Longitudinal bipolar montage.

amplitude. They can be so prominent as to be confused with epileptiform activity.

While there is room for experience and judgment in differentiation of juvenile vertex activity from epileptiform activity, some general guidelines are that *juvenile vertex waves*

- Are prominent during sleep without any signs of abnormal vertex activity during the awake state,
- Disappear during deeper stages of sleep,
- Are associated with spindles,

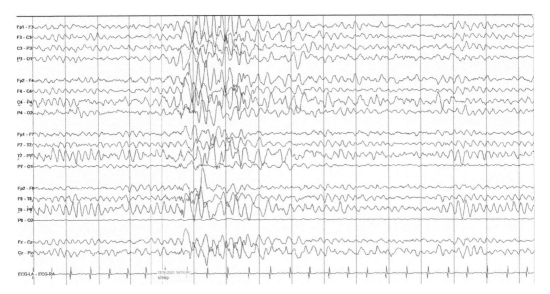

FIGURE 6.1.9 Hypnagogic hypersynchrony in 5-year-old boy. Longitudinal bipolar montage.

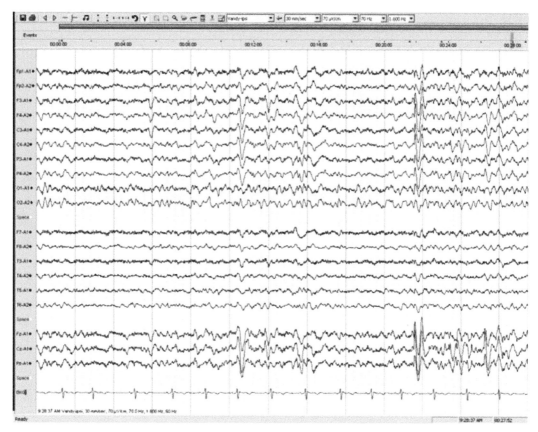

FIGURE 6.1.10 Vertex waves. Ipsilateral ear reference montage.

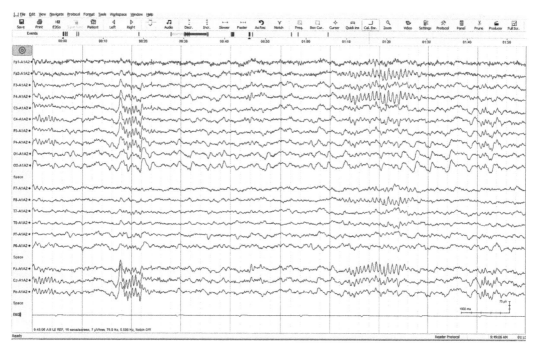

FIGURE 6.1.11 K-complex, on the left side of the image. Linked ear reference montage.

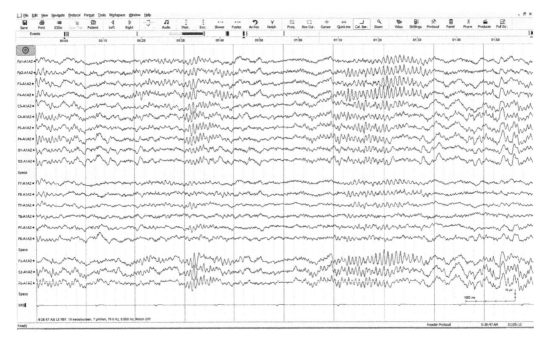

FIGURE 6.1.12 Synchronous sleep spindles. Linked ear reference montage.

- Are associated with K-complexes that have a vertex component similar to the waves in question.

Regarding these guidelines, prominence of vertex activity in sleep without a waking correlate is different from augmentation of epileptiform activity during sleep. Occasionally, interictal or ictal activity will appear during sleep when there is no sign during the awake state. However, total absence during the awake state with prominence during light sleep is not impossible but is unexpected.

Disappearance of vertex waves during deeper sleep cannot be observed in most routine office studies because sleep beyond Stage 2 is rarely obtained. Video monitoring for longer time intervals (usually overnight EEG) would then be required to capture all sleep stages.

Association with spindles is a good clue to the identity of vertex activity, although even this is imperfect since high-frequency rhythmic epileptiform activity can occasionally be seen. This pattern is most common in younger patients, so the chance occurrence of vertex epileptiform plus central alpha-range rhythmic activity is quite uncommon.

K-complexes (Figure 6.1.11) are the fusion of a vertex with a sleep spindle. If K-complexes are seen and the vertex component has the same general appearance as the midline waves under question, the activity is more likely to be vertex than epileptiform.

Sleep Spindles

Sleep spindles (Figure 6.1.12) are not present at birth but begin to appear consistently at about 2 months. Early sleep spindles are often prolonged and have an appearance different from adult spindles in that they have a sharp negative peak and rounded base. Given brain immaturity and incomplete myelination, left and right spindles appear asynchronously. By 18 months of age, however, the majority of spindles should be synchronous with both hemispheres. By 2 years of age, the general appearance of the sleep spindles is the same as in adults.

6.2

Abnormal Pediatric EEG

KEVIN C. ESS

NEONATAL EEG ABNORMALITIES

Neonatal electroencephalogram (EEG) abnormalities usually fall into one of the following groups:

- Background abnormality,
- Abnormality of maturation,
- Epileptiform activity.

These are defined in Table 6.2.1 and will be described subsequently in more detail.

Background Abnormality

Neonates typically cycle through wakefulness and sleep many times per day, usually once per hour. For this reason, neonatal EEG should at least be 60 min in duration to capture all stages. This will allow an assessment of state change which might not be seen during the 20–40 min of a "routine" EEG, but, for longer duration recordings can be reasonably interpreted as normal versus abnormal.

Excessive slow activity is difficult to identify in neonates since delta is normally such a prominent part of the record. Abnormal delta tends to be unilateral or diffuse, whereas normal delta is symmetrically regional (e.g., anterior). Abnormal delta tends to not respond to stimulation with attenuation, but this lack of reactivity is also normal in very young premature infants.

Amplitude asymmetries are abnormal if greater than 50% and consistent. Usually there are differences in frequency composition associated with

---

TABLE 6.2.1 NEONATAL ELECTROENCEPHALOGRAM (EEG) ABNORMALITIES

Type	Pattern	Description
Background abnormality	Excessive slow activity	Excessive slow activity can be difficult to diagnose with already-prominent delta. Pathologic delta is more widespread and lacks reactivity.
	Low voltage background	Low voltage suggests global cortical dysfunction. At the extreme of this, an isoelectric EEG can be a confirmatory test for brain death.
	Burst suppression pattern	Burst suppression can be difficulty to differentiate from a trace discontinu pattern, but when seen indicates severe cerebral functional disturbance.
	Asymmetric background	Asymmetry in background suggests a functional or structural lesion usually affecting the side with the lower and less rich activity. Amplitude asymmetries are usually only significant for a difference of 50% or more. Intracranial and extracranial fluid collections are a common cause.
Abnormality of maturation	Dysmature	EEG background appears that of a younger conceptional age. Suggests encephalopathy.
Epileptiform abnormality	Focal discharges	Consistent localization of sharp waves, as opposed to normal sharp transients. Often occur in trains.
	Multifocal discharges	Multifocal sharp waves or spikes with an abnormal background, as opposed to normal multifocal transients.
	Rhythmic activity	Rhythmic activity in the alpha or theta range is usually abnormal and can be epileptiform even in the absence of a sharp component.
	Pseudo-beta-alpha-theta-delta	Ictal discharge beginning in the beta range and slowing to the delta range.

amplitude asymmetry as well. Note that both intracranial and extracranial pathology can result in amplitude asymmetry; for example, subdural, subgaleal, or scalp hematomas can all produce attenuation of EEG over the affected area.

Low-voltage EEG in non-rapid eye movement (non-REM) sleep usually indicates a global abnormality in cortical function. Note that REM sleep might also be associated with a low-voltage background, so recording of all stages of sleep is important. Also, bilateral subdural hematomas can produce symmetric attenuation and therefore may be missed on EEG.

Isoelectric EEG can be a confirmatory test for brain death in neonates, but there are special considerations concerning diagnosis of brain death in neonates.

Burst suppression can be difficult to differentiate from a normal discontinuous Tracé discontinu (TD) pattern. If truly present however, the implication is usually the result of a global cerebral process such as ischemia and anoxia. Burst suppression is differentiated from a normal discontinuous pattern usually by knowledge of conceptional age with an expectation of the degree of discontinuity, reactivity of the background if the patient is old enough, and clinical information.

There can be a disconnect in the appearance of the EEG and clinical evaluation of premature infants. Preterm infants can manifest a markedly abnormal neurologic exam with little or no abnormality in EEG and vice versa. Suffice it to say that the EEG and the examination are evaluated independently and then should be interpreted in concert.

MATURATION

Abnormalities of Maturation

Dysmature pattern is typically an EEG appearance that is "younger" than expected for conceptional age.

For example, a discontinuous pattern with an interburst interval of more than 1 min would be considered normal at 26 weeks but would be distinctly abnormal at 36 weeks. A dysmature pattern is usually interpreted as a neonatal encephalopathy, but no specific etiology can be inferred from such findings.

Persistent dysmaturity is associated with poor neurologic outcome, but transient dysmaturity can be associated with no long-term neurologic sequelae.

Abnormalities Dependent on Maturation

Maturation of the EEG requires that the EEG reader's expectation of background be able to change commensurate with the age of the patient. Posterior slow waves of youth are normal in a child through to early adult life, but similar waves in middle or advanced age are likely physiologically different and pathologic. A discontinuous pattern is still seen in a normal term infant, to a certain extent, but would be distinctly abnormal at 6 months of age.

Certain EEG rhythms can look remarkably similar yet be of totally different implication depending on age. Sleep spindles in young children can be prolonged yet are normal when they first appear. Almost identical patterns in preterm infants are not sleep spindles and can represent an ictal pattern.

A markedly discontinuous pattern is normal in a very premature infant but in an older child or adult an almost identical appearance can be a burst suppression pattern, indicative of severe cerebral dysfunction. Similarly, this burst suppression pattern can be due to a cerebral destructive process or to medication-induced coma, with the distinction between these on EEG basis alone difficult if not impossible to make in some circumstances.[1]

EPILEPTIFORM ACTIVITY

Epileptiform abnormalities in neonates can have markedly difference appearance from epileptiform abnormalities in older children and adults. The abnormalities are usually focal or multifocal but seldom generalized since pathways facilitating spread and generalization are not fully developed.

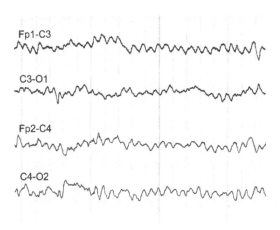

FIGURE 6.2.1 Rhythmic discharge in a neonate.

Focal discharges can be midline/vertex, right, or left. Differentiation from normal sharp transients is usually by a consistent localization of pathologic sharp waves and occurrence of abnormal sharp activity in trains; normal sharp transients usually do not occur in trains with consistent interval. Trains of discharges can have an unimpressive sharp component so that they appear like a run of fast activity in the alpha or theta range, but rhythmic activity in neonates is not normal, helping with differentiation from normal activity. Differentiation of rhythmic fast activity from a normal delta brush is by absence of the underlying delta wave and longer duration

of the rhythmic train with seizure activity (Figure 6.2.1).

Focal discharges often correlate with focal seizures, but the correlation between discharge location and clinical motor manifestation is not as good as in older children and adults. Also, focal discharges in neonates do not always have as strong a correlation with focal structural lesions, as in older individuals. Most epileptiform discharges are surface-negative, as in older individuals. Surface-positive discharges are seen in some infants with intracerebral hemorrhage, but this correlation is far from being highly sensitive or specific. Restricted spread patterns are sometimes

TABLE 6.2.2 PEDIATRIC EPILEPTIC ENCEPHALOPATHIES

Disorder	Clinical	Electroencephalogram (EEG)
Early infantile epileptic encephalopathy (EIEE or Ohtahara syndrome)	Early seizures, even in utero. Tonic spasms especially but also tonic-clonic, clonic, myoclonic, atonic, absence, focal impaired awareness. May progress to West or Lennox-Gastaut syndrome.	Burst suppression in waking and sleep states, often asymmetric.
Early myoclonic encephalopathy (also known as neonatal myoclonic encephalopathy	Myoclonus which can be subtle or pronounced, often shifting in location. Onset in first months. May have subtle partial seizures, tonic seizures. Epileptic spasms may develop. Developmental delay.	Burst suppression, often asymmetric. Eventually hypsarrhythmia.
Infantile spasms and West syndrome	West syndrome is a triad of infantile spasms, developmental delay, and hypsarrhythmia.	Hypsarrhythmia.
Severe myoclonic epilepsy of infancy (SMEI or Dravet syndrome)	Initially clonic seizures with fever in the first year. Often focal but may be generalized. Status epilepticus common. Later afebrile, with myoclonic seizures and photosensitivity. Often developmental slowing with worsening seizures.	Normal early, later polyspike and spike-wave discharges, focal or generalized. Some show a photoparoxysmal response.
Childhood epileptic encephalopathy (Lennox-Gastaut syndrome or LGS)	Multiple seizure types with developmental regression. May have especially tonic, atonic, and/or absence seizures. May also have myoclonic, generalized tonic-clonic, or partial-onset seizures.	Slow spike-and-wave discharges at 1.5–2 Hz. Slow background in most, becoming more disorganized in sleep
Acquired epileptic aphasia (AEA, Landau-Kleffner syndrome)	Progressive regression of language function in previously normal children, usually both receptive and expressive but one may predominate. Seizures in most, especially focal impaired awareness with atypical absence appearance or generalized.	Spike-and-wave discharges of high amplitude, especially temporal bilaterally, but also may be multifocal or generalized, especially in non-rapid eye movement (REM) sleep.

seen as well, with only a single electrode appearing to be involved with seizures. This is likely again due to immature myelination but such findings should be carefully reviewed for artifacts, such as intermittent poor contact with a single electrode on the scalp.

Multifocal discharges are differentiated from normal multifocal sharp transients by an otherwise abnormal background, occurrence of the discharges in trains, and associated clinical seizures. The seizures may be subtle but are usually clonic and also frequently involve eye movements.

Pseudo-beta-alpha-theta-delta is descriptive pattern of a discharge that starts at high frequency and slows. Beginning frequency is usually at least 8–12/sec, and the frequency slows to 0.5–3/sec. The appearance can be smooth or sharp. Associated seizures are clonic, myoclonic, or subtle, and, as such, this is an ictal pattern. The most common cause is perinatal asphyxia, often with a poor prognosis. The decrease in frequency can have the appearance of dropping to a harmonic of an original frequency.

Seizures in neonates, as in older patients, occasionally are associated with no EEG abnormality on scalp recording. In these circumstances, the generator is presumed to be subcortical or at least not involving cortex close to the scalp. Seizures of subcortical origin in neonates usually indicate severe damage, with the failure of cortical projection being a manifestation of this damage. A careful review of semiology is needed as most neonatal seizures are stereotypical. Alternative nonepileptic diagnoses such as movement disorders and normal physiological movements of neonates should also be considered.

Many of the abnormalities seen in the pediatric population are discussed in the broad presentation of epileptiform and nonepileptiform abnormalities. Some findings are shared between children and adults (e.g., focal and generalized spikes or slowing). But some are specific to a pediatric population (e.g., central temporal sharp waves associated with benign epilepsy with centrotemporal spikes, hypsarrhythmia).

Young children may develop progressive encephalopathies associated with epileptic and/ or myoclonic seizures. These have been classified by International League Against Epilepsy as *epileptic encephalopathies*.[2] In general, they tend to be refractory to many anti-seizure medications. Some of the most important types are discussed in Table 6.2.2. The genetic underpinnings of these disorders are increasingly being discovered.

6.3

Pediatric Seizures

KEVIN C. ESS

NEONATAL SEIZURES

Preterm and term infants often have seizures due to multiple etiologies. A large multicenter study reported the most common clinical associations being hypoxic ischemic encephalopathy (HIE) (33%) and intracranial hemorrhage (ICH) (27%).[1] This same study found that subclinical seizures were seen more often in preterm (24%) compared to term infants (14%).

Preterm neonatal seizures tend to be associated with a higher mortality than term neonates with seizures. Also, they tend to be less responsive to anti-seizure medications (ASMs),[2] which may reflect in part immaturity of the gamma-aminobutyric acid (GABA) transport system. Seizures in these patients can have varied clinical manifestations including tonic seizures, tonic gaze deviation, and clonic activity of individual limbs. Subclinical or subtle seizures are also seen, although infrequently, and may only manifest with changes in vital signs.

EPILEPTIC ENCEPHALOPATHY

Epileptic Spasms

Epileptic spasms (ES) are historically termed *infantile spasms* (IS) and are classically diagnosed when a child with clonic/flexion spasms has hypsarrhythmia on electroencephalogram (EEG). *West syndrome* is a subset of ES with developmental delay and regression.[3] Classification is made complex because some patients have delay and regression before they have spasms, and many children with either adequately or inadequately treated ES ultimately will have an intellectual disability, consistent with an overall diagnosis of epileptic encephalopathy. For an EEG diagnosis, frank hypsarrhythmia is usually seen with advanced untreated cases, but some patients on the other end of the spectrum can have normal EEG while awake but multifocal epileptiform patterns and characteristic electrodecrement patterns emerging only during sleep. Figures 6.3.1 and 6.3.2 show examples.

Historically, first-line management of ES in the United States was intramuscular adrenocorticotropic hormone (ACTH). High-dose oral glucocorticoids can also be used, with some studies suggesting a lower response rate. Vigabatrin is used in much of the world and increasingly so in the United States. Other drugs are sometimes used such as valproate, topiramate, or zonisamide. However, there is considerably less clinical data to support the use of these drugs. Side effects with ACTH/glucocorticoids can be extreme, with marked irritability, hypertension, and insulin resistance. Vigabatrin can cause permanent peripheral visual loss and also can lead to white matter abnormalities seen on brain magnetic resonance imaging (MRI).

Lennox-Gastaut Syndrome

Lennox-Gastaut syndrome (LGS) is an epileptic encephalopathy with a characteristic EEG pattern and types of seizures (Figure 6.3.3). Patients ultimately have cognitive deficits with drug-resistant seizures, often of multiple types.[4] These include atonic (drop) seizures as well as tonic, tonic-clonic, and absence-type seizures. Many experts require tonic seizures for the diagnosis as well as an intellectual disability and onset before the age of 10 years. Functional neuroimaging suggests LGS is from "secondary network epilepsy" with complex brain dysfunction involving cortical and subcortical structures, with the distinctly abnormal pattern of increased activity of both the resting (default mode) network as well as the "attention" network.[5]

The causes of LGS are varied and cannot always be identified. LGS is associated with multiple etiologies including HIE, meningoencephalitis, tuberous sclerosis complex, and other chromosomal, genetic, and metabolic disorders. Emerging evidence suggests that both ES and LGS are epileptic

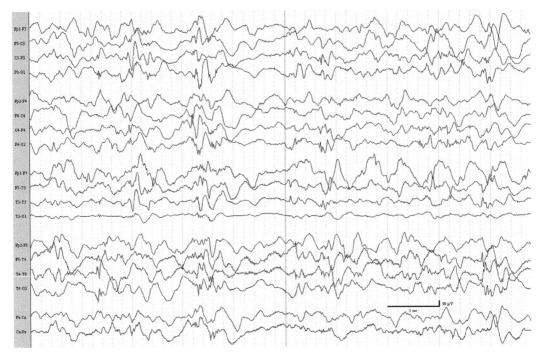

FIGURE 6.3.1 Hypsarrhythmia. Longitudinal bipolar montage.

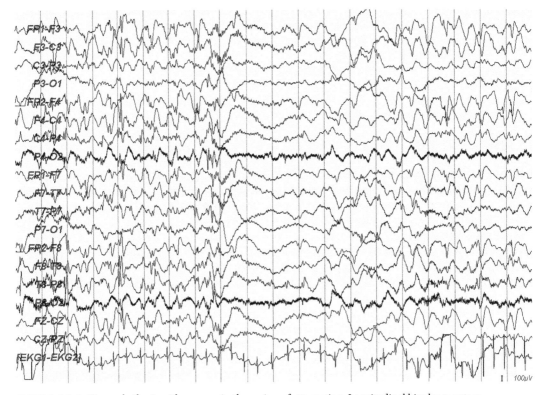

FIGURE 6.3.2 Hypsarrhythmia with a spasm in the region of attenuation. Longitudinal bipolar montage.

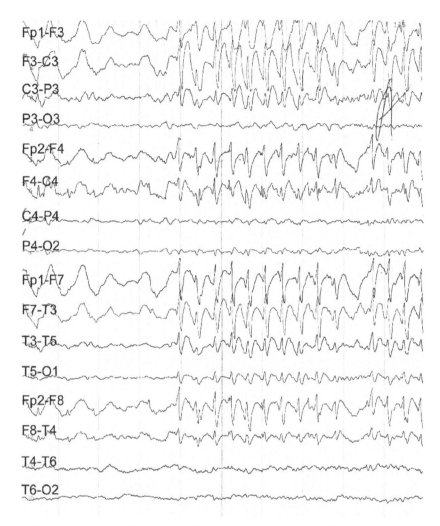

FIGURE 6.3.3 Lennox-Gastaut syndrome. Atypical absence seizure. Longitudinal bipolar montage.

encephalopathies with age-dependent clinical and EEG manifestations because many patients with ES go on to have LGS syndrome when older.

EEG in LGS classically features *slow spike-wave* (SSW) complexes (Figure 6.3.4). Frequency is less than 2.5 Hz. Some but not all slow waves are associated with a spike or sharp wave. Tonic seizures in LGS are associated with overall voltage attenuation and are reminiscent of the electrodecrement patterns seen in ES but, again, with age-dependent clinical manifestations.

Management of the seizures in LGS is typically with valproate, topiramate, or lamotrigine but other agents are also used including levetiracetam, clobazam, rufinamide, zonisamide, and cannabinoids. Nonpharmacologic therapy includes ketogenic diet, corpus callosotomy, or vagal nerve stimulation (VNS). Treatment does not alter the poor functional prognosis but may reduce the debilitating nature of the seizures, particularly the atonic/drop seizures which often lead to secondary head and facial injuries.

Rasmussen Encephalitis

Rasmussen encephalitis, also known as Rasmussen syndrome is an inflammatory disorder affecting one hemisphere and producing focal seizures and hemiparesis. The etiology is unknown, and although there is an inflammatory component, no focused interventions to target the presumed underlying pathophysiology has proved effective.[6] The initial presentation is usually focal-onset seizures with or without hemiparesis which initially may seem mild and controllable with medications. With progression over time, there is worsening hemiparesis and seizures, with about half

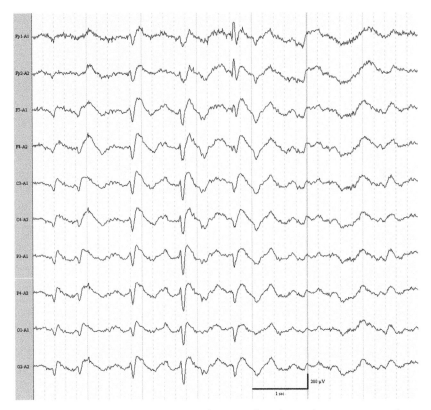

FIGURE 6.3.4 Slow spike-wave in Lennox Gastaut syndrome. Ipsilateral ear reference, parasagittal portion.

developing *epilepsy partialis continua* (EPC). Figure 6.3.5 shows the interictal EEG from a child with Rasmussen encephalitis. Figure 6.3.6 shows an ictal recording from the same patient.

MRI early on may be normal but subsequent studies reveal hemiatrophy, initially seen as enlargement of one lateral ventricle, with more diffuse atrophy then seen.

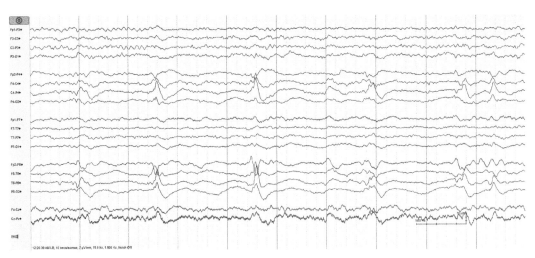

FIGURE 6.3.5 Electroencephalogram (EEG) of child with Rasmussen encephalitis (interictal). Longitudinal bipolar montage.

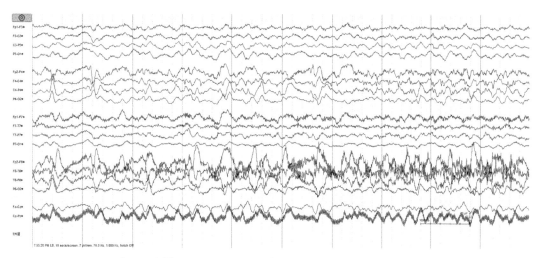

FIGURE 6.3.6 Figure of same child as in Figure 6.3.5, with Rasmussen encephalitis (seizure). Longitudinal bipolar montage.

EEG can show a variety of findings, but slowing over the affected hemisphere is common with localized interictal discharges, but eventually with more frequent discharges, EPC, and frank electrographic seizures. Interictal discharges can be seen over the contralateral unaffected hemisphere with further progression.

Management with multiple ASMs alone or in combination is often suboptimal with refractory seizures, especially EPC. Given the presumed pathophysiology, immune-modulating therapies have been tried but there is minimal evidence of efficacy for seizures or slowing the progression of hemiparesis. Surgical approaches are often employed, with the best successes seen with either anatomical or functional hemispherectomy. This dramatic intervention has the potential to stop seizures, particularly the spread of seizures to the contralateral hemisphere. Hemiparesis is often already present at time of surgery and weakness may stabilize or worsen depending on the age of the patient, seizure duration, and other factors that influence brain plasticity. For select younger patients, language centers of the left hemisphere can shift to the right side of the brain due to the frequent left hemispheric seizures or can be relearned following a left hemispherectomy.

Severe Myoclonic Epilepsy of Infancy: Dravet Syndrome

Severe myoclonic epilepsy of infancy (SMEI) or *Dravet syndrome* is characterized by recurrent tonic-clonic or hemi-convulsive seizures, often myoclonic or atypical absence seizures,

exacerbation by hyperthermia, and initial normal physical and intellectual development. Many patients present with febrile status epilepticus. As a syndrome, the diagnosis was initially made on clinical features alone without a confirmatory genetic test. However, loss of function mutations in the *SCN1A* gene account for almost all cases. MRI is usually normal. EEG shows no specific features. Intellectual disability develops between 18 months and 5 years. Motor deficits develop by 3–4 years with hypotonia, poor coordination, and abnormal gait.

An excellent consensus report by Wirrell et al.[7] should be consulted by providers evaluating and managing these patients.

EEG shows background slowing with focal and generalized interictal discharges. Photoparoxysmal response are common. Figures 6.3.7 and 6.3.8 show ictal and interictal examples from a patient with Dravet.

First-line management of the seizures is often with clobazam or valproate, and if one does not produce adequate control they are often used together. Second-line agents include stiripentol, topiramate, levetiracetam, zonisamide, and rufinamide. Newer drugs that are approved by the US Food and Drug Administration (FDA) for Dravet syndrome include cannabinoids and fenfluramine.

ABSENCE EPILEPSY

Childhood absence epilepsy (CAE) is characterized by typical staring type "absence" seizures and usually seen in children with normal physical,

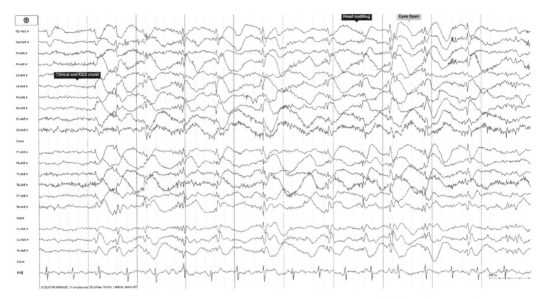

FIGURE 6.3.7 Severe myoclonic epilepsy of infancy. Dravet patient with seizure of high amplitude. Right peri-vertex more than left; discharges with clinical correlate of head nodding. Average reference montage.

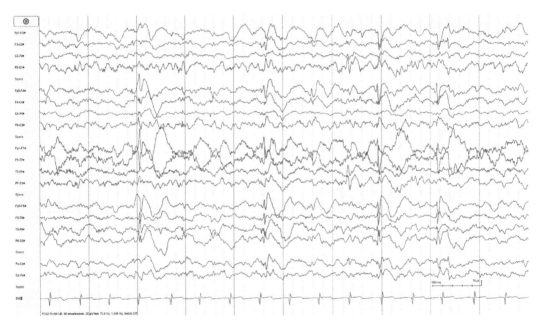

FIGURE 6.3.8 An interictal example from same patient as in Figure 6.3.7. Generalized discharges. Longitudinal bipolar montage.

intellectual, and behavioral development. Females are more often affected than males. Typical absence seizures are subdivided into *simple* and *complex*.

Simple absence seizures are characterized by an abrupt loss of activity and response, often with the appearance of a staring spell. There is no loss of posture. There is also no aura, and there is no

post-ictal confusion. After the event, patients usually immediately resume what they were doing prior to the episode.

Complex absence seizures are characterized by similar staring spells but with positive findings which can be diverse, such as twitching of the mouth or arms, eye blinks, some loss of postural tone, and occasionally incontinence in the absence of generalized motor activity.

EEG of patients with typical CAE shows the iconic *3-per-second spike-and-wave discharges* with an abrupt onset and offset. Frequency of the discharge, however, often starts a bit faster than 3 Hz and slows slightly during the discharge, with a common progression being approximately 4 Hz reducing to 2.5 Hz (Figure 6.3.9). After cessation of the discharge, the pre-ictal background is restored. Brief discharges, perhaps 5 sec or less, may be accompanied by no clinical event although active engagement with the patient may reveal a clinical accompaniment to even brief (2–3 sec) discharges. Events are often precipitated by hyperventilation, hence when absence epilepsy is suspected, sustained hyperventilation should be performed during the EEG. Hypoglycemia can augment the discharge, but this is not specific for absence epilepsy since hypoglycemia can also augment and precipitate focal discharges.

Some patients will develop absence status which has a clinical appearance quite different from typical brief absence seizures. This is seen most commonly in adults.

The clinical onset of CAE is approximately 5–7 years of age, with most patients remitting by age 10–14 years although some may remit sooner. Multiple medications can be used, with ethosuximide, levetiracetam, lamotrigine, and valproic acid seemingly the most effective and well-tolerated. Drugs for focal seizures such as carbamazepine and oxcarbazepine should be avoided as they may exacerbate generalized seizures.

Juvenile absence epilepsy (JAE) can be very similar in seizure semiology as well as EEG patterns as CAE. However, this group of patients usually starts having seizures around age 10–14, a time when patients with CAE are usually remitting. Furthermore, patients with JAE often do not grow out of their seizures and may have lifelong epilepsy. Many patients with JAE go on to develop more than just absence seizures, particularly myoclonic seizures, and they often will ultimately meet criteria for juvenile myoclonic epilepsy (JME).

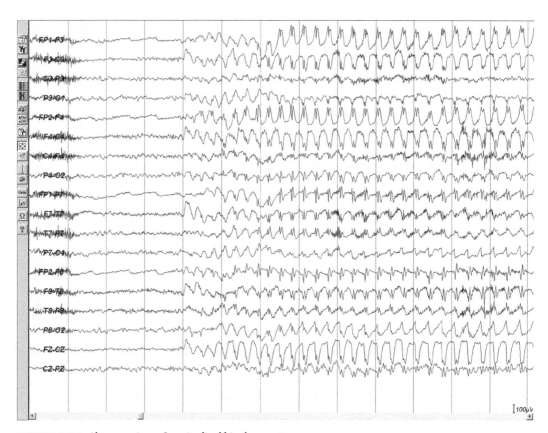

FIGURE 6.3.9 Absence seizure. Longitudinal bipolar montage.

JUVENILE MYOCLONIC EPILEPSY

JME presents with seizures of various types usually around puberty. Myoclonic seizures are common and required for diagnosis.[8] Absence seizures can occur and, as detailed earlier, can be the presenting seizure type for years. Generalized tonic-clonic seizures are also common in these patients. The myoclonic seizures can be unilateral or bilateral, involving multiple muscle groups. Consciousness may or may not be disturbed, and there may be brief unresponsiveness similar to absence seizures.

EEG in JME usually has a normal background with superimposed 3–6 Hz spike-wave discharges which are generalized but with a frontal predominance (Figures 6.3.10 and 6.3.11). Myoclonic events are associated with irregular polyspike discharges, usually generalized. A minority of patients exhibit focal or significantly lateralized generalized discharges or fragments of generalized discharges which can make interpretation difficult.

SELF-LIMITED FOCAL EPILEPSIES OF CHILDHOOD

With the revised classification of epilepsies, what used to be termed *benign focal epilepsies* are now called *self-limited focal epilepsies of childhood*.

Benign epilepsy with centrotemporal spikes (BECTS) was previously termed *benign rolandic epilepsy*, but this term had fallen out of favor even before the new classification.

Typical clinical presentation is of a 7- to 10-year-old child with normal intellectual and motor development who presents with nocturnal episodes of unilateral sensory and motor symptoms. A common report, if the child recalls, is of tingling and then later clonic activity of one side of the face. This are often accompanied by guttural sounds and vocalizations leading to much parental/caregiver anxiety. The seizures are usually not frequent, and some providers may opt to not start daily ASM, reasoning that infrequent seizures that will spontaneously remit are less of an overall risk than side effects of years of daily medications. This decision needs to be individualized with each patient. The seizures abate by adolescence.

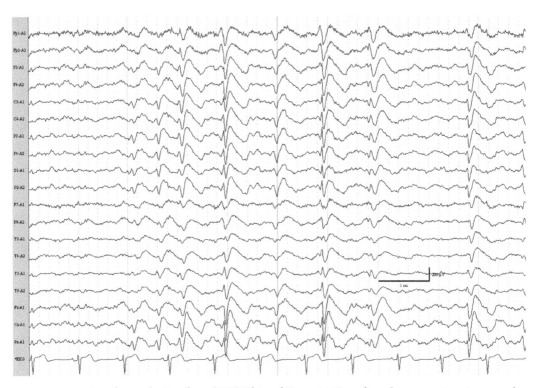

FIGURE 6.3.10 Juvenile myoclonic epilepsy (JME). This and Figure 6.3.11 are from the same patient. Average reference montage.

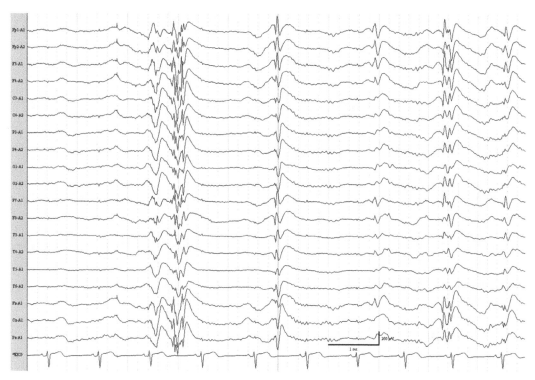

FIGURE 6.3.11 Juvenile myoclonic epilepsy (JME). Same patient as in Figure 6.3.10, with polyspikes. Average reference montage.

EEG shows central to mid-temporal high-voltage sharp waves, sometimes extending to parietal sharp waves which are activated during sleep (Figure 6.3.12). They have a distinctive morphology and have a lateral dipole, with positive polarity seen in the anterior leads and negative polarity in the central/temporal (rolandic sulcus) region. Many patients have either left or right discharges on any individual routine EEG, but longer EEG or subsequent studies can reveal independent discharges involving both hemispheres.

Benign occipital epilepsy has been studied in depth by Panayiotopoulos.[9] Patients most commonly present with emesis but also visual or ocular motor symptoms. EEG discharges are occipital predominant, but they commonly extend into adjacent posterior temporal and parietal regions (Figure 6.3.13). As patients get older, the interictal discharges can move more anterior and even can take on a generalized appearance. The diagnosis of benign occipital epilepsy then can still be made in an older child who no longer has occipital discharges but a compatible history.

Panayiotopoulos syndrome typically is associated with normal MRI and normal neurologic development. Treatment is with a variety of commonly used agents, and the disorder seems to be quite responsive to pharmacologic therapy. Most patients remit having seizures by 16 years of age.

LANDAU-KLEFFNER SYNDROME (LKS)

Landau-Kleffner syndrome (LKS) is also called *acquired epileptic aphasia.* Patients present with regression in language, often with apparent deafness, associated with behavioral abnormalities.[10] More than half, but not all, develop clinical seizures. The seizures can have a variety of manifestations, including focal clonic, focal to bilateral tonic-clonic, absence, and atonic.

EEG often shows interictal focal discharges, usually in midtemporal regions, while in the awake state (Figure 6.3.14). In the sleep state, *continuous spike-and-wave during sleep* (CSWS) can be seen, but bilateral focal discharges can also be seen along with focal temporal discharges.[11] MRI is typically normal.

A variety of medications have been used including clobazam and ethosuximide, but large series examining efficacy are lacking. Some patients recover language function but others

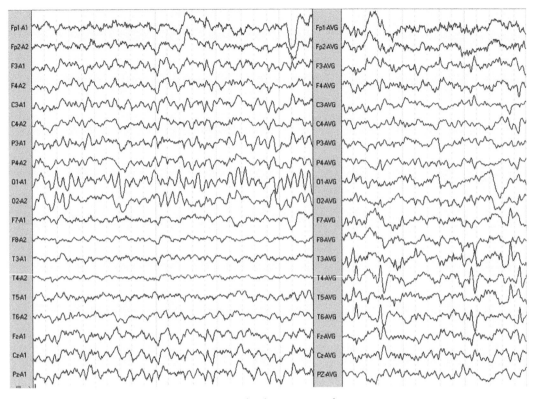

FIGURE 6.3.12 Benign epilepsy with centrotemporal spikes. Average reference montage.

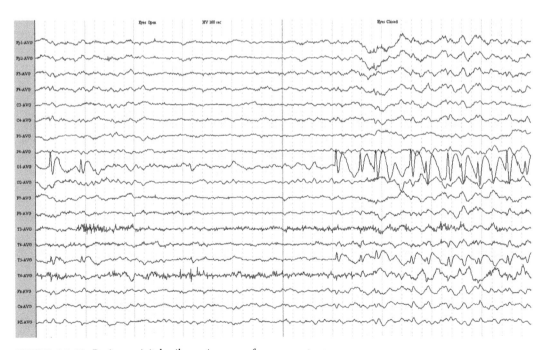

FIGURE 6.3.13 Benign occipital epilepsy. Average reference montage.

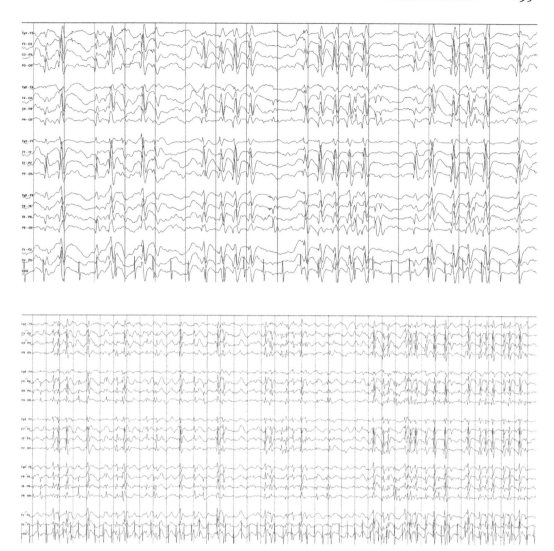

FIGURE 6.3.14 Landau-Kleffner patient. (Top: normal timebase; Bottom: compressed timebase) This 8-year-old boy started having language regression at age 6. Despite treatment with corticosteroids, he had no improvement. Language improvement was seen after nightly high doses of diazepam with electroencephalogram (EEG) improvement as well. Weaning of diazepam was associated with worsening language and return of floridly abnormal sleep EEG. High-amplitude discharges seen with compression of EEG time course to better appreciate frequency of generalized discharges. Longitudinal bipolar montage.

are left with language deficit. Of note, the initial patients described were not actually deaf, but their epileptic receptive aphasia was so severe that they seemed to be unable to hear.

CONTINUOUS SPIKE-AND-WAVE DURING SLEEP

This is a diagnosis made by EEG findings. Patients usually already have a diagnosis of epilepsy. There is very often development of cognitive deficits and often language deterioration with elements of aphasia. Myoclonic or absence seizures or even focal seizures may develop during the day. During sleep there are pathognomonic generalized spike and slow wave activity especially during deeper Stages 3 and 4 of slow-wave sleep (Figure 6.3.15). The electrographic events can be prolonged and take up most of the sleeping record. The discharges may be absent during an awake and light sleep (Stage 1–2) office recording, so the diagnosis may be missed in a routine office evaluation.

Medications for seizures with CSWS are multiple and include valproate, levetiracetam, clobazam, and ethosuximide.[12] Steroids and/or

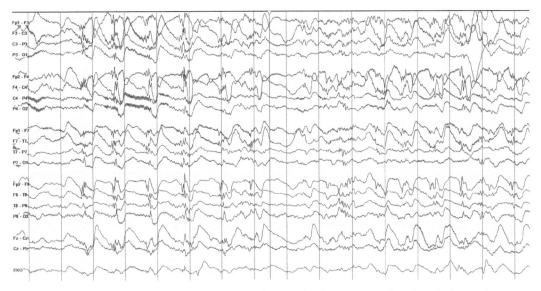

FIGURE 6.3.15 Continuous spike wave in sleep (CSWS). Generalized-appearing epileptiform discharges during Stage 3 sleep. Longitudinal bipolar montage.

intravenous immunoglobulin (IVIG) are used by some, but this should generally be managed only by a pediatric epilepsy specialist. An alternative term commonly used is *electrical status epilepticus during sleep* (ESES).

ATYPICAL BENIGN PARTIAL EPILEPSY

Atypical benign partial epilepsy (ABPE) is a very rare condition characterized by multiple types of seizures, focal or generalized. CSWS is often seen.[13] There are often neurocognitive and language deficits looking clinically like LKS. Few patients have been studied in depth to determine if this is a distinct syndrome or a variant of LKS.

FEBRILE SEIZURES

Febrile seizures are a common condition evaluated by pediatricians and neurologists. By definition, it is a seizure secondary to fever which is not associated with infection of the central nervous system (CNS) (e.g., meningitis or metabolic disorder caused by systemic illness such as hyponatremia or hypoglycemia). Between 2% and 5% of children have at least one febrile seizure with some variability seen in different racial backgrounds. Age range for children with febrile seizures is usually between 5 months and 5 years, but occasional patients younger and older than this range are seen. The first febrile seizure, however, should be seen at less than 3 years of age. Peak incidence is 18–24 months.[14]

Ictal manifestations are varied and can be generalized tonic-clonic or tonic or other symptomatology which may or may not have been an actual seizure. For the purpose of prognostication, febrile seizures are divided into *simple* and *complex*. *Simple febrile seizures* are single generalized seizures of less than 15 min duration associated with fever. *Complex febrile seizures* are otherwise, in that they can be longer than 15 min, recur within 24 hours, or have focal features.

EEG if obtained soon after the seizure is typically normal but may show slowing. Focal findings are uncommon and when present suggest injury or an underlying structural abnormality. Most neurologists do not consider EEG essential for children with simple febrile seizures but usually recommend them for complex febrile seizures. Even here the yield is low as almost all children, even those with complex febrile seizures, "grow out" of this condition.[15] It is uncommon for children, in general, with febrile seizures to later have afebrile seizures but this can be seen in genetic epilepsies, for example mutation of the *SCN1A* gene causing generalized epilepsy with febrile seizures plus (GEFS+) or Dravet syndrome.[16,17]

The principal reasons for neurologic consultation are to advise on risk of recurrence and need for treatment, if any. The overall risk of subsequent unprovoked afebrile seizures is approximately 2–5%. This risk is higher than that seen for the general population but usually by itself does not warrant treatment with ASMs. The risk of future unprovoked afebrile seizure is increased in patients with febrile status epilepticus, complex febrile seizure, and neurologic abnormality in exam or development. ASMs are generally not warranted, and do not lower the risk for subsequent unprovoked seizures. Phenobarbital has been shown to decrease the likelihood of future febrile seizures but adverse events from this medication are not thought to be worth the benefit. In addition, benzodiazepines have also been employed for bridge therapy during febrile episodes by some neurologists but is generally not recommended; it is again generally accepted that adverse event risk exceeds benefit for most children.

PART 7

Differential Diagnosis

7.1

Overview

KARL E. MISULIS AND HASAN H. SONMEZTURK

The differential diagnosis of seizures includes a host of nonepileptic events, physiological as well as psychological. The most common conditions in the differential diagnosis vary somewhat with age: transient ischemic attacks (TIAs) and transient global amnesia (TGA) are important conditions in the differential diagnosis in advanced age, but less likely in younger individuals. Psychogenic nonepileptic events, syncope, and some sleep disorders imitate epilepsy through much of the lifespan.

In this book, we have been using the term *nonepileptic events* rather than *nonepileptic seizures* and will continue to use this terminology here. The term "psychogenic nonepileptic events" (PNE) is the former "psychogenic nonepileptic seizure." *Physiologic nonepileptic events* include conditions which could be mistaken for seizures yet are not psychogenic, such as syncope, movement disorders, cataplexy, narcolepsy, TIA, TGA, and others.

Table 7.1.1 lists some common disorders that can be mistaken for seizures.

TABLE 7.1.1 DISORDERS OFTEN MISTAKEN FOR SEIZURES

Disorder	Features
Psychogenic nonepileptic events	Psychogenic events resembling clinical seizure without abnormalities in electroencephalogram (EEG) activity. Majority of these patients suffer from a true psychiatric disorder such as conversion disorder and often are nonmalingerers
Syncope	Syncope is episodic loss of consciousness due to hypoperfusion of the brain. About 80% of syncopes occur with associated variable level rhythmic or isolated but repeating clonus in upper and lower extremities and torso.
Cardiac arrhythmia	Many patients with cardiac arrhythmia may experience loss of consciousness events with similar clinical characteristics as syncope.
Dementia	Particularly patients with episodic altered mental status (sundowning) or hallucinations.
Parkinson disease	Particularly patients with freezing episodes.
Hyperventilation/Panic attacks	Acute short-lasting anxiety or panic attacks can mimic certain seizure types, particularly insular lobe seizures.
Complicated migraines	Particularly patients with episodic motor or sensory symptoms.
Transient ischemic attacks	These cause episodic and temporary motor, speech, visual, or other sensory symptoms which often can be interpreted as seizures.
Transient global amnesia	Sudden unexplained confusional state and memory impairment.
Various metabolic disorders	Electrolyte imbalances, hypo- or hyperglycemia.
Sleep myoclonus	Periodic jerks of the legs during sleep. Interferes with quality of sleep.
Parasomnia	Include confusional arousals, narcolepsy, night terrors, sleep-walking, and some cases of nocturnal bed-wetting. Can be mistaken for ictal or post-ictal effect.

TABLE 7.1.1 CONTINUED

Disorder	Features
Chorea and other paroxysmal movement disorders	Irregular stereotypic movements of the extremities.
	Due to disorder of the basal ganglia.
	Can be so pronounced that EEG may be required for differentiation.
Sandifer syndrome (reflux)	Torsional dystonia mainly involving the neck and shoulders.
	Associated with hiatal hernia or esophageal reflux.
Behavioral, staring, or motor events in patients with cognitive disabilities	Repetitive movements can develop in children with mental retardation.
	Can resemble seizure activity because of repetitive stereotypic movements.
Breath-holding spells	Children may hold their breath until they lose consciousness.
	Subsets include pallid and cyanotic breath-holding spells.
Cough syncope	Loss of consciousness associated with decreased cerebral perfusion.
	Most often seen in individuals with chronic obstructive pulmonary disease (COPD), asthma, or other causes of chronic cough.
Nonepileptic myoclonus	Myoclonus during the day but not associated with EEG changes.
	Essential myoclonus is a common etiology. Subcortical or spinal myoclonus can occur in various disorders unrelated to epilepsy.
Startle	Startle can be seen in patients with certain types of epilepsy but also can be present in patients without seizures.
	Startle is present to a limited extent in normal subjects but also is enhanced by some psychological and neurologic disorders and is enhanced by some medicines.
Drug-induced encephalopathy (e.g., tiagabine)	Patients with seizures sometimes develop encephalopathy from their anti-epileptic medications, often but not invariably at high levels.
	Tiagabine encephalopathy may be mistaken for focal impaired awareness status epilepticus or post-ictal somnolence.
Violence	Directed violence is almost never epileptiform.
	Nondirected violence can be epileptiform, but usually is not.

7.2

Psychogenic Nonepileptic Events

KARL E. MISULIS

Psychogenic nonepileptic events (PNE) are emotionally triggered attacks that resemble seizures, but are not associated with epileptic seizure activity.[1] Approximately 20% of patients presenting to an epilepsy center with intractable epilepsy are found to have nonepileptic events. The term *pseudoseizures* should phased out in writing and practice. The incidence of PNE in the general population can reach up to 5 per 100,000 persons per year. There is a higher prevalence in women, who represent 70–80% of those affected.

Up to 10–15% of patients have both epileptic seizures and nonepileptic events.[2,3] Distinguishing the two can be difficult. We often have to teach the patient or family how to distinguish between them and ask for the frequency of each type of event.

CLINICAL PRESENTATIONS

A major role of epilepsy monitoring units is the differentiation of epileptic seizures from PNE, and video-electroencephalographic (EEG) monitoring has helped analyze the semiology of nonepileptic events. The spectrum of clinical presentations of nonepileptic events is almost as broad as that of epileptic seizures. PNE semiology can be classified into three categories[4,5]:

- PNE with generalized shaking,
- PNE with minor motor activity,
- PNE with motionless unresponsiveness or collapse.

Generalized shaking is the most common manifestation of PNE in adults and adolescents. Staring spells can occur as well, with clinical features that could be mistaken for absence or focal impaired awareness seizures. In children, prolonged staring and unresponsiveness was the most common pattern. Although there are many features that PNE have in common with epileptic seizures, there are some differentiating features.[6,7,8,9,10]

Clinical features that may suggest PNE, as opposed to generalized tonic-clonic seizure, include

- Responsiveness during a generalized convulsive seizure;
- Event usually precipitated by suggestion;
- Pelvic thrusting;
- Large-amplitude, side-to-side head movements;
- Asynchronous or alternating jerking of the two sides (as opposed to synchronous jerking);
- Absence of whole-body rigidity before generalized jerking;
- Event can be terminated by the examiner by nonpharmacological means such as suggestion.
- Abrupt termination of the event, without a post-ictal period;
- Eyes closed during an event, particularly if there is resistance to eye opening;
- Shallow rapid respiration (as opposed to stertorous respiration).

No single clinical feature is sufficient for a diagnosis of PNE; a combination of features increases their value. Many of the listed clinical features can be seen frontal lobe focal impaired awareness seizures; however, PNE tend to be prolonged in duration, while frontal focal impaired awareness seizures are short in duration.

PNE usually do not start out of sleep. Seizures that clearly arise out of sleep are usually epileptic. However, PNE may arise out of a waking state, as evidenced by EEG, while the patient clinically appears asleep (pseudosleep).

Other features that favor PNE include:

- Discontinuous clinical seizure activity;
- Prolonged seizure duration (pseudostatus epilepticus);
- Eye fluttering;

- Dramatic vocalizations of choking, gagging, or gasping;
- Stuttering;
- Weeping and other emotional display;
- Excessive variability in seizure manifestations.

Despite these general guidelines, experienced neurophysiologists are commonly wrong in the clinical diagnosis of seizures because of the broad spectrum of how epileptic seizures and nonepileptic events can manifest. Vagal nerve stimulation (VNS) has even been placed in patients in whom PNE was ultimately documented.[11] Video-EEG monitoring with recording of typical attacks is crucial for the definitive diagnosis of PNE.

Suggestion may help trigger PNE; hyperventilation and photic stimulation are preferred suggestion techniques since they are usually in standard use for most patients in the EEG lab. If other suggestion methods are used, they should not involve patient deception. It is also important to be aware that some individuals are suggestible, so suggestion may precipitate events which are not typical of those under question. Family members may have to view the recorded events and verify that they are typical attacks.

It is important to keep in mind that some epileptic seizures may have no scalp EEG correlate; examples include cingulate or orbitofrontal focal impaired awareness seizures, supplementary motor seizures, and motor focal aware seizures. It is often necessary to record multiple attacks to evaluate if events are stereotyped. Frontal lobe seizures tend to be very stereotyped. In addition, they may demonstrate increased severity in association with anti-seizure medication (ASM) withdrawal. Secondary generalization is usually definitive proof that the initial manifestations are epileptic.

Urinary incontinence has been considered by some to be a differentiating feature between epileptic and nonepileptic events, but this is not the case if one depends on history; urinary incontinence has no significant differentiating value between epileptic, nonepileptic, and syncopal events.[12]

Tongue biting occurs more commonly with epileptic generalized tonic-clonic seizures but is also frequently reported by patients with PNE. Epileptic seizures are associated with biting the side of the tongue, while PNE are more likely to be associated with biting the tip of the tongue or the lip.

EEG MANIFESTATIONS

EEG Artifactual Patterns

EEG during a PNE is normal, although muscle and movement artifact may obscure the recording. Evaluation of the recording may depend on observing the EEG background immediately before and after the clinical seizure. Epileptic seizures have a slow and/or suppressed background after the seizure, whereas nonepileptic events show an EEG background that returns to normal immediately after the seizure artifact subsides (see Figure 7.2.1).

The patient in Figure 7.2.1 shows movement and muscle artifact, but there is no electrocerebral discharge associated with the clinical seizure activity. Movement during an epileptic or nonepileptic event can obscure the EEG, so that visualization or nonvisualization of electrographic seizure activity is not possible. The EEG activity immediately before and after the clinical seizure activity is evaluated to determine whether there is an abnormality that makes it more or less likely to be epileptic. This differentiation is described in Table 7.2.1 (see also Figures 7.2.2 and 7.2.3).

Evolution of EEGs of Nonepileptic Event with Tremor

Figures 7.2.4 are the recordings of a 26-year-old woman with recurrent PNE. The rhythmic activity represents artifact due to rhythmic coarse tremor.

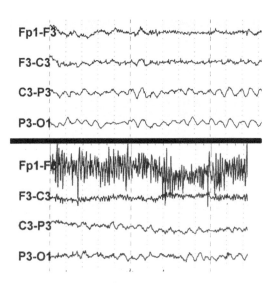

FIGURE 7.2.1 Nonepileptic event.

TABLE 7.2.1 DIFFERENTIATION OF EPILEPTIC FROM NONEPILEPTIC EVENT

Electroencephalogram (EEG) feature	Epileptic event	Nonepileptic event
EEG before event	May be normal or show focal or generalized discharges prior to the clinical seizure	Normal EEG
EEG during event	Electrocerebral discharge during the seizure	No electrocerebral discharge during the episode Muscle and movement artifact may obscure the recording
EEG after event	Slowed and often suppressed after the seizure	Normal, no post-ictal slowing or attenuation

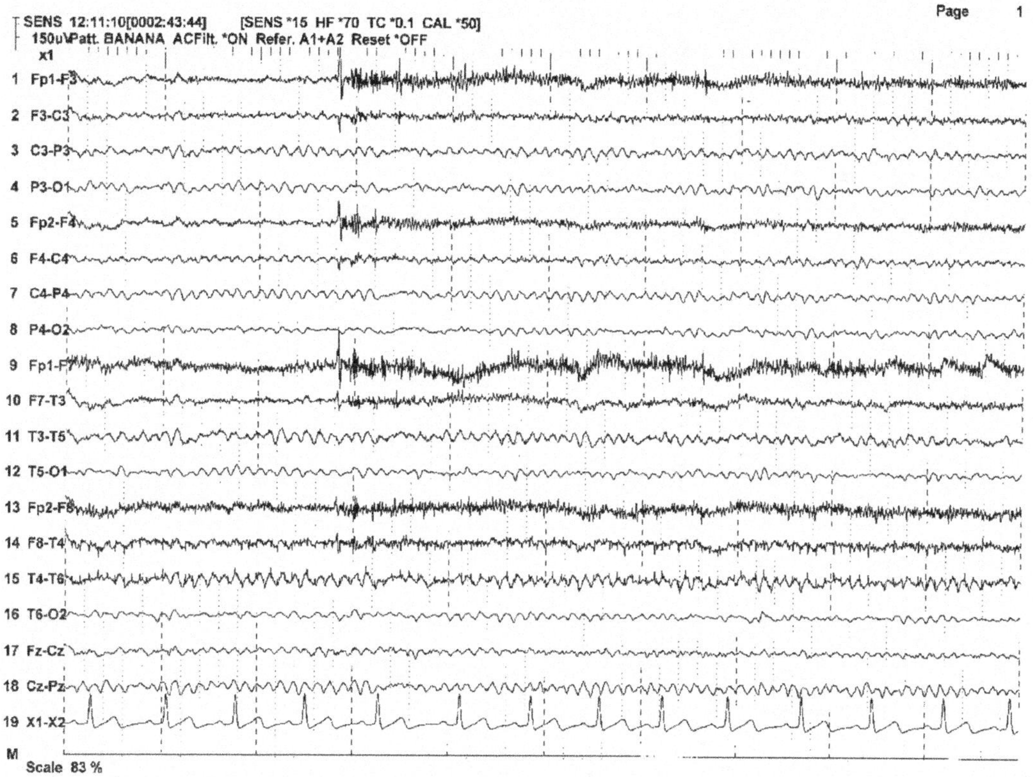

FIGURE 7.2.2 Nonepileptic event. Longitudinal bipolar montage.

Figure 7.2.4 shows rhythmic activity associated with clinical convulsive activity, which could easily be confused with epileptiform activity. The normal background is replaced by growing artifact from movements. There are no spikes in association with the slow activity. In addition, the frequency does not evolve during the course of the activity.

The page shown in Figure 7.2.5 directly follows the page shown in Figure 7.2.4. The repetitive slow activity continues at a constant frequency, without evolution in appearance of rhythm.

The last epoch of EEG (Figure 7.2.6) shows the end of the event, where the amplitude of the activity reduces until normal background returns. There is neither background slowing

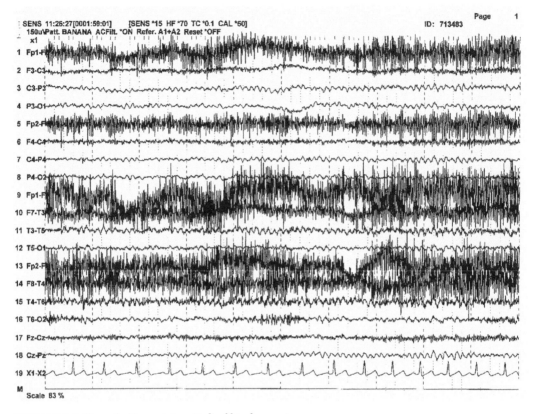

FIGURE 7.2.3 Nonepileptic event. Longitudinal bipolar montage.

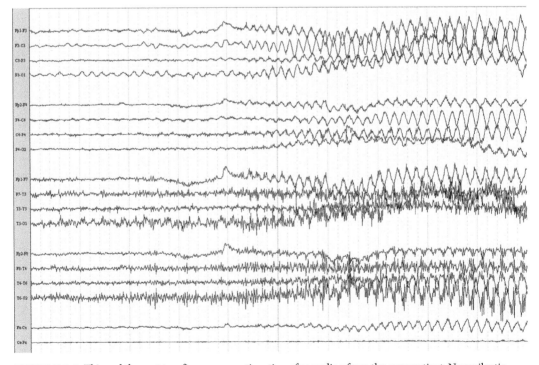

FIGURE 7.2.4 This and the next two figures are continuation of recording from the same patient. Nonepileptic event. Longitudinal bipolar montage.

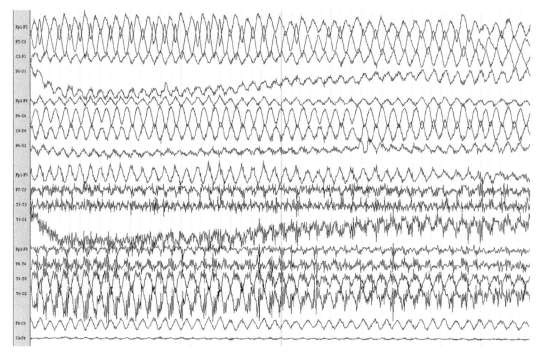

FIGURE 7.2.5 Nonepileptic event. Longitudinal bipolar montage.

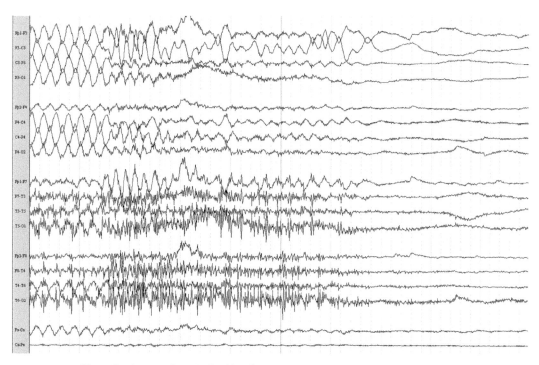

FIGURE 7.2.6 Nonepileptic event. Longitudinal bipolar montage.

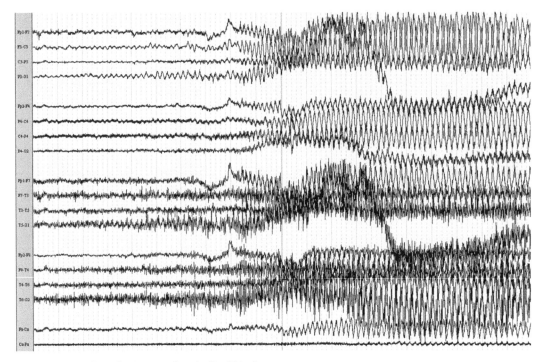

FIGURE 7.2.7 Nonepileptic event. Longitudinal bipolar montage.

nor attenuation, although reduction in amplitude results in an appearance of attenuation, especially if gain was reduced during the episode.

Termination of the event is associated with restoration of the normal background.

Observation of the same event at a slower time base (Figure 7.2.7) shows the monorhythmic character of the clinical seizure, quite different from the appearance of an epileptic seizure.

7.3

Syncope

KARL E. MISULIS

OVERVIEW

Syncope is transient loss of consciousness due to loss of brain perfusion, but the differential diagnosis of this final common path is wide. This is a form of *physiologic nonepileptic event*.

CAUSES OF SYNCOPE

The causes of syncope are multiple, some of which include:

- Cardiac arrhythmia,
- Orthostatic hypotension,
- Vasovagal ("neurocardiogenic") syncope,
- Orthostatic hypotension,
- Migraine,
- Vertebrobasilar insufficiency.

Most causes of syncope are preceded by a sensation of lightheadedness. However, the duration of this may not be long enough for it to be remembered. Syncope due to cardiac arrhythmia may also be more abrupt with no preceding lightheadedness. Among the cardiac causes are both brady- and tachyarrhythmias. Orthostatic hypotension is characterized by lightheadedness and syncope when the patient rises to a stand.[1] Basilar migraine is commonly associated with dizziness that is more akin to true vertigo than presyncopal sensation. Migraine, in general, can be associated with syncope due to autonomic instability.[2] Likewise, vertebrobasilar insufficiency can be associated with syncope as a component of the symptoms, but dizziness and ataxia are more common symptoms.

EEG MANIFESTATIONS OF SYNCOPE

Electroencephalogram (EEG) is most helpful if there are typical epileptiform discharges during the clinical event. However, with syncope, no discharges are seen. If the syncope is due to orthostatic hypotension, video-EEG during the tilt-table testing is particularly helpful. Changes in EEG were seen in only 43% of patients with syncope and in 9% of patients with orthostatic tachycardia although the numbers were small.[3] EEG findings during the syncope were diffuse slowing and one episode of flattening.

DIFFERENTIATION OF SYNCOPE FROM SEIZURE ACTIVITY

Differentiation of syncope from seizures is often a focus of neurologic consultation. While syncope is best recognized by loss of consciousness, loss of tone, and loss of posture, many individuals will have brief multifocal arrhythmic myoclonus, which is a common source of misdiagnosis of epileptic seizures. Syncope with myoclonus has been called "convulsive syncope", but the myoclonus is of brainstem origin, not cortical in origin. In addition to myoclonus, patients with syncope may have posturing, head turning, lateral or upward eye deviation, or oral automatisms.

The incidence of convulsive activity during syncope is low but significant. Estimates vary between series, with up to 6% of patients with syncope during tilt-table testing having convulsive activity and up to 12% of patients who have syncope during blood donation having convulsive activity.[4] Part of the variability in reported convulsive frequency is undoubtedly due to observer attention: motor activity is more likely to be identified if looked for.

Some differentiating features are:

- Syncope can be triggered by certain activities, which is unexpected with seizures. Examples include intense pain, intense emotion, standing for prolonged periods of time in hot crowded places, sudden standing from sitting or lying position, urination, defecation, and cough. In addition, presence of dehydration, known heart disease, and prior syncope should favor of syncope.

- Syncope often has warning presyncopal sensation, such as nausea, cold sweat, lightheadedness, graying of vision, and sounds becoming more distant, which are different from common seizure auras.
- The myoclonus associated with syncope is of much shorter duration (usually <15 sec) than tonic-clonic activity (usually >15 sec)
- Prominent pallor described by witnesses favors syncope although it may also be an autonomic manifestation of some seizures.
- Seizures result in post-ictal confusion or lethargy, not expected with syncope.

However, if the fall from syncope results in concussion, there could be more confusion than expected.

- Recollection of loss of consciousness favors syncope.[5]
- Reduced tone with the event is suggestive of syncope rather than seizure disorder.[6]

Complicating the differentiation between seizure and syncope is that syncope due to bradycardia or even asystole can occur as a complication of epileptic seizure. In a review of multiple case series, ictal bradycardia or asystole was uncommon but identified especially in patients with focal seizures with impaired awareness.[7] Focus was most commonly left temporal.

7.4

Other Disorders Mistaken for Seizures

KARL E. MISULIS

MOVEMENT DISORDERS

Some movement disorders can have sufficient fast components that they might be confused with seizure activity. This is especially true for myoclonus but also for others, including dyskinesias and hemiballismus.

Nonepileptic Myoclonus

Myoclonic seizures, seen in a number of epileptic syndromes, particularly juvenile myoclonic epilepsy (JME), are generated in the cortex and usually associated with an electrical discharge at the scalp. However, myoclonus can also be non-epileptic and can be generated at any level of the central nervous system (CNS). *Essential myoclonus* is episodic jerking not associated with other epileptic or degenerative disease. There are either no other neurologic signs, or there may be dystonia or tremor. Inheritance can be dominant or sporadic. The dominant essential myoclonus usually presents before the age of 20 years. The movements disappear in sleep. Treatment of benign myoclonus is usually not needed.

Nocturnal Myoclonus

Nocturnal myoclonus is a normal phenomenon. However, if excessive, it may interfere with the quality of sleep. Nocturnal myoclonus is commonly seen as a primary disorder or with restless legs syndrome (RLS) but can also be secondary to a variety of other medical and neurologic conditions.

Chorea and Paroxysmal Dyskinesia

Chorea can occasionally be confused with seizure activity because of the repetitive and stereotyped writhing, twisting movements.

Differentiation of chorea from seizure is aided by the following features:

- Chorea is associated with maintained ability to move the limbs, even during the episode of involuntary limb movement.

- Chorea is present only in the waking state and disappears during sleep.
- Chorea is not associated with post-ictal weakness.
- Chorea is not associated with cognitive changes.

When chorea is paroxysmal, it is more likely to be confused as epileptic.

Paroxysmal dyskinesia is characterized by combinations of chorea, athetosis, ballism, and a dystonic posture, occurring in attacks. It is classified into two broad categories: *kinesigenic* and *nonkinesigenic*. Both conditions are usually familial.

Kinesigenic dyskinesia: The attacks of paroxysmal kinesigenic dyskinesia are very brief, lasting seconds, and are brought on by a sudden movement, particularly after inactivity. The movements may or may not be stereotyped and can be bilateral or alternate sides. This is helpful in distinguishing them from epileptic seizures which, if lateralized, tend to consistently affect the same side. As with other movement disorders, consciousness is always preserved, and there is no post-ictal change. However, the condition responds very well to anti-seizure medications (ASMs), which are effective in preventing recurrence of attacks.

Nonkinesigenic dyskinesia: The attacks in paroxysmal nonkinesigenic dyskinesia are longer, lasting minutes to hours. They are not precipitated by movement but can be brought on by a variety of factors such as stress, fatigue, excitement, alcohol, or caffeine. This condition does not usually respond to ASMs.

Paroxysmal dyskinesias can also be misdiagnosed as psychogenic, especially when the preservation of cognitive function is appreciated.[1]

Hemiballismus

Hemiballismus is violent movements of one side of the body. The movements are most marked in the proximal muscles. The flailing of the limbs can result in injury to the patient. Hemiballismus can be mistaken for seizure activity but can be differentiated by preservation of consciousness and movement of the affected side, normal electroencephalogram (EEG) during the movement, and irregular appearance of the movements. Hemiballismus is due to damage to the subthalamic nucleus, with stroke being the most common cause. Hemiballismus is often misdiagnosed as psychogenic because of the dramatic presentation and relatively rare occurrence.

Hyperekplexia

Hyperekplexia is a startle syndrome with myoclonic movements triggered by a variety of stimuli. The response, including the myoclonic movements, is more prominent than would be expected by normal startle. The exaggerated startle can be mistaken for a startle-evoked seizure. The myoclonic movements are more generalized than normally expected. Hyperekplexia is an inherited disorder, most often with autosomal dominant transmission. Some patients can have seizures and cognitive impairment associated with the exaggerated startle.[2]

Tremor

The most common tremors are seldom confused with seizure activity, including essential tremor and Parkinson's tremor. However, some other tremors do not have the correlation with rest and activity, and the associated clinical profile of these entities and can be confused with seizure activity. Prominent among these is *midbrain tremor*, also called *rubral tremor* or *Holmes tremor*. When this occurs in the setting of previous stroke, the tremor plus the neurologic deficit can raise concern for post-stroke seizure activity.[3]

SLEEP DISORDERS

Parasomnias

Parasomnias are disorders of sleep characterized by undesirable physical events or experiences that occur during entry into sleep, within sleep, or during arousals from sleep.[4] They can be subdivided into disorders of arousal from non-rapid eye movement (non-REM) sleep, parasomnias associated with REM sleep, and other parasomnias (see Table 7.4.1).

In general, parasomnias tend to occur in children and young adults. Some have a familial basis. Parasomnias can be mistaken for seizures, particularly frontal lobe seizures which often arise

TABLE 7.4.1 PARASOMNIAS

Disorder	Features
Restless legs syndrome	Motor restlessness sometimes with twitching. Violent jerking might suggest seizure to some.
Sleep myoclonus	Jerking of the legs which can cause arousal. Differentiated from seizure in part by occurrence of single jerk and arousal.
Hypnic jerks	Brief jerks at sleep inception. Differentiated from seizures in part because they are single jerks and not seen in deep sleep.
Head banging	Rocking of the body especially in young children, often misinterpreted as seizure activity.
Sleep walking	Occasionally confused with seizure because of the patient may appear confused as if post-ictal.
Sleep talking	Seldom confused with seizures in the absence of other symptoms.
Sleep terrors and nightmares	Abrupt awakening with fright, sleep terrors are from non-rapid eye movement (REM) sleep, nightmares are from REM sleep.
REM behavioral disorder	Motor activity during dreaming can be vigorous and even violent but differ from stereotyped movements of seizures.
Enuresis	Losing control of bladder at night can suggest seizure but this would seldom be the only sign.

out of sleep. Differentiation depends on careful history and observation. Video-EEG monitoring can aid in the differential diagnosis, although this is seldom needed.

Sleep walking, sleep terror, and confusional arousals are *arousal parasomnias* that occur with partial awakening out of slow wave sleep, the deepest non-REM sleep, usually within 1–3 hours after sleep onset. With all arousal parasomnias, the patient, usually a child, typically has no memory of the events. These parasomnias cause concern in family members.

Sleep walking is characterized by patients being found walking or standing. The eyes are open and there may be partial responsiveness. When the patient is stimulated, arousal is often accompanied by confusion and disorientation for a brief time.

Confusional arousals present typically with the child being found seated in bed with eyes open, appearing alert, but unresponsive. As with sleep walking, if awakened, the child will be confused and frightened.

Sleep terrors have more extreme manifestations, with screaming, crying, facial expression of terror, agitation, and thrashing. There is often associated sweating, tachycardia, and tachypnea. The duration is a few minutes, and the patient then goes back to sleep. Sleep terrors are more common in children and become less prevalent with increasing age.

The distinction between arousal parasomnias and nocturnal frontal lobe seizures is based on the following clinical features[5]:

- Arousal parasomnias tend to have an earlier age at onset than nocturnal frontal lobe seizures and tend to resolve with increasing age, unlike frontal lobe seizures.
- Arousal parasomnias typically occur once in a night, infrequently, while frontal lobe seizures are more frequent, often with several in one night.
- Arousal parasomnias last several minutes, while frontal lobe seizures usually last less than 1 min.
- Episodes in arousal disorders can vary in clinical manifestations, while frontal lobe seizures are very stereotyped.
- Posturing is not usually present in arousal parasomnias while common in nocturnal frontal lobe focal impaired awareness seizures.

REM parasomnias arise out of REM sleep and include nightmares and REM behavior disorder. These are more likely in the last half of the night, when REM sleep predominates. *Nightmares* are frightening dreams, the details of which are recalled, an important distinguishing feature from sleep terror. Nightmares often result in awakening from sleep with anxiety. Upon awakening there is full alertness, with no confusion or disorientation, unlike the case with night terrors. While single nightmares are common in normal individuals, recurrent nightmares represent a disorder. *REM behavior disorder* is motor activity during dreaming. The physiology is thought to be pathological absence of normal sleep paralysis that should be present during REM. The behavior can be quite violent, including punching, kicking, and running movements. REM behavior disorder is more

likely in the second half of the night when REM is more prevalent. It is more common after age 50 years, with strong male predominance. It may be seen in some normal patients, particularly as a transient effect of some medications or medication withdrawal. When it is a chronic disorder, it is more common in some neurologic disorders, particularly Lewy Body dementia and Parkinson's disease.

The distinction of REM behavior disorder from frontal lobe seizures is based on the following features:

- The age at onset of REM behavior disorder is usually older than 50, later than usual for nocturnal frontal lobe epilepsy.
- The REM behavior disorder episodes occur in association with dreams, usually in the second half of the night. Frontal lobe seizures occur at any time during sleep.
- The patients remember their dreams, and the behaviors in sleep are consistent with dream content.
- After arousal from REM behavior disorder, the patient is lucid and oriented.

Sleep talking is a common disorder which affects normal people and is increased in incidence with certain disorders, including dementia and especially in Lewy Body dementia, where it also tends to be loud.[6,7] Sleep talking is seldom confused with seizure activity in the absence of other symptoms.

Other parasomnias include a large number of conditions, only of some of which are potentially confused with seizures. *Enuresis* is seldom confused with seizure activity, although this, along with finding blood on a pillow, make the thoughtful patients or parents have concern over unobserved nocturnal seizure activity. These findings, however, are not commonly due to seizure in the absence of other findings.

Sleep-Related Movement Disorders

RLS is motor restlessness of the legs which can affect patients day or night but is worse in the evening or night. The main criterion for diagnosis is an urge to move the legs caused by uncomfortable sensations. The manifestations worsen or start during inactivity and are relieved by movement. In the differential diagnosis of seizure, patients may report twitching of the legs and may emphasize violent jerking which could suggest seizure activity. Sleep myoclonus is often seen in patients with RLS.

Sleep myoclonus is episodic jerking of lower leg muscles. The jerks can interfere with not only the sleep of the patient but also with that of the sleeping partner. Sleep myoclonus is often familial and often seen in patients with RLS. Sleep myoclonus is differentiated from seizure by the occurrence only during sleep, single and irregular nature of the jerks, and absence of ictal or interictal abnormalities on EEG.

Hypnic jerks are the brief jerks which interfere with descent into sleep. They may involve a single limb or the entire body. They are differentiated from seizure activity by the single nature of the jerks and absence of occurrence in awake state or deep sleep. This is a common condition which is considered normal.

Sleep-related rhythmic movement disorder is a stereotyped rhythmic movement disorder affecting the head, body, or extremities, which can occur with the patient either supine or prone or even on hands and knees. The rocking can cause movement of the bed or actual banging of the head into the headboard, which may be mistaken for seizure activity. The behaviors may result in injury. Young children are most commonly affected. Head banging and other sleep-related rhythmic movement disorder may occur during any stage of sleep. Parents may have difficulty awakening the children, solidifying their concern over seizure activity. The behavior usually lasts less than 15 min at a time but may repeat through the night. Differentiation from seizure activity is mainly by description of the activity. Video-EEG monitoring or polysomnography are rarely necessary for diagnosis.

Migraine and Migraine Equivalent

Migraine can rarely cause episodic symptoms that can be mistaken for seizure activity. The most common migraine types that can be confused with seizures are listed here.

- *Classical migraine with visual aura* can be difficult to distinguish from occipital lobe seizures, which may be followed by a migraine-like headache. Distinguishing features include
  - The migraine aura is longer than visual seizures (5–60 min as compared to <30 sec).
  - The visual aura in migraine is most commonly a fortification spectrum or scintillating scotoma, whereas the most occipital lobe seizure aura is colored circles.
- *Classical migraine with sensory aura*. Both sensory seizure and migraine can have a sensory march, but the sensory march is much shorter in duration in sensory seizures.
- *Acute confusional migraine*.
- *Migraine without headache*, or migraine equivalent.
- *Basilar migraine*.

Episodic vertigo and syncope can be a sign of basilar migraine. One example is shown in Figures 7.4.1 and 7.4.2. These are from a 9-year-old girl with episodes that occurred about every other day. She would become irritable and whiny, and this was followed by development of ataxia. She used to become unresponsive, but treatment with levetiracetam resulted in improvement in this manifestation. Duration was 30–45 min.

The first sample, shown in Figure 7.4.1, is the baseline normal EEG. This is followed by high-voltage bursts of delta activity (Figure 7.4.2). Note the sensitivity of 30 μV/mm.

Reflux

Sandifer syndrome is torsional dystonia of the neck and upper arms which can trigger extensive neurologic evaluation, especially for seizure.[8] This is due to reflux, although the exact pathophysiology is not known. Children with reflux can present with apnea, with or without motor activity that can suggest seizure activity. More commonly, reflux presents with episodic vomiting, poor feeding, and weight loss.

Diagnosis of reflux often depends on cooperative consultation by neurology and gastroenterology. Observation during an episode is key to the diagnosis. These episodes are so common that observations are multiple.

BEHAVIORAL DISORDERS

Behavioral disorders can be mistaken for seizure activity. This activity can include directed violence or nondirected violence.

Directed Violence

Seizure activity has been used as a legal defense for directed violence.[9] Most physicians believe that directed violence does not occur as a result of seizure activity. Plotting, traveling to a crime scene, and attacking an individual would not be expected from epileptic seizure activity.

Nondirected Violence

Nondirected violence can be occasionally seen as a component of seizure activity. Motor activity

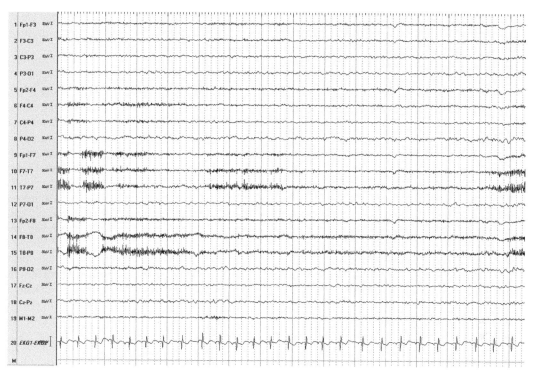

FIGURE 7.4.1 Basilar migraine baseline. Longitudinal bipolar montage.

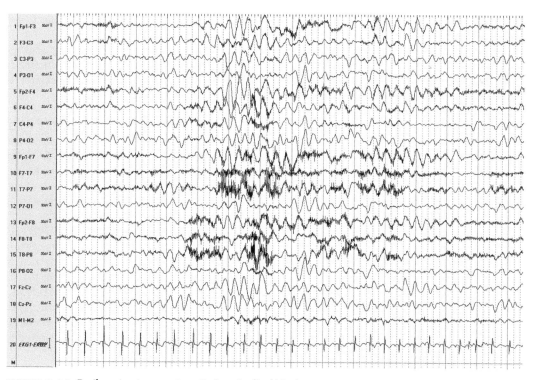

FIGURE 7.4.2 Basilar migraine symptomatic. Longitudinal bipolar montage.

associated with focal impaired awareness seizures may appear violent. Biting, hitting, kicking, and scratching are uncommon with epileptic seizures and, when present, are nondirected, affecting only those restraining the patient or in proximity.

Post-ictal states can be associated with agitation and confusion, resulting in nondirected violence, again especially when trying fight restraints. Violence may have an increased incidence in patients with post-ictal psychosis, especially with seizures of temporal origin.[10]

BREATH-HOLDING SPELLS

Breath-holding spells can be frightening to parents and can be mistaken for seizures or even cardiac arrest. They can affect up to 4.6% of young children, although most estimates are much lower.[11] There are two types of breath-holding: *cyanotic* and *pallid*. Both have a duration of 5–60 sec.

Cyanotic breath-holding spells are characterized by a brief cry, followed by apnea in end-expiration. The child becomes cyanotic and unconscious because of hypoxia. Shortly thereafter, the child awakens.

Pallid breath-holding spells are characterized by little or no cry, followed by bradycardia or even asystole, resulting in the pallid appearance. The child is pale and lifeless. The child becomes awake and normal in color in minutes.

Diagnosis of breath-holding spells depends on observation, and the spells can be frightening even to experienced clinicians. EEG can help differentiation. In both types of spells, the EEG becomes suppressed and, depending on duration, virtually flat.

Breath-holding spells of both types tend to disappear by about age 5 years.

STARTLE

All of us normally have alerting reactions in response to stimuli that we consider to be novel and important. In *startle syndrome*, the alerting response is enhanced. This can be present in some patients for unknown reasons, can be inherited, or can be acquired due to CNS disease.

Hyperekplexia was discussed briefly earlier and is an inherited disorder in which there is exaggerated startle. An unexpected, even relatively minor stimulus results in transient stiffness followed by a fall. Hyperekplexia must be distinguished from epilepsy.

Startle-induced seizures occur in some epilepsies, particularly frontal lobe epilepsy originating in the supplementary motor area. Stimulation induces seizure activity with a startle-like stiffening of the body. In contrast to other startle conditions, there is an electrographic discharge evident with this event.[12]

COUGH SYNCOPE

During prolonged coughing, intrathoracic and intra-abdominal pressures are transmitted via the great veins to the intracranial compartment, causing transient elevated intracranial pressure. The resulting reduction of cerebral perfusion pressure may cause a critical impairment of cerebral blood flow (CBF).[13]

During coughing, patients show a transient cerebral circulatory arrest, which coincides with loss of consciousness. EEG shows slowing and attenuation (see Figure 7.4.3).

Obstructive airway disease seems to be a prerequisite to build up the intrathoracic and intracranial pressures to a degree sufficient to compromise CBF and cause cough syncope.

TRANSIENT ISCHEMIC ATTACK

Transient ischemic attack (TIA) is transient neurological deficit caused by interruption in blood flow in a vascular distribution. This is seldom confused with seizure activity, but seizure is considered if there are recurrent episodes and especially if they are stereotyped.

EEG during confirmed TIA usually does not produce ictal discharges but rather reduction in faster (alpha and beta) activity and increase in slower (theta and delta) activity.[14]

TRANSIENT GLOBAL AMNESIA

Transient global amnesia (TGA) presents with loss of the ability to acquire new memories, *anterograde amnesia*. Historical recollection is preserved. Most patients are at least 50 years of age. Duration is usually a few hours, seldom more than 12 hours, and not more than 24 hours.

EEG may be ordered when a patient with TGA presents to the emergency department because of concern for focal impaired awareness seizure or absence seizure. EEG is usually normal, though there are reports of epileptiform discharges in a minority of patients, typically left-sided or bilateral, but not right-sided.[15] TGA is not believed to be epileptic, and EEG is probably not indicated unless there are repeated episodes.

PEAK TOXICITY OF ASMs

Patients taking ASMs may misinterpret symptoms of peak-level toxicity as seizures. This is more likely with some ASMs, particularly those acting

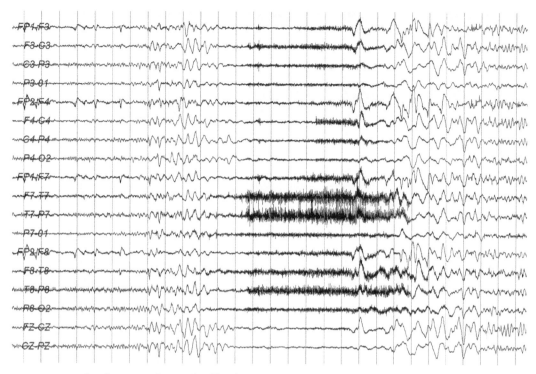

FIGURE 7.4.3 Cough syncope. Longitudinal bipolar montage.

on the sodium channel. Symptoms may include blurred vision, double vision, dizziness, unsteadiness, and confusion.

These manifestations can be distinguished from seizures by the following:

- Longer duration (usually >10 min).
- Manifestations of blurred vision or double vision, which are unlikely during seizures.
- The symptoms are temporally related to ASM intake.
- The symptoms are more likely with taking the ASM on an empty stomach and less likely if the ASM is taken with food.
- The symptoms subside with reducing or dividing the dose, or after switching to an extended-release preparation.

DRUG-INDUCED ENCEPHALOPATHY

Encephalopathy is the most common cause for neurological consultations in most hospitals. Patients have confusion, memory loss, or other cognitive deficits. Occasional patients may have myoclonic activity and others may have tremor, but it is unlikely that this could be confused with seizure activity.

Cefepime Neurotoxicity

Cefepime neurotoxicity is a common occurrence in hospital neurology.[16] Common symptoms are encephalopathy, myoclonus, and seizures. These can develop with appropriate doses, but are more common with renal insufficiency, especially when doses are not adequately adjusted for the renal impairment. Cases of status epilepticus have been reported with cefepime, especially in children.[17] Figure 7.4.4 shows the EEG of a patient with cefepime toxicity.

Opiate-Induced Myoclonus

Myoclonus that can be mistaken for seizures has been seen with institution, maintenance, or withdrawal of opiates.[18, 19] Opioid-induced myoclonus is more common in patients on other agents, especially antipsychotics or antidepressants.

Antidepressant-Induced Myoclonus

Selective serotonin reuptake inhibitors (SSRIs) and tricyclic antidepressants (TCAs) can both produce myoclonus which can be focal, multifocal, or generalized. The pattern can be positive or negative myoclonus. Drugs of these classes used in

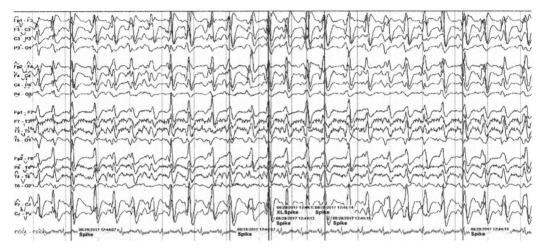

FIGURE 7.4.4 Cefepime toxicity. Longitudinal bipolar montage.

combination seem to be associated with a higher incidence of myoclonus.

Tiagabine Encephalopathy

Tiagabine is an uncommonly used ASM, especially for partial seizures. Some patients treated with tiagabine may develop episodes of altered responsiveness and awareness, lasting up to hours. It is not totally clear if this is an encephalopathy or a type of nonconvulsive status epilepticus of the absence variety. Recent reports have shown generalized slow activity in association with the encephalopathy. Reduction in dose of the tiagabine results in disappearance or decreased severity of the episodes.[20]

Recreational Drugs

A host of recreational drugs have been associated with activity that resembles seizure but is more likely to be a drug-induced movement disorder.[21]

Crack cocaine can produce chorea or myoclonus which can be mistaken for seizures. This has been seen with acute intoxication, in which case it is of limited duration, a few hours. However, less-severe movement disorders have been observed with cocaine withdrawal, and these last much longer.

Amphetamines can produce repetitive and stereotyped movements which can be mistaken for seizures, especially when seen in the context of encephalopathy.

PART 8

Seizure Management

8.1

Management of Pediatric Seizures

KEVIN C. ESS

MEDICAL MANAGEMENT ISSUES IN THE PEDIATRIC POPULATION

Absence Epilepsy

Medications typically used for absence epilepsy include ethosuximide, levetiracetam, lamotrigine, and valproic acid (VPA). Medications commonly used for focal-onset seizures, such as carbamazepine and oxcarbazepine, should not be used and may exacerbate seizures.

Juvenile Myoclonic Epilepsy

Juvenile myoclonic epilepsy (JME) is most commonly treated with valproate; however VPA should be avoided in women of childbearing potential, if possible. If no other good options are available, VPA has been used at low doses and with some assurance that pregnancies will be planned so that medication changes can be considered.

Alternatives include mainly lamotrigine and levetiracetam. There is also some evidence for effectiveness of topiramate, zonisamide, and, recently, perampanel, although none of these is perfectly safe in pregnancy.[1]

Landau-Kleffner Syndrome

About 75% of Landau-Kleffner syndrome (LKS) patients have clinical seizures. We are aware of no large controlled studies, so almost every anticonvulsant used in children and some surgical therapies have been tried. In addition, intravenous immunoglobulin (IVIG) and corticosteroids have been tried.

Lennox-Gastaut Syndrome

Lennox-Gastaut syndrome (LGS) is also treated with a wide variety of anti-seizure medications (ASMs), commensurate with the refractory nature of the seizures in many patients. VPA, lamotrigine, topiramate, rufinamide, felbamate, cannabidiol, and clobazam have been reported to be effective in some patients.

Benign Focal Epilepsy of Childhood

Treatment is not always needed. When ASMs are used, they typically reduce mainly the number of secondarily generalized seizures, but not so much the focal seizures. The best data, though still very limited, are with levetiracetam, valproate, carbamazepine, and oxcarbazepine.

Status Epilepticus

Almost any type of seizure can present with or develop into status epilepticus, and this neurological emergency is a common occurrence. Seizures with fever are the most frequent cause of pediatric status epilepticus, which is not the case for adults.[2] First-line treatment is usually with benzodiazepines, and a variety of routes can be used. Rectal diazepam is commonly used, but diazepam or midazolam can also be given by nasal spray.

Fosphenytoin is commonly used as the first conventional ASM and can be given intramuscularly as well as intravenously; it has an advantage over phenytoin in its faster rate of administration. Historically, phenobarbital has been the next agent to be used, but because of sedation and other concerns, valproate and levetiracetam have assumed more prominent roles. Note that doses used are often greater than those listed in prescribing information approved by the US Food and Drug Administration (FDA).

Up to 25% of status epilepticus can be refractory to first lines of therapy and therefore intubation and sedation along with escalation of ASM therapy is needed. Continuous electroencephalogram (EEG) monitoring is warranted. This is an especially important point as some patients who were thought to be post-ictal after status epilepticus had actually transitioned from convulsive to nonconvulsive status epilepticus, a fact that would not have been apparent without EEG.[3]

Patients with a history of absence epilepsy should also be investigated with EEG for any prolonged episodes of altered mental status because nonconvulsive status epilepticus is possible; in these cases, treatment with benzodiazepines and other agents is similar to that described earlier.

DIETARY MANAGEMENT IN THE PEDIATRIC POPULATION

The *ketogenic diet* is an important treatment option for patients with epilepsy. Its use has become increasing common over the past 20 years and is backed up by well-designed clinical studies of ketogenic diet efficacy and tolerability. Young children with epilepsy are an important group to consider for dietary therapy, especially the full ketogenic diet, which is less tolerated by older children and adults. The diet's tolerability in young children is due to control of food intake by parents, motivation of parents, and less developed preferences for tastes and textures in young children. Children with a gastronomy tube or gastrostomy-jejunostomy (GJ) tube are further accessible for application of the ketogenic diet. Many families perceive the ketogenic diet as a "natural" approach and a pathway to avoid medications. Counseling for diet initiation should include information that this is not a natural diet, and that a high-fat low-carbohydrate diet has its own risks and benefits and must be closely managed by experienced neurologists and dieticians. Most patients will require concomitant ASM but one of the goals for using the ketogenic diet is better seizure control with less total medication. Ketogenic diet therapy is usually initiated during inpatient stays, given the need to closely monitor for hypoglycemia while the patient transitions to a carbohydrate-predominant to lipid-predominant ketogenic diet. Many patients also experience nausea and vomiting with diet initiation, and the inpatient stay also allows the extensive teaching required for family/caregivers to safely administer the diet at home. More information can be found at The Charlie Foundation, a patient advocacy organization that promotes the ketogenic diet.[4]

Because the full ketogenic diet is challenging to maintain in older children and adults, other forms of the diet have become popular. They share low carbohydrate intake but are not as strict as the ketogenic diet. These include Modified Atkins Diet as well as the Low Glycemic Diet. There is scientific support for these interventions, and they can also be used as an adjunctive approach to epilepsy in addition to medications.

SURGICAL MANAGEMENT IN THE PEDIATRIC POPULATION

Optimal management of epilepsy in children requires use of all modalities to achieve the aspirational clinical goals of no seizures and no side effects. While medications are often effective, seizures in up to 30% of patients are refractory, and other modalities including diet and epilepsy surgery, should be considered.

The field of epilepsy surgery has advanced greatly over the past 20 years with advanced neuroimaging, EEG, and neurosurgical techniques allowing precise localization and resection of discrete portions of cerebral cortex that are causing seizures. As children are more likely to have epilepsy due to cortical malformations and other focal lesions, identifying a structural lesion as a cause of seizures provides a surgical option if medications or diet therapies are ineffective and/or cause intolerable side effects. Details of the surgical management of pediatric epilepsy is outside the scope of this book, but to ascertain whether patients are good candidates for surgery, the clinician should include tests such as high-quality brain magnetic resonance imaging (MRI), nuclear imaging with positron emission tomography/single positron emission computed tomography (PET/SPECT), invasive EEG monitoring, functional mapping of eloquent cortex, and neuropsychology assessments. Focal resections can often produce excellent results with patients who were thoroughly evaluated. Less good results are achieved when brain MRI findings are normal ("nonlesional") or when there is more than one area of seizure onset.

While outwardly drastic, some patients with hemispheric lesions (e.g., Sturge-Weber syndrome, hemimegalencephaly) will ultimately require an extensive procedure involving one-half of the brain. This can be an *anatomic hemispherectomy* (removal of all of one hemisphere) or a *functional hemispherectomy* (removal of a portion of the hemisphere with disconnection of the rest). Functional hemispherectomy is currently used at most centers because this approach helps decreases complications previously seen with anatomic hemispherectomy.

Patients can also be considered for surgical approaches that do not involve resection of the cerebral cortex. Corpus callosotomy is often used for patients with intractable tonic seizures and atonic seizures/drop attacks. This procedure can interrupt the spread pattern of seizures, and, while patients still have seizures, they can maintain posture during them and not suffer trauma from frequent and violent falls. Either the entire corpus callosum can be divided or just the anterior two-thirds portion. This procedure minimizes corpus callosum disconnection syndrome, more likely to be seen following a full procedure.

Other surgical approaches include the *vagal nerve stimulator* (VNS), which is often considered for patients who have medically intractable seizures but don't have other surgical options. VNS is more of a palliative approach and should only be considered if a more definitive surgery (e.g., focal resection) is not possible. Other devices are being developed, with *responsive neurostimulation* (RNS) becoming an option in recent years. Unlike the VNS, the RNS is targeted specifically to each patient and can detect seizure activity and then counter it with injected current to mitigate seizures. This can be an option if the epileptogenic cortex is eloquent, especially if involved with language or primary motor function.

Other approaches to surgery include subpial transection, but this approach to disconnect discrete areas of cerebral cortex is now rarely used.

COMORBIDITIES IN PEDIATRIC EPILEPSIES

Comorbidities are prominent issues in pediatric patients as well as in adults. Some of these are discussed with special relevance to pediatrics here; elsewhere in this book comorbidities are discussed in more general terms.

Anxiety and depression are considerably more common in children with epilepsy than in the general population.[5] The causes are multifactorial, with some contributing factors being the biological etiology of the epilepsy also causing mental health problems, the psychosocial stigma of having epilepsy in the patient as well as in family and friends, the family's reaction to the disorder, the necessity of regular medical care for a chronic disorder, and the logistics and chemistry of ASM therapy. Assessment and management of anxiety and depression is essential for full treatment of the patient.[6] Anxiety and depression can still be present even if seizures are under excellent control and should be screened for at every clinical encounter.

Cognitive disturbance is present in many patients with pediatric epilepsies. In general, this is likely related to underlying causes and syndromes rather than to individual seizures themselves. While worse seizure control does correlate with worse cognitive outcome, the reason is more likely the neuropathologic substrate than the seizures themselves. However, patients with high seizure burdens (e.g., undiagnosed and untreated absence) usually struggle with school performance and may be inappropriately considered to have a primary memory, attention, or cognitive disorder.

Behavioral disturbances are common in some children with epilepsy. The cause can be multifactorial, including the social stigma of having epilepsy, medication side effects, the underlying neuropathology of the epileptic disorder, and the background of the social support structures.[7] These need to be addressed specifically because management of epilepsy, including seizure control, does not seem to correlate with the severity of these behavioral problems. Moreover, some children who have recently achieved seizure freedom may present with worsening behavior. This is usually attributed to a lifting of a state of encephalopathy ("epileptic fog") that was previously caused by frequent cycling between ictal and post-ictal states. The successful treatment of seizures then paradoxically is associated with worsening behavior if the child's mental state is no longer impaired from the seizures and their "true" behavior and personality comes out.

Migraine and epilepsy frequently coexist in the pediatric population just as they do in adults. Either can develop first. There is even some laboratory data supporting commonalities in brain biology.[8] Coexistence of migraine and epilepsy in a patient can aid ASM selection, since topiramate, valproate, and several others have been shown to have benefit in migraine prevention. The severity of migraine in children up until adolescence is usually less than that seen in adults. Symptomatic treatment of migraine with ibuprofen, for example, is often successful with younger patients as long as the medication is taken soon after headaches begin and at an appropriate dose for weight (10 mg/kg).

PROGNOSIS IN PEDIATRIC EPILEPSIES

Prognosis of children with epilepsy depends more on the underlying cause than on the seizures themselves, so seizure control does not significantly affect ultimate outcome.[9] Therefore, epilepsy control can be measured in multiple ways, including seizure number, need for ASM, neurologic function, quality of life, and behavior function. Expected prognosis for a few of the epilepsy syndromes is discussed briefly here.

Absence epilepsy: At least 80% of patients with absence epilepsy are able to discontinue medication without seizure recurrence and have normal neurological and cognitive function.[10]

Dravet syndrome/severe myoclonic epilepsy in infancy (SMEI): These patients are almost always afflicted lifelong with developmental and intellectual disabilities. Seizures may lessen/stabilize with transition to adulthood though they rarely abate, and they require continued treatment. These patients almost always need guardianship when they reach 18 years because they are unable to manage financial and medical decisions. The legal process varies from state to state in the United States and should be started at least 1 year before the child turns 18 years old.

Febrile seizures: Children with febrile seizures have a 5% or less risk of subsequent unprovoked seizures. In the absence of other pathology, patients with simple febrile seizures should have normal development. Patients with complex febrile seizures have a slightly higher rate of developing epilepsy with afebrile seizures, but still the vast majority have no further seizures and enjoy normal development.

Epileptic spasms (ES): ES has a very poor prognosis with, at best, 15% of patients with ES of unknown etiology having normal development.[11] Seizures persisted after treatment in 67% of patients in this same report. Patients with known causes (e.g., hypoxic-ischemic encephalopathy [HIE], tuberous sclerosis complex) will have abnormal outcomes due to their underlying disorders as well as from the impact of ES during critical windows of brain development. As mentioned before, many patients also go on to have LGS.

JME: Most patients (up to 85%) have seizure control with ASMs though multiple trials may be needed. With transition to adult life, ongoing seizures are common but up to 60% can be seizure-free on medications, and, in one study, 28% were seizure-free as adults without ASM therapy.[12] However, patients with JME should be counseled that they are unlikely to grow out of this condition.

LKS: Numbers are small for follow-up, so exact percentages cannot be presented. The language manifestations of LKS can improve, but most patients are left with persistent elements of aphasia and intellectual disabilities in adult life. Similarly, a subset have complete seizure control but very few have normal independent lives.[13]

LGS: LGS is characterized by seizures which are typically difficult to treat, and complete control is seldom achieved. Multiple ASMs and the ketogenic diet are often tried, as well as surgical approaches such as corpus callosotomy and implantation of the VNS. Patients typically reach adult years with cognitive and behavioral deficits as well as refractory seizures.[14] The same anticipatory concerns about legal guardianship apply to this patient population.

8.2

Management of Adult Seizures/Epilepsy

BASSEL ABOU-KHALIL

IF AND WHEN TO INITIATE THERAPY

Anti-seizure medications (ASMs) are prescribed for most but not all patients with seizures. Some of the clinical scenarios that may not require medical treatment include

- Single unprovoked seizures,
- Provoked seizure(s),
- Benign epilepsy of childhood with centrotemporal spikes (BECTS) with infrequent seizures,
- Juvenile myoclonic epilepsy (JME) with myoclonic seizures only.

A single unprovoked seizure has a relatively low risk of recurrence with a normal neurologic exam, normal magnetic resonance imaging (MRI), and normal electroencephalogram (EEG) (Figure 8.2.1). Observation without treatment may be warranted in such cases, provided a seizure recurrence does not involve undue risk to the patient or to the patient's career. Risk of recurrence after a single unprovoked seizure is about 40–50% overall at 2 years. However, patients with normal neurological examination, normal imaging, and normal EEG have a significantly lower rate of approximately 25%.

In 2015, the American Academy of Neurology (AAN) and the American Epilepsy Society (AES) released guidelines on management of patients with a first unprovoked seizure.[1] They began with the conclusion that, from available evidence, the risk of recurrence in the first 2 years after a single unprovoked seizure is 21–45%. The risk of recurrence is increased with epileptiform abnormalities on EEG, prior brain injury such as from stroke or trauma, significant abnormality on brain imaging, or nocturnal seizure. Treatment does reduce the risk of recurrent seizure in the 2 years following the seizure, but does not seem to reduce the risk of epilepsy in the long term.

Single provoked seizure due to metabolic derangement/toxic exposure, acute head injury, or other limited central nervous system (CNS) insult does not necessarily demand ASM therapy. If the seizures recur, then initiation of therapy appropriate to the seizure type is warranted. The duration of treatment depends on how quickly the provoking factor can be reversed. It can be for only a few days. If the provoking factor cannot be immediately reversed, as in the case with an inflammatory process, the duration of treatment may be as long as several months.

Recurrent Unprovoked Seizure

Recurrent unprovoked seizures usually deserve treatment with an ASM. With more than one unprovoked seizure, more than two-thirds of individuals will have a seizure recurrence. However, there are some exceptions to this rule. For example, juvenile myoclonic epilepsy (JME) in selected patients might be relatively mild, manifesting with only myoclonic seizures. It may be managed by self-help guidelines (e.g., avoid sleep deprivation, alcohol binges, and certain medications), without ASMs. Some patients with focal epilepsy may have only mild subjective focal aware seizures and may not even seek a medical opinion or choose to be treated.

Treatment is usually initiated with a single ASM. It is preferable to start at a low dose and titrate slowly, unless there is a reason for urgency. The initial target dose is usually the smallest dose found effective in clinical trials. However, for some ASMs, an even smaller dose has been found effective after marketing. For example, lamotrigine 125–200 mg/d was sufficient for seizure control in most patients with new-onset epilepsy, while the smallest dose found effective in add-on trials was 300 mg/d.[2] If the initial target dose is not sufficient to control seizures, the dose can then be increased gradually until seizure control is achieved or adverse effects appear. There is an

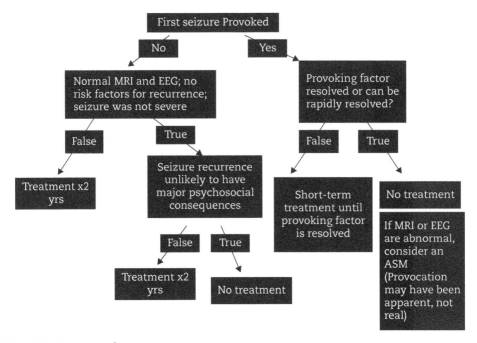

FIGURE 8.2.1 First seizure therapy.

important exception to this guideline in patients with infrequent seizures. For these patients, it is best for the initial target dose to be a "middle of the road" dose. The following sections discuss the recommended initial treatment options depending on seizure classification.

Focal-Onset Seizures

Focal-onset seizures have traditionally been treated with carbamazepine or phenytoin. However, these older agents have been largely replaced by some of the newer ASMs, which have pharmacokinetic and tolerability advantages (see Table 8.2.1). Among the new ASMs, US Food and Drug Administration (FDA) approval has been given for oxcarbazepine, topiramate, lacosamide, and eslicarbazepine as first-line treatments based on clinical trials. However, good clinical evidence supports the effectiveness of lamotrigine, levetiracetam, and gabapentin. Lamotrigine seems to be particularly attractive due to favorable tolerability (particularly less effect on cognition and alertness), but the slow titration is a limiting factor when rapid onset of action is needed. However, even in this situation, it is worthy of consideration for later transition. The large Standard and New Antiepileptic Drug (SANAD) trial comparing lamotrigine,

carbamazepine, gabapentin, oxcarbazepine, and topiramate in partial epilepsy favored lamotrigine for the primary outcome measure, balancing efficacy and tolerability.[3] Topiramate also requires a slow titration, and it has important cognitive potential adverse effects. As a result, it is usually not a first-choice treatment, unless there is comorbidity such as migraine and obesity. When rapid onset of action is needed, the new ASMs to be considered as first-line treatment are levetiracetam and oxcarbazepine. In 2016, the FDA adopted a policy that a drug's efficacy as adjunctive therapy in adults can be extrapolated to efficacy in monotherapy. This extrapolation requires data demonstrating that the drug has equivalent pharmacokinetics between its original approved use and its extrapolated use. Based on this, perampanel, brivaracetam, and cenobamate received broad approval covering adjunctive and monotherapy use. However, they are not appropriate for initial monotherapy use in the absence of comparative trials.

Generalized-Onset Seizures

Absence seizures: Ethosuximide is the drug of choice for initiating therapy in most patients with generalized absence seizures. If the patient

TABLE 8.2.1 ANTI-SEIZURE MEDICATIONS (ASMS)

Drug	FDA-approved indications
Brivaracetam (Briviact)	Focal seizures ≥4 years
Cannabidiol (Epidiolex)	Seizures associated with Lennox-Gastaut syndrome, Dravet syndrome, or tuberous sclerosis complex age ≥1 year
Carbamazepine (Tegretol)	Focal-onset, generalized-onset tonic-clonic, but not absence or myoclonic seizures
Cenobamate (Xcopri)	Focal-onset seizures in adults
Clonazepam (Klonopin)	Lennox-Gastaut, absence type, akinetic, and myoclonic seizures as adjunctive or monotherapy
Clobazam (Onfi)	Seizures with Lennox-Gastaut syndrome in children age ≥2 years as adjunctive therapy
Eslicarbazepine acetate (Aptiom)	Focal-onset seizures in age ≥4 years
Ethosuximide (Zarontin)	Absence seizures
Felbamate (Felbatol)	Focal-onset seizures, but only if failed alternatives Adjunctive therapy for generalized seizures in children with Lennox-Gastaut
Fenfluramine (Fintepla)	Dravet syndrome
Gabapentin (Neurontin)	Adjunctive therapy for focal seizures in adults and children >3 years
Lacosamide (Vimpat)	Focal-onset seizures and adjunctive therapy for generalized-onset tonic-clonic seizures in those >4 years
Lamotrigine (Lamictal)	Adjunctive for focal-onset, generalized-onset tonic-clonic, generalized seizures of Lennox-Gastaut Monotherapy for focal-onset seizures as conversion from phenytoin, carbamazepine, phenobarbital, primidone, valproate
Levetiracetam (Keppra)	Adjunctive therapy for focal-onset seizures >1 month, myoclonic seizures of juvenile myoclonic epilepsy in those >12 years old, generalized-onset tonic-clonic seizures in patients with idiopathic generalized epilepsy IV formulation for patients >16 years with focal-onset, myoclonic, and generalized-onset tonic-clonic seizures
Methsuximide (Celontin)	Absence seizures refractory to other ASMs
Oxcarbazepine (Trileptal)	Focal-onset seizures as monotherapy or adjunctive in adults, and in children of specific ages
Perampanel	Focal-onset seizures in patients ≥4 years alone or adjunctive Generalized-onset tonic-clonic seizures in patients ≥12 years as adjunctive therapy
Phenobarbital (Luminal)	Broad range of seizures except absence
Phenytoin (Dilantin)	Focal-onset, generalized-onset tonic-clonic, postoperative
Primidone (Mysoline)	Broad range of seizures including focal-onset, generalized-onset tonic-clonic
Pregabalin (Lyrica)	Focal-onset seizures in adults as adjunctive therapy
Rufinamide (Banzel)	Lennox-Gastaut as adjunctive therapy
Stiripentol (Diacomit)	Seizures associated with Dravet syndrome in patients ≥2 years taking clobazam, not as monotherapy
Tiagabine (Gabitril)	Focal-onset seizures in adults and children >12 years, as adjunctive therapy
Topiramate (Topamax)	Initial monotherapy for focal-onset or generalized-onset tonic clonic seizures, age ≥2 years Adjunctive therapy for focal-onset or primary generalized tonic clonic seizures age ≥2 Adjunctive therapy for seizures associated with Lennox-Gastaut syndrome, age ≥2
Valproate (Depakote, Depakene, Depacon iv)	Focal-onset seizures, absence seizures
Vigabatrin (Sabril)	Adjunctive therapy for adults with refractory focal-onset seizures, who have tried several alternatives and in whom the potential benefits outweigh the potential loss of vision
Zonisamide (Zonegran)	Focal-onset seizures in adults as adjunctive therapy

has coexistent generalized tonic-clonic or myo-clonic seizures, then valproate is a better choice. Lamotrigine was found to be less effective than ethosuximide and valproate for absence seizures in a large comparative trial.[4] Nevertheless, it is an important option in a woman of childbearing potential (due to valproate teratogenicity) or in a man with comorbidities that prohibit the use of valproate (such as obesity).

Idiopathic generalized epilepsy with generalized tonic-clonic seizures: Valproate appears to be the most effective agent and is the drug of choice for men, but because of the risk of birth defects and other developmental abnormalities, lamotrigine and levetiracetam are preferable first-choice options for women with childbearing potential.

Generalized myoclonic seizures: Valproate is likely the most effective agent as monotherapy. Levetiracetam is approved for adjunctive therapy but may also be effective in monotherapy. Other agents have weaker evidence for efficacy and no FDA indication. Lamotrigine may be effective in some individuals but may also exacerbate myoclonic seizures in others. Topiramate, zonisamide, perampanel, and benzodiazepines may also be effective in some individuals (see Table 8.2.2).

CONSIDERATIONS IN THERAPY

Age

Age plays a complex role in drug selection, mainly in relation to medication tolerability and safety. For example, valproate-associated hepatic failure most commonly occurs in children younger than 2 years. Also more common in children are rash from lamotrigine and behavioral adverse effects of some medications such as phenobarbital and levetiracetam. On the other hand, children younger than 13 do not seem at risk of aplastic anemia from felbamate.

Older age predisposes to hyponatremia from carbamazepine and particularly oxcarbazepine. Seniors also are more likely to experience the common adverse effects of somnolence and ataxia. Also, seniors are more likely to be on multiple drugs, hence a predisposition to drug–drug interactions. Last, seniors are more likely to have reduced hepatic and renal clearance, requiring consideration in dosing. In general, lamotrigine and gabapentin are better tolerated in the elderly than is immediate-release carbamazepine.[5] However, administering carbamazepine in an extended-release preparation improves its tolerability.

Pregnancy and Childbearing Potential

Women of childbearing age are often taking ASMs for uses other than epilepsy, including migraine prophylaxis and psychiatric indications. When a woman considers pregnancy or becomes pregnant, cessation of medications is considered, but this is potentially unsafe when ASMs are given for epilepsy: there are considerable risks to the mother as well as potential deleterious effects of uncontrolled seizures to the fetus. In addition, by the time the patient is found to be pregnant, much of the teratogenicity on major organs has already taken effect, so cessation of the ASM at that point does not protect against major organ birth defects.

To lower the incidence of birth defects in women with epilepsy and to optimize pregnancy outcome, it is essential to have a discussion of changes in ASM therapy prior to planned pregnancy.

No drug is without risk during pregnancy. However, some medications, particularly lamotrigine, levetiracetam, oxcarbazepine, gabapentin, and zonisamide, are associated with minimal risk during pregnancy. On the other hand, valproate is associated with a dose-dependent increased risk of birth defects. While major malformations are determined during exposure in the first 6 weeks of gestation, valproate is also associated with adverse cognitive and behavioral adverse effects that may be related to exposure during later stages of pregnancy. As a result, valproate should be avoided at all stages of pregnancy if possible.[6] Phenobarbital and topiramate also have increased risk of major malformations. Phenytoin and carbamazepine have only slight increased risk of malformations. Most ASMs do not have sufficient data to assess safety in pregnancy. It should be noted that even for ASMs deemed safe during pregnancy, the risk of malformation increases with higher doses so that the lowest effective dose should be used.[7] Registration of patients in pregnancy registries is needed to assess safety in pregnancy. The two largest registries are EURAP, launched in Europe and later extended to several other nations worldwide, and the North American AED Pregnancy Registry, organized through Massachusetts General Hospital (MGH). Patients continue to be enrolled, so physicians of all specialties prescribing ASMs in women of childbearing potential should advise patients to enroll in the registry if they become pregnant.

Before Pregnancy

Managing ASMs in a woman with childbearing potential should be proactive when at all

TABLE 8.2.2 SPECTRUM OF EFFICACY

Antiseizure medication	Seizure type indication/Epilepsy type indication						
	Focal-onset	Generalized tonic-clonic	Generalized Absence	Generalized Myoclonic	Lennox-Gastaut syndrome	Dravet syndrome	Tuberous sclerosis
Phenobarbital	FDA		–	+			
Primidone	FDA		–	+			
Phenytoin	FDA		–	–			
Methsuximide	+	–	FDA	–			
Ethosuximide	-	–	FDA	–			
Clonazepam,	+	+	FDA-A	FDA-A	FDA-A		
Carbamazepine	FDA		–	–			
Valproate	FDA-M	++	FDA-M	++	++		
Vigabatrin*	FDA-A	–	–	–			
Felbamate	FDA-A/MC	+	–	–	FDA-A		
Gabapentin	FDA-A	–	–	–			
Lamotrigine	FDA-MC/A ++ MI	FDA- A	+	+/–	FDA-A		
Topiramate	FDA-MI/A	FDA- A	+/–	+	FDA-A		
Tiagabine	FDA-A	–	–	–			
Levetiracetam	FDA-A ++ MI	FDA- A	+	FDA-A	+		
Oxcarbazepine	FDA-MI/A	–	–	–			
Zonisamide	FDA-A ++ MI	+	+	+	+		
Pregabalin	FDA-A	–	–	–			
Lacosamide	FDA	FDA-A	–	–			
Rufinamide	+	–	–	–	FDA-A		
Clobazam	+	+	+	+	FDA-A		
Perampanel	FDA	FDA-A	+	+			
Eslicarbazepine acetate	FDA	–	–	–			
Brivaracetam	FDA	+	+	+			
Cannabidiol	+	+			FDA	FDA	FDA
Stiripentol						FDA-A	
Cenobamate	FDA						
Fenfluramine						FDA	

+ Evidence for efficacy without specific US Food and Drug Administration indication.
++MI- evidence to support initial monotherapy use without FDA indication.
FDA = FDA approved, without specification as to monotherapy or adjunctive therapy.
FDA-A = FDA approved as adjunctive therapy.
FDA-M = FDA approved as monotherapy.
FDA-MC = FDA approved for conversion to monotherapy.
FDA-MI = FDA approved as initial monotherapy.

possible, and there should be counseling prior to pregnancy. There should be discussion of which medications are most appropriate for the seizure type, which ASMs place the fetus at higher risk for adverse outcomes, and risk of seizures for the fetus. Because of the imperfect data and complexity of the decision-making process, each case must be individualized, and the ultimate decision is made by the patient and physician together. There should certainly be an effort to reduce the medication load in women taking multiple ASMs. If the patient has pure absence or pure subjective focal aware seizures, withdrawal of seizure medications can be considered. If a patient is on valproate, then a change to an alternative, such as lamotrigine, should be considered.

Some examples follow:

- A 19-year-old woman with absence epilepsy has been seizure-free on ethosuximide for

2 years. She has never had another type of seizure besides generalized absence. After discussion with the physician, she decides to discontinue ethosuximide before pregnancy. She is not expected to develop any seizures that would be dangerous to the child. She decided to remain off the drug even if absence seizures recur.

- A 25-year-old woman with generalized tonic-clonic seizures is well controlled on valproate, given for both seizures and migraines. Considering the high risk of birth defects and cognitive as well as developmental risks of valproate, it was recommended that she should switch to another ASM. After discussion with the physician, she transitions off valproate to lamotrigine.

Folate and multivitamin supplementation reduce the incidence of birth defects associated with ASMs. Folate use is also associated with higher IQ in children exposed to ASMs in utero. We recommend supplementation at prenatal doses for women with any reasonable risk of pregnancy, particularly those who are actively trying to get pregnant.

During Pregnancy

Management is more complex when the patient presents after she is already pregnant. All of the same factors just discussed will be considered, but there is a sense of concern that a substantial portion of the risk of major malformations has already been experienced. In addition, a trial off ASMs during pregnancy is riskier than one before pregnancy. Simplification of ASM polytherapy is still appropriate. In addition, patients who become pregnant on valproate should be changed to an alternative agent if possible. Although exposure to valproate in the beginning of pregnancy is associated with risk of major malformation, later exposure also can result in lower IQ and other developmental abnormalities, and adverse outcomes.[8] All patients who are pregnant should be on multivitamin supplementation, including prenatal doses of folate.

ASM blood levels have to be monitored more closely during pregnancy than before, because of changes in metabolism and volume of distribution. In particular, lamotrigine level is lowered by estrogen in the second trimester, with a higher risk of breakthrough seizures, so the dose usually has to be increased. Following delivery, the dose has

to be decreased. It is recommended that the dose be brought back to its pre-pregnancy level in two steps: half the reduction the day of delivery and the other half after 1 week. The clearance of several other medications can also be increased during pregnancy, though with less important impact on seizure control; these include levetiracetam, oxcarbazepine active metabolite, topiramate, and zonisamide. There is great variability between women, so that monitoring of serum concentration is needed for management of dosing during pregnancy.[9]

After pregnancy, while breastfeeding, the risk to the child from ASM transmission appears to be low and arguably less than the benefits of breastfeeding.[10]

Comorbid Conditions

Numerous comorbid conditions alter potential ASM selection and dose management. Some comorbid conditions are effectively treated with certain ASMs, which makes these preferable. ASMs with FDA-approved nonepileptic indications include:

- Topiramate for migraine prophylaxis;
- Valproate for migraine prophylaxis and acute treatment and maintenance for mania/bipolar disorder;
- Lamotrigine for maintenance for bipolar disorder;
- Clonazepam for panic disorder;
- Carbamazepine for trigeminal neuralgia and acute manic and mixed episodes associated with bipolar disorder (Equetro extended-release capsules);
- Gabapentin for postherpetic neuralgia and restless leg syndrome (extended-release gabapentin enacarbil);
- Pregabalin for diabetic peripheral neuropathy, postherpetic neuralgia, fibromyalgia, and neuropathic pain associated with spinal cord injury.

In addition, several ASMs are used without official FDA indication in the treatment of headaches (particularly gabapentin), insomnia (gabapentin and pregabalin), restless leg syndrome (gabapentin and pregabalin), and essential tremor (primidone and topiramate). On the other hand, some comorbid conditions can be exacerbated by certain ASMs, which makes them less desirable. For example, patients with obesity should avoid valproate, carbamazepine, and pregabalin, which can cause weight gain. Topiramate and zonisamide, which can cause weight loss, may then be favored. Topiramate and zonisamide are relatively contraindicated in individuals with kidney stones. Patients with psychosis should avoid topiramate, zonisamide, and levetiracetam. While we cannot be complete in this discussion, we present here some general guidelines.

Migraine: The coexistence of epilepsy and migraine is common. Topiramate and valproate both have FDA indications for migraine and could be considered if the frequency of migraine attacks justifies prophylactic therapy. There have been reports of multiple other ASMs being used for migraine, but efficacy and clinical utility have yet to be proved.[11,12]

Bipolar disorder: Valproate and lamotrigine have FDA indications for bipolar disorder. The former is favored for predominant mania and the latter for predominant depression. Carbamazepine also has an FDA indication with an extended release preparation. Oxcarbazepine and topiramate have also been used off-label for bipolar disorder.

Hepatic insufficiency: Valproate and other agents with principal hepatic metabolism should be avoided if possible. If used, dose adjustment is needed.

Renal insufficiency: Renal insufficiency reduces the clearance of many drugs with renal elimination so that lower doses have to be used. In addition, patients on hemodialysis may need to be redosed after dialysis.

Chemotherapy and immune modulators: Some chemotherapeutic agents and anti-rejection medications have their metabolism altered by enzyme-inducing ASMs. For some of these medications, this reduces the efficacy of treatment or makes the cost of therapy substantially higher.

Etiology

Epilepsy etiology does not generally influence the choice of medical therapy, with the exception of autoimmune etiology, which is increasingly recognized as a cause of seizures and epilepsy. Recurrent seizures related to autoimmune limbic encephalitis often respond poorly to ASMs. In addition, patients have more frequent allergic reactions to these medications. On the other hand, immunotherapy is very effective, particularly when used early. Immunotherapy should be considered when there is evidence of an autoimmune etiology. In such cases, treatment with ASMs can often be discontinued after a shorter latency than with other etiologies.

Epileptic Syndrome and Genetics

At present, the seizure type is the main predictor of response, and epileptic syndrome plays limited role. However, there are exceptions. For example, autosomal dominant sleep-related hypermotor epilepsy (previously called *nocturnal frontal lobe epilepsy*) responds particularly well to carbamazepine and oxcarbazepine.

There are also instances where the epileptic syndrome diagnosis makes a particular ASM undesirable. For example, lamotrigine and other sodium channel-blocking ASMs are known to aggravate severe myoclonic epilepsy of infancy (Dravet syndrome). Fenfluramine is effective for Dravet syndrome, but for no other epilepsy conditions. Several other less common pediatric genetic syndromes have specificity for certain medications. Phenytoin is contraindicated in progressive myoclonic epilepsies because it can worsen progressive ataxia and cause dementia. It is expected that genetics and syndrome diagnosis will have a greater role in medication selection in the future as the pathophysiology of epilepsy is better understood.

Adverse Effects

Adverse effects of ASMs as well as other drugs can be easily accessed through online references (e.g., dailymed.nlm.nih.gov) as well as product-specific websites. Note that there are some common reported adverse effects such as dizziness, gait difficulty, nausea, headache, rash, and somnolence. Comparing the frequency of these symptoms in patients treated with active drug compared with patients treated with placebo can give us a good indication of how often these can be attributed to the drug.

Expense of Medications

In an ideal universe, we would not have to be sensitive to price in medication selection, but we do not practice in that world. Many electronic health record systems have the ability to show the cost to the patient of a medication before we prescribe it. The effects of high cost include reduced compliance and stress due to financial burden.

Cost is one of the principal reasons for noncompliance.[13] Cost sensitivity should be a part of medication selection process.

Limitations of Data

Glauser et al.[14] summarized much of the efficacy of ASMs with the level of studies performed. For JME, there are no Class I studies and no Level

TABLE 8.2.3 LIMITATIONS OF DATA

Seizure type or epilepsy syndrome	Class I studies	Class II studies	Class III studies	Level of efficacy and effectiveness evidence (in alphabetical order)
Adults with partial-onsets seizures	4	I	34	Level A: CBZ, LEV, PHT, ZNS Level B: VPA Level C: GBP, LTG, OXC, PB, TPM. VGB Level C: CZP, PRM
Children with partial-onset seizures	1	0	19	Level A: OXC Level B: None Level C: CBZ, PB, PHT, TPM, VPA, VGB Level D: CLB, CZB, LTG, ZNS
Elderly adult with partial-onset seizures	1	1	3	Level A: GBP, LTG Level B: None Level C: CBZ Level D: TPM, VPA
Adults with generalized onset tonic-clonic seizures	0	0	27	Level A: None Level B: None Level C: CBZ, LTG, OXC, PB, PHT, TPM, VPA Level D: GBP, LEV, VGB
Children with generalized onset tonic-clonic seizures	0	0	14	Level A: None Level B: None Level C: CBZ, PB, PHT, TPM, VPA Level D: OXC
Children with absence seizures	1	0	7	Level A: ESM, VPA Level B: None Level C: LTG Level D: None
Benign epilepsy with centrotemporal spikes (BECTS)	0	0	3	Level A: None Level B: None Level C: CBZ, VPA Level D: GBP. LEV, OXC, STM
Juvenile myoclonic epilepsy (JME)	0	0	1	Level A: None Level B: None Level C: None Level D: TPM, VPA

CBZ, carbamazepine; CLB, clobazam; CZB, clorazepate dipotassium; ESM, ethosuximide; GBP, gabapentin; LEV, levetiracetam; LTG, lamotrigine; OXC, oxcarbazepine; PB, phenobarbital; PHT, phenytoin; STM, sulthiame ; TPM, topiramate; VPA, valproic acid; ZNS, zonisamide.

A, B, or C data, only Level D data. There are no Level A or B data for children and adults with generalized-onset tonic-clonic seizures (see Table 8.2.3).

Limitations of FDA Indications

Medical professionals understand that the FDA approves medications for specific indications only if evidence supporting efficacy satisfies regulatory requirements and also if someone files for the indication. This is an expensive process, so FDA-approved indications are not expanded unless some company finds potential profit worth the application fee and internal costs. Hence indications seldom expand after generic formulations are approved. However, providers are not bound by FDA-approved indications when ordering an agent. Nevertheless, many patients do not understand this system, and some insurance companies use lack of FDA indication as a rationale for noncoverage.

DOSING FOR FIRST-LINE THERAPY

The dosing for first-line therapy is described for each ASM in Table 8.2.4.

TABLE 8.2.4 DOSING FOR ANTI-SEIZURE MEDICATIONS (ASMs) APPROPRIATE AS INITIAL MONOTHERAPY IN ADULTS

ASM	Starting daily dose	Titration	Initial target daily dose	Schedule
Phenobarbital	30–60 mg	Increase by 30–60 mg as needed	100 mg	Once daily dosing at bedtime reduces sedation and is justified by long half-life
Phenytoin	200–400 mg	Not needed	200–400 mg	Once daily at bedtime; bid or tid if drug-resistant
Ethosuximide	500 mg	250 mg every week as needed	750–1,000 mg	Bid or tid (for tolerability)
Carbamazepine	200 mg	200 mg every 3 days	400–800 mg	Bid or tid
Valproate	500 mg	optional	1,000 mg	Bid for DR, once daily for ER
Gabapentin	300–400 mg	Increase by 300–400 mg daily	1,200 mg	Bid or tid
Lamotrigine	25 mg	Double every 2 weeks	200 mg	Bid (once daily for ER)
Topiramate	25 mg	Add 25 mg every week	100 mg	Once daily at bedtime or bid (once daily for ER)
Levetiracetam	500–1000 mg	If starting at 500 mg, add 500 mg after one week if needed	1,000 mg	Bid (once daily for ER)
Oxcarbazepine	300–600 mg	If starting at 300 mg, add 300 mg after one week	600 mg	Bid (once daily for ER)
Zonisamide	100 mg	Add 100 mg after 1–2 weeks	200 mg	Once-daily dosing at bedtime is justified by long half-life
Eslicarbazepine Acetate	400 mg	Add 400 mg after one week	800 mg	Once daily at bedtime
Lacosamide	100 mg	Add 100 mg after one week	200 mg	Bid

Bid, twice daily; DR, delayed release; ER, extended release; tid, three times daily.

It is essential to be familiar with the pharmacokinetics of these ASMs for best use and particularly for dosing schedule (Table 8.2.5).

DRUG-LEVEL MONITORING

Serum levels are measurable for most ASMs. ASM serum levels should only assist in clinical decision-making and should not be the primary basis for dosing decisions. A "therapeutic range" has been suggested for some ASMs. This is best established for the older agents phenytoin, carbamazepine, and valproate and is also helpful for lamotrigine and oxcarbazepine. The range is only a useful guide, and a value outside the range should not be the only reason to change the dose. Routine ASM level monitoring is not necessary.

ASM levels are most helpful in the following situations:

- As a reference value once a clinically effective dose has been reached.

- Verifying that the ASM level is within the effective range for a patient with infrequent seizures, for whom ascertainment of effective seizure control may take a very long time. In this case, the neurologist would aim for a level in the middle of the range.

- Monitoring phenytoin level during titration in a patient with difficult to control seizures. Because of nonlinear kinetics, the level may increase excessively with a small increment in the dose. The level may need to be checked intermittently during the process of titration. At a serum level near 20 μg/mL, additional titration may result in toxicity.

- Verifying stability of ASM level for phenytoin, which has nonlinear kinetics. The phenytoin level can fluctuate widely with a small change in dose or small change in absorption.

TABLE 8.2.5 PHARMACOKINETIC PROPERTIES OF ANTI-SEIZURE MEDICATIONS (ASMs) APPROPRIATE AS INITIAL MONOTHERAPY

ASM	Oral absorption/ bioavailability High: ≥90 % Intermediate: ≥70% to <90% Low: <70%	Half-life (hours) Short: ≤10 Intermediate: >10–30< Long: ≥30	Extended release preparation	Intravenous preparation	Metabolism + <50% ++ ≥50% to ≤90% >90%
Phenobarbital	High	Long	–	Yes	++ Liver
Phenytoin	Intermediate	Intermediate	Yes	Yes	+++Liver
Ethosuximide	High	Long	–	–	++Liver
Carbamazepine	Intermediate	Intermediate	Yes	Yes	+++Liver
Valproate	High	Intermediate	Yes	Yes	+++Liver
Gabapentin	Low	Short	–*	–	None
Lamotrigine	High	Intermediate	Yes	–	+++Liver
Topiramate	Intermediate	Intermediate	–**	–	+Liver
Levetiracetam	High	Short	Yes	Yes	+Blood
Oxcarbazepine	High	Intermediate¶	–**	–	+++Liver
Zonisamide	High	Long	–	–	++Liver
Eslicarbazepine Acetate	High	Intermediate	–	–	++Liver
Lacosamide	High	Intermediate	–	Yes	++Liver

* Not approved for epilepsy.
¶ Combination of parent drug and active metabolite monohydroxy derivative.

- After a breakthrough seizure occurs, to determine if the breakthrough seizure was related to a drop in the serum level.
- To help explain lack of ASM efficacy at what appears to be a high dose. A low level despite a high dose may indicate that the patient is a high metabolizer or is not compliant. A low level may encourage repeat measurements to verify stability. Large variability may suggest inconsistent compliance. If the patient is compliant, a low level indicates room for further increases in dosing if needed for seizure control, even at the maximal dose recommended in the prescribing information. Undetectable levels despite a high dose suggest noncompliance.
- To help explain appearance of adverse effects at a relatively low dose. A high level may suggest that the patient is a slow metabolizer, and a lower dose may be indicated.
- To watch for pharmacokinetic interactions after introduction of another medication that may affect the baseline ASM.
- To monitor ASM level during pregnancy, which is known to reduce some ASM levels.
- To monitor stability of ASM level when switching to a different formulation or a different brand.

For highly protein-bound ASMs such as phenytoin and valproate, the protein-free portion is responsible for efficacy and toxicity. When these ASMs are used in monotherapy in an otherwise healthy individual, the total serum level is a good predictor of the protein-free level. However, measuring protein-free levels will be important in physiological states that may change the proportion of binding such that the total level is no longer a predictor of the protein-free level. These clinical situations include low-protein states such as renal failure, hepatic failure, malnutrition, and old age, pregnancy, or concomitant use of phenytoin and valproate, with resultant competition for protein binding. Phenytoin and valproate are both approximately 90% protein-bound. Protein-binding of valproate can be saturated at high doses, at which point the free level may be much higher than predicted by the total serum level.

ASM levels should generally assist therapy rather than direct it. With some exceptions, it is generally not appropriate to drive the ASM dose to achieve a level in the "therapeutic range" because the definition of the therapeutic range is arbitrary to a certain extent. If there is a good clinical response, then measurement of the level can show what an effective level is for that patient. One exception to this rule is in the patient with very infrequent seizures. In such a case, it may take a very long time to determine if the treatment has been successful. It is then recommended to titrate to a middle-range dose or a middle-range level.

If the seizures are not controlled on what would normally be a reasonable target dose, then measurement of the level can determine whether there is room to increase the dose further. Toxicity is usually determined by clinical symptoms rather than levels. However, if the drug level is significantly higher than the published upper limit of "therapeutic range," then further increase in dose is likely not warranted. On the other hand, if good seizure control is achieved by a level that is somewhat higher than the "therapeutic range," yet there are no symptoms or signs of toxicity, then the dose should usually not be reduced despite the high level.

If a patient has loss of seizure control, one of the possible reasons is reduction in blood level, either due to missing doses or change in metabolism. Missing doses is a major cause of reduced drug level. Altered metabolism can be from exposure to a new drug (e.g., antibiotic) or alcohol.

Some drugs have nonlinear kinetics, so small changes in dose can produce large changes in levels. Phenytoin is currently the only ASM with proven nonlinear kinetics. At low levels, small dose changes produce small changes in level, whereas at higher levels (e.g., mid to high therapeutic) small dose changes can produce large changes in level. As phenytoin is being pushed to maximal therapeutic levels, careful monitoring of the level is warranted (see Table 8.2.6).

SECOND-LINE THERAPY

If an ASM is not tolerated, it should be replaced with another. However, if an ASM trial fails due to lack of efficacy, there are more options. Before an ASM trial has been declared a failure, it is important to review a number of questions.

- Has the medication been titrated to the maximum tolerated dose?
- Has the patient been compliant with the medication?
- Are the breakthrough seizures provoked by factors that can be corrected, such as sleep deprivation, alcohol or drug abuse, or concomitant use of a medication known to reduce the seizure threshold?

If it is determined that the ASM has truly failed due to lack of efficacy, the physician can choose to replace it with another ASM in monotherapy or add another ASM. Studies do not show a difference in efficacy and side effects between these two options, although there is a slight trend favoring adjunctive therapy with another medication.[15,16,17,18] From a commonsense perspective, replacement monotherapy is the best choice if the first ASM was completely ineffective. However, if the first ASM was partially effective, adding a second ASM may be a better consideration. Other considerations may favor substitution versus add-on therapy (Table 8.2.7).

Replacing the first ASM usually requires first adding the new ASM before withdrawing the old one. It is acceptable and sometimes advantageous to reduce the dose of the first ASM as the new ASM is titrated. An overnight switch is possible for some ASMs, provided the doses are

TABLE 8.2.6 ANTISEIZURE MEDICATION (ASM) LEVELS THAT ARE MOST USEFUL IN PRACTICE

ASM	Lower end of range (µg/mL) Breakthrough seizures more likely below this value	Higher end of range (µg/mL) Toxicity more likely above this value
Phenytoin	Total level: 10 Free level: 1	Total level: 20 Free level: 2
Carbamazepine	4	12
Valproate	Total level: 50 Free level: 5	Total level: 100 Free level: 10
Lamotrigine	2	20
Oxcarbazepine (level measures MHD metabolite)	10	35

MHD, monohydroxy derivative.

TABLE 8.2.7 CONSIDERATIONS FAVORING SUBSTITUTION VERSUS ADD-ON THERAPY AFTER FAILURE OF FIRST ANTI-SEIZURE MEDICATION (ASM)

Favoring substitution monotherapy	Favoring add-on therapy
First ASM not tolerated	First ASM partially effective and well-tolerated
First ASM totally ineffective	First ASM effective, but with complete seizure control only at doses that are not well tolerated; well-tolerated at lower doses
Woman of childbearing potential contemplating pregnancy Patients with compliance challenges Financial limitations	Add-on ASM not well-tested in monotherapy

not high (see Figure 8.2.2). An overnight switch has been well tested for carbamazepine to oxcarbazepine conversion using a 2:3 dose ratio, provided the dose of carbamazepine is 800 mg or less. Based on some similarity in properties and mechanism (but without supportive published evidence), one of the authors also switches gabapentin to pregabalin using a 6:1 ratio (if the gabapentin dose is 1,800 mg or less) and topiramate to zonisamide (using a 1:1 ratio for a dose of 200 mg or less).

All ASMs are FDA-approved for adjunctive therapy. Table 8.2.8 outlines the pharmacokinetic properties of ASMs that are not appropriate for initial therapy in adults.

Adding a new ASM to an old one should consider interactions between the two. The interaction can be pharmacokinetic (e.g., a change in the serum level of the old drug as the new one is added) or pharmacodynamic (e.g., no change in the level of the old ASM, but increased toxicity because of additive adverse experiences). Some pharmacodynamic interactions are favorable, with evidence of synergy. Such beneficial additive effects are best demonstrated for the combination of lamotrigine and valproate. Another combination that seems to be particularly helpful is that of lamotrigine and levetiracetam, but it has less support in the literature. In general, there is a suggestion that an ASM combination with different

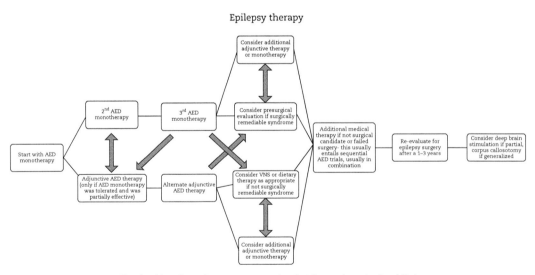

Epilepsy therapy

The algorithm shows the next step assuming that the previous step has failed

FIGURE 8.2.2 Approach to epilepsy therapy.

TABLE 8.2.8 PHARMACOKINETIC PROPERTIES OF ANTI-SEIZURE MEDICATIONS (ASMs) NOT APPROPRIATE AS INITIAL MONOTHERAPY

ASM	Oral absorption/ bioavailability High: ≥90 % Intermediate: ≥70% to <90% Low: <70%	Half-life (hours) Short: ≤10 Intermediate: >10-30< Long: ≥30	Extended release preparation	Intravenous preparation (USA)	Metabolism + <50% ++ ≥50% to ≤90% >90%	Comments
Primidone	High	Intermediate[a]	–	–	++Liver	
Clonazepam	High	Long	–	–	++Liver	
Methsuximide[b]	High	Long	–	–	+Liver	
Felbamate	High	Intermediate	–	–	++Liver	
Tiagabine	High	Short	–	–	+++Liver	
Pregabalin	High	Short	–	–	None	
Rufinamide	Intermediate	Short	–	–	+++Liver	
Vigabatrin	High	Short[c]	–	–	None	
Clobazam	High	Long	–	–	+++Liver	
Perampanel	High	Long	–	–	+++Liver	
Brivaracetam	High	Short	–	Yes	++Liver	
Cannabidiol	Low	Long	–	–	+++Liver	
Cenobamate	Intermediate	Long	–	–	+++Liver	

[b] Applies to active metabolite N-desmethylmethsuximide.
[a] Long for the metabolite phenobarbital.
[c] The duration of effect is longer than expected from T1/2 because the drug works through irreversible inhibition of gamma-aminobutyric acid (GABA) transaminase enzyme.

mechanisms may be more efficacious than a combination of two ASMs with the same mechanism (see Table 8.2.9). For the ASMs recommended as second- and third-line therapy, please refer to Table 8.2.10.

DRUG INTERACTIONS

Pharmacokinetic interaction implies that the addition of an ASM to another results in a change in serum level. Factors that make a drug more likely to interact are enzyme induction or inhibition, liver metabolism, and high protein binding. Table 8.2.11 shows the potential of ASMs to interact based on these properties.

ASM Interactions

The most common pharmacokinetic interactions are a result of enzyme induction resulting in increased clearance and lower serum level, or enzyme inhibition resulting in decreased clearance with resulting accumulation and increased serum level.[19]

Some ASMs, such as carbamazepine, phenytoin, and phenobarbital, produce profound and widespread enzyme induction and result in

reduced levels of other ASMs that are metabolized by the liver. The greater the liver metabolism of an ASM, the more it is affected by enzyme inducers. This is why it can be very difficult to achieve a therapeutic level of valproate in the presence of carbamazepine or phenytoin. The increased metabolism can also increase the production of toxic metabolites that mediate some types of valproate toxicity. Other ASMs have more modest and more selective enzyme induction. For example, oxcarbazepine enzyme induction is more specific for hepatic enzymes responsible for the metabolism of some calcium antagonists, oral contraceptives, and cyclosporin. However, oxcarbazepine does not affect valproate or warfarin levels, which are markedly affected by carbamazepine.

Valproate is a hepatic enzyme inhibitor and markedly reduces the metabolism of lamotrigine and rufinamide so that titration rates and target dose of these latter medications is considerably reduced in the presence of valproate. If valproate is added to lamotrigine or rufinamide, the doses of these medications have to be reduced by at least 50% to prevent toxicity. Felbamate is also an

TABLE 8.2.9 KEY KNOWN ANTI-SEIZURE MEDICATION (ASM) MECHANISMS OF ACTION

ASM	Sodium channel blocking	Enhancing GABA	Glutamate receptor antagonism	Blocking high-voltage activated calcium channels	Blocking T-calcium channels	Binding alpha-2-delta subunit of voltage-activated calcium channels	Binding SV2A	Comment
Phenobarbital		X	X	X				
Primidone		X	X					
Phenytoin	X							
Methsuximide†	X							
Ethosuximide					X			
Clonazepam and clobazam		X						
Carbamazepine	X							
Valproate	X	X			X			NMDA receptor antagonism
Felbamate	X	X	X	X				
Gabapentin						X		
Lamotrigine	X			X				
Topiramate	X	X	X					Kainate and AMPA Receptor antagonism
Tiagabine		X						Inhibition of GABA reuptake
Levetiracetam							X	
Oxcarbazepine	X							
Zonisamide	X		X		X			
Pregabalin						X		
Lacosamide	X							Selective enhancing of slow inactivation of voltage-gated sodium channels
Rufinamide	X							
Vigabatrin		X						Irreversible inhibition of GABA transaminase
Perampanel			X					selective noncompetitive antagonism of the AMPA receptor
Eslicarbazepine acetate	X							
Brivaracetam							X	
Cannabidiol		X						
Cenobamate	X	X						Also modulates intracellular calcium

AMPA, alpha-amino-3-hydroxy-5-methyl-4-isoxazole propionic acid; GABA, gamma-aminobutyric acid; NMDA, N-methyl-D-aspartate.

TABLE 8.2.10 ANTI-SEIZURE MEDICATIONS (ASMs) FOR FIRST THROUGH LATER LINES OF THERAPY

	Focal-onset	Generalized tonic-clonic	Generalized absence	Generalized myoclonic	Generalized tonic-atonic in Lennox-Gastaut syndrome (LGS)
First-line	Lamotrigine Levetiracetam Oxcarbazepine Eslicarbazepine acetate Lacosamide Topiramate Zonisamide Carbamazepine Phenytoin Valproate Phenobarbital Gabapentin	Valproate Lamotrigine Levetiracetam Topiramate	Ethosuximide Valproate Lamotrigine	Valproate Levetiracetam	Valproate
Second- and third-line	All above Pregabalin Brivaracetam Cenobamate Tiagabine Clobazam Perampanel Methsuximide Clonazepam	All above Zonisamide Clonazepam Lacosamide Rufinamide Clonazepam Clobazam	All above Levetiracetam Zonisamide Clonazepam Clobazam Methsuximide	All above Zonisamide Topiramate Lamotrigine[a] Clonazepam Clobazam	Rufinamide Lamotrigine Topiramate Clobazam Clonazepam Cannabidiol
Late consideration	Vigabatrin Felbamate Primidone	Phenytoin[b] Carbamazepine[b] Phenobarbital Primidone Methsuximide Felbamate	Topiramate[c] Felbamate	Primidone Felbamate	Zonisamide Levetiracetam Brivaracetam Lacosamide Felbamate

[a] May worsen myoclonic seizures in some patients.
[b] May activate myoclonic and absence seizures in some patients.
[c] Effective in case series, but ineffective in one controlled trial.

important inhibitor of liver enzymes, so that doses of several ASMs have to be reduced in conjunction with its addition. Valproate and felbamate both inhibit the clearance and cause accumulation of carbamazepine epoxide, which is a metabolite of carbamazepine responsible for some important carbamazepine toxic adverse effects. Awareness of this interaction is important since toxicity may occur in the presence of low carbamazepine levels. Carbamazepine epoxide levels must be measured on request and sent to a central laboratory. Several ASMs are selective inhibitors of specific liver enzymes. For example, oxcarbazepine can inhibit the liver enzyme responsible for phenytoin metabolism and can produce an elevation of phenytoin level.

Another type of interaction is competition for protein binding, which can play a role in ASMs that are highly protein bound. In particular, the competition of phenytoin and valproate for protein binding is clinically relevant because therapeutic decisions are often made based on total serum levels, while the free levels determine efficacy and toxicity. For example, in the presence of valproate competing for protein binding, the protein-free portion of phenytoin may rise from 10% to 30%.

TABLE 8.2.11 PHARMACOKINETIC INTERACTIONS

Antiseizure medication	Hepatic enzyme induction	Autoinduction	Hepatic enzyme inhibition	Affected by enzyme inducers	Affected by enzyme inhibitors	Protein-binding
	+ minimal (usually selective) ++ intermediate +++ pronounced − absent			+ affected − not affected		High ≥85% Low<85%
Phenobarbital	+++	−	−	+	+	Low
Primidone	+++	−	−	+	+	Low
Phenytoin	+++	−	−	+	+	High
Methsuximide[b]	+	−	−	+	−	Low
Ethosuximide	−	−	−	+	−	Low
Clonazepam	−	−	−	−	−	High
Carbamazepine	+++	+++	−	+	++	Low
Valproate	−	−	+++	+	+	High
Felbamate	+	−	++	+	+	Low
Gabapentin	−	−	−	−	−	None
Lamotrigine	+	+	−	+	++	None
Topiramate	+[a]	−	+[a]	+	−	Low
Tiagabine	−	−	−	+	−	High
Levetiracetam	−	−	−	+/−	−	Low
Oxcarbazepine[b]	++[c]	−	+[c]	+	−	Low
Zonisamide	−	−	−	+	+	Low
Pregabalin	−	−	−	−	−	None
Lacosamide	−	−	−	+	−	Low
Rufinamide	+	−	+	+	++	Low
Vigabatrin	+	−	−	−	−	None
Clobazam	+	−	+	−	++§	Intermediate
Perampanel	+	−	+	+	+	High
Eslicarbazepine acetate	++	−	+	+	−	Low
Brivaracetam	−	−	+	+	−	Low
Cannabidiol	−	−	++	+	+	High
Cenobamate	+	−	++	+	+	Low

[a] At doses ≥200 mg.
[b] Parent drug and metabolite.
[c] At doses ≥900 mg.
[d] Applies to active metabolite N-desmethylclobazam.

A phenytoin total level of 15 μg/mL may be associated with severe toxicity because the free level is 4.5 μg/mL, equivalent to a total level of 45 μg/mL in an individual with the expected 10% unbound fraction. Thus, when valproate and phenytoin are used together, free levels should be measured if needed for therapeutic decision-making. Tiagabine and perampanel are also highly protein bound, but because of their low dose and small concentration, they are less likely to affect phenytoin or valproate protein binding. In addition, their dosing is almost never based on serum level.

Pharmacodynamic interactions do not involve a change in serum concentration of the involved ASM. They are most often related to the additive toxicity of ASMs that have the same mechanism of action. Pharmacodynamic interactions are often seen when combining ASMs that act on the sodium channel. For example, dizziness, blurred vision, diplopia, and unsteadiness are often seen when combining lamotrigine, lacosamide, carbamazepine, or oxcarbazepine. Thus, mechanism of action is currently more relevant to tolerability than to efficacy of ASMs.

Interactions between ASM and non-ASM medications are potentially bidirectional and are most likely with the oldest ASM. The enzyme-inducing ASMs may reduce the efficacy of many medications metabolized by the liver, such as warfarin, oral contraceptives, many chemotherapeutic agents, etc. Similarly, ASM levels are affected by inducers or inhibitors of their metabolism. Carbamazepine and phenytoin levels can be elevated by many non-ASM medications. The long list of agents that inhibit carbamazepine metabolism and result in carbamazepine accumulation includes cimetidine, diltiazem, erythromycin, clarithromycin, fluoxetine, isoniazid, propoxyphene, ketoconazole (and related agents), verapamil, and grapefruit juice. Oxcarbazepine, which is related to carbamazepine, is not subject to this type of interaction.

One important interaction is between estrogen, an inducer of glucuronidation, and ASMs that are metabolized by glucuronidation. Lamotrigine is the most susceptible, but valproate and oxcarbazepine are also affected to a lesser degree. Estrogen-containing oral contraceptives can reduce the lamotrigine serum level considerably, with associated increase in seizure frequency.

SUCCESS OF ASM THERAPY

Effectiveness of medical therapy is strongly dependent on epilepsy syndrome and underlying pathology. Patients with idiopathic generalized epilepsy are much more likely to have complete seizure control than are patients with focal epilepsy or structural/metabolic generalized epilepsy. For those with focal epilepsy, specific lesions, such as hippocampal sclerosis or dual pathology, are associated with a lower chance of seizure control.

Drug-Resistant Epilepsy

Despite the proliferation of ASMs, approximately one-third of patients with epilepsy have persistent seizures.[20] Early response to treatment is an important predictor of drug resistance. Patients started on a first monotherapy trial have a roughly 50% chance of seizure freedom. If the first ASM is failed due to side effects, the chance of seizure freedom with next monotherapy remains roughly 50%. However, if the first drug is failed due to lack of efficacy, the chance of the second drug achieving total seizure control becomes much less, approximately 11%. After failure of two ASMs, few patients become seizure-free in the long term, whether with a third monotherapy or with combination therapy. One study that related the chances of seizure control to the number of failed ASMs found 0% of seizure control after failure of 6 or 7 ASMs.[21]

Definition of Drug Resistance

What failed treatment is sufficient for the patient to qualify as drug-resistant? The International League Against Epilepsy (ILAE) defined drug resistance as failure of adequate trials of two tolerated, appropriately chosen and used ASM schedules (whether as monotherapy or in combination) to achieve sustained seizure freedom.[22] Failure of an ASM must be because of lack of efficacy and not intolerance. Epilepsy cannot be considered drug-resistant if the ASM is underdosed or inappropriate for seizure type, or if the diagnosis of epilepsy is wrong (e.g., nonepileptic events).

Management Options for Drug-Resistant Epilepsy

Patients with drug-resistant epilepsy should have a re-evaluation of the diagnosis. As always, the possibility of a diagnosis other than epilepsy should be considered when seizures do not respond to appropriate medications. The most common alternative diagnoses are psychogenic nonepileptic events and syncope. If the diagnosis of epilepsy is confirmed, evaluation for epilepsy surgery is warranted. Epilepsy surgery is appropriate if the patient has a surgically remediable syndrome with a high chance of complete seizure freedom. Examples of "surgically remediable syndromes" include epilepsy with unilateral hippocampal sclerosis and epilepsy with a well-defined small epileptogenic lesion, such as cavernous malformation or benign tumor. For these patients, the chances of seizure freedom with epilepsy surgery are approximately 70%, which is much better than could be expected with any subsequent planned medication trial.

Patients who do not have a surgically remediable syndrome should have trials of additional ASMs, most probably combination therapies. However, dietary therapy and vagus nerve stimulation (VNS) can be considered in individuals who are tired of ineffective ASM therapies or are experiencing adverse effects from ineffective therapies. VNS should not be implanted without first confirming the diagnosis of epilepsy; a considerable number of patients subjected to this procedure have nonepileptic events, and we must be excessively vigilant to confirm the epilepsy diagnosis.

If a patient is not an optimal candidate for epilepsy surgery, trials of additional ASMs alone or in combination are appropriate before consideration of a surgical procedure that has a lower yield or that is palliative. An algorithm for identifying and managing drug-resistant epilepsy is provided in Figure 8.2.3.

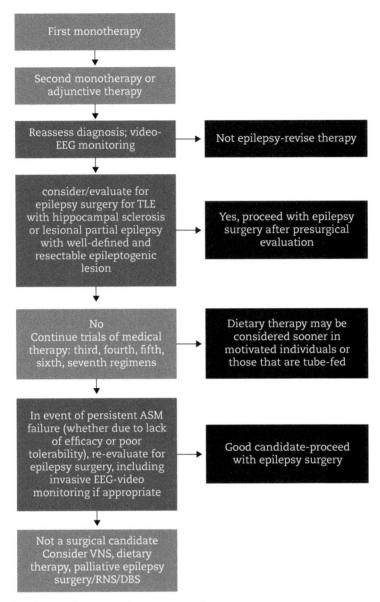

FIGURE 8.2.3 Identifying and managing drug-resistant epilepsy.

AUTOIMMUNE EPILEPSY

Epilepsy can be a long-term outcome of auto-immune encephalitis, particularly when immunotherapy treatment is delayed or not used. In addition, epilepsy can have an underlying autoimmune basis even without a prior acute autoimmune encephalitis. The most common antibody in these patients is anti-GAD. Patients with autoimmune epilepsy are frequently resistant to ASMs, and immunotherapy should be considered as a treatment option. The best response to immunotherapy is seen when antibodies are directed to cell membrane targets. With antibodies directed against cytoplasmic or nuclear targets, including anti-GAD antibodies, worthwhile improvement is less likely but is still seen in approximately one-third of patients. First-line immunotherapy includes intravenous or oral steroids, intravenous immunoglobulin (IVIG), and plasmapheresis. Second-line immunotherapy includes rituximab, mycophenolate mofetil, and cyclophosphamide. Immunotherapy is usually given in consultation with a neuro-immunologist.

DISCONTINUATION OF MEDICAL THERAPY

When patients enter into long-term remission, discontinuation of ASM therapy may be considered in some individuals. However, it is not possible to determine if the remission will persist after medication withdrawal. While there are indicators to help predict successful ASM withdrawal, there is no way to be absolutely sure that seizures will not recur. When deciding to withdraw medications, one must consider both the consequences of seizure recurrence (loss of driving privileges, risk to employment, possibility that seizures may be harder to control after recurrence) and the benefit of eliminating medication side effects and medication cost.

Children have a lower risk of seizure recurrence than adults, in general, although it depends on seizure type and etiology. This means that a trial of ASM withdrawal can be considered sooner in children (1–2 years of seizure freedom) than in adults (4–5 years of seizure freedom).

ASM withdrawal is more likely to be successful in

- Patients with pure genetic epilepsy syndromes as compared to those with epilepsy of a structural-metabolic etiology;
- Patients with epilepsy onset in adolescence as compared to epilepsy starting in childhood;
- Patients with a normal EEG as compared to those with abnormal EEG;
- Patients with focal-onset seizures who became seizure-free quickly as compared to those who needed more than 5 years to become seizure-free;
- Adults with shorter duration of active epilepsy and a longer duration of seizure remission as opposed to adults with longer duration of active epilepsy and shorter seizure remission;
- Patients with normal psychiatric examination as compared to those with abnormal psychiatric examination;
- Patients with normal IQ as compared to those with an IQ of less than 70;
- Patients with normal MRI as compared to patients with MRI showing hippocampal sclerosis.

Abrupt discontinuation of ASMs is never recommended. Severe seizures may occur during withdrawal of some ASMs, particularly benzodiazepines, carbamazepine, and oxcarbazepine. It is generally best to withdraw medications slowly.

8.3

Management of Status Epilepticus

HASAN H. SONMEZTURK

TREATMENT AND PROGNOSIS OF STATUS EPILEPTICUS

There have been several Class I randomized controlled trials testing first-line agents for in-hospital and outside hospital treatment of generalized convulsive status epilepticus (GCSE).[1] SE treatment starts with stabilization therapies including ABCs (airway, breathing, circulation), timing seizure from onset, continuous vital sign monitoring, oxygenation, metabolic parameters check (e.g., blood gases), establishing intravenous (IV) access, and sending blood chemistry for electrolytes, toxicology, and hematology (Box 8.3.1).

After initial stabilization, which should take 0–5 min initial medical therapy should be initiated at 5 min. Benzodiazepines such as lorazepam IV, diazepam IV and midazolam IM all have Level A scientific evidence as first-line agents for the treatment of GCSE (Box 8.3.2). Phenobarbital IV also has Level A evidence as initial therapy. If treatment is taking place in the field (outside hospital), rectal diazepam and intranasal midazolam can be used and, both of these agents have Level B evidence for initial treatment of SE.

If GCSE cannot be stopped with first-line agents, the second-line agents are initiated usually around minute 20. However, many scholars recommend ordering the second-line agents while trying first-line agents so they are ready for timely administration if first-line agents fail. A recent randomized controlled trial provided Level A evidence for three nonsedating anti-seizure medications (ASMs) as second-line agents for the treatment of GCSE.[2] These were fosphenytoin, valproate, and levetiracetam. Each of these agents led to seizure cessation and improved alertness by 60 min in approximately half the patients, and the three drugs were associated with similar incidences of adverse events. There were no differences between efficacy and adverse events (Box 8.3.3).

Evidence-based treatment for GCSE or any other kind of SE lasting beyond 40 min is scarce at best. However, there are general recommendations and conventional approaches. If second-line agents fail, preparations should be made for IV general anesthesia with the administration of third-line agents. An additional dose of IV fosphenytoin can be given at 5–10 mg/kg (max

---

BOX 8.3.1 STATUS EPILEPTICUS PHASES OF CARE: 0–5 MINUTES (STABILIZATION PHASE)

Stabilize patient (airway, breathing, circulation, disability: neurologic exam).

Time seizure from its onset, monitor vital signs.

Assess oxygenation, give oxygen via nasal cannula/mask, consider intubation if respiratory assistance is needed.

Initiate electrocardiogram (EKG) monitoring.

Collect finger stick blood glucose. If glucose <60 mg/dL then

Adults: 100 mg thiamine IV followed by D50 (50 ml IV) and start second IV with D5NS

Children ≥2 years: 2 mL/kg D25W IV

Children <2 years: 4 mL/kg D12.5W IV

Attempt IV access and collect electrolytes, hematology, tox screen (if appropriate), and anticonvulsant drug levels. Use normal saline to keep IV lines open.

BOX 8.3.2 STATUS EPILEPTICUS PHASES OF CARE: 5–20 MINUTES (INITIAL THERAPY PHASE)

If seizures continue:

A BZD is the initial therapy of choice (Level A):

Choose *one* of the following three equivalent first-line options following recommended dosing and frequency:

- IM Midazolam (10 mg for >40 kg, 5 mg for 13–40 kg, single dose, Level A)
- IV Lorazepam (0.1 mg/kg/dose, max: 4 mg/dose, may repeat dose once, Level A)
- IV Diazepam (0.15–2 mg/kg/dose, max 10 mg/dose, may repeat once, Level A)

If none of these three options is available, choose one of the following:

- IV phenobarbital (15 mg/kg/dose, single dose, Level A)
- Rectal diazepam (0.2–0.5 mg/kg, max: 20 mg/dose, single dose, Level B)
- Intranasal midazolam (Level B), buccal midazolam (Level B)

---

30 mg/kg) before the initiation of sedation with intubation. The third-line anesthetic agents most commonly used are infusions of pentobarbital, midazolam, and propofol (Box 8.3.4). All three agents are generally acceptable choices for the first 24 hours of treatment; however, if seizures persist beyond 24 hours, it is recommended to switch to pentobarbital coma as propofol runs the risk of propofol infusion syndrome and midazolam runs the risk of tachyphylaxis.[3]

In one retrospective study by Ferlisi and Shorvon, the outcome of 1,168 refractory and super-refractory SE cases were reviewed and anesthetic therapy outcomes were reported (Table 8.3.1).

It is recommended that IV sedation be tapered off every 24–48 hours to reassess and, if seizures recur, adjust the nonsedating ASMs and resume anesthesia. In selected patients who have only focal or multifocal electrographic and clinical seizures and were intubated only for airway protection, not resuming generalized anesthesia can be considered. These patients should not have generalized convulsions or generalized bihemispheric bisynchronous electrographic ictal discharges. This approach can provide real-time assessment of response to nonsedating ASM optimization and faster seizure control. Patient's awakening can also change the perspective of family members and care providers, avoiding premature withdrawal of care, which is not an uncommon cause of death in refractory SE (RSE) and super-refractory SE (SRSE) patients.[4] According to one study by Sutter et al. 2014, anesthetic use in SE was associated with a 2.9-fold increase in death independent of possible confounders.[5]

BOX 8.3.3 STATUS EPILEPTICUS PHASES OF CARE: 20–40 MINUTES (SECOND THERAPY PHASE)

If seizures continue:

Choose *one* of the following second-line options and give as a single dose:

- IV fosphenytoin (20 mg Phenytoin Equivalent [PE]/kg, max: 1,500 mg PE/dose, single dose, Level A)
- IV valproic acid (40 mg/kg, max: 3,000 mg/dose, single dose, Level A)
- IV levetiracetam (60 mg/kg, max: 4,500 mg/dose, single dose, Level A)

If none of these options is available:

- IV phenobarbital (15–20 mg/kg, max dose, Level B)

BOX 8.3.4   STATUS EPILEPTICUS PHASES OF CARE: 40 MINUTES–24 HOURS (THIRD-LINE THERAPY)

If seizures continue:

- Pentobarbital 5–15 mg/kg load, 0.5–5 mg/kg/h maintenance
- Midazolam 0.2 mg/kg load, 0.05–0.5 mg/kg/h maintenance
- Propofol 1 mg/kg over 5 min, repeat ×1 if necessary, 2–4 mg/kg/h to start maintenance, adjust to 1–15 mg/kg/h

The use of nonsedating ASMs for the treatment of SRSE is also experimental at best. However, high doses of phenobarbital IV with blood levels reaching as high as 100–150 µg/mL can be an option. This agent will prevent withdrawal seizures while anesthetic agents are tapered off, and it can be given IV and tapered over a very long time, thus providing smooth transition from anesthesia to awake state. It can also be continued via oral administration after the patient is extubated or discharged. Several small retrospective studies showed more favorable outcomes when patients used phenobarbital to transition out of sedation.[6,7,8]

There are case reports and case series reporting the benefit of using very high doses of nonsedating ASMs for RSE and SRSE. These are levetiracetam (4 gm IV load and maintain at 6 g/d) lacosamide (800 mg IV load and maintain at 400 mg/d), perampanel at 24–36 mg/d, topiramate at 400–800 mg/d, and clobazam at 40–60 mg/d. Other agents/methods that can be tried for SRSE after all of the earlier mentioned therapies fail are lidocaine (100 mg IV load followed by 1.5 mg/min IV infusion for 24 hours), ketamine, etomidate, ketogenic diet, hypothermia (24–48 hours), immunosuppressive or immunomodulatory agents (if etiology is unknown), and plasmapheresis for autoimmune encephalitis cases.

SE continues to be a serious condition with high mortality rate. One study[9] showed a 27% death rate in GCSE (overt) and a 67.7% death rate in nonconvulsive SE (NCSE) (subtle GCSE). High but variable rates of mortality have been reported for RSE and SRSE, mostly with grave prognoses: mortality rates run to 33–39% with only 15–22% of patients returning to their baseline functionality.[10]

MEDICATIONS USED FOR STATUS EPILEPTICUS

Note that some of the doses and methods of ASM administration just discussed are accepted medical practice yet not FDA-approved. Consult current scientific and regulatory information before prescribing these agents. Off-label use is appropriate when supported by good rationale and data.

The paucity of rigorous data regarding treatment of SE is problematic considering the number of patients seen with this condition. There are Level A data for SE for only phenytoin, valproate, phenobarbital, and lorazepam. Yet there are other convincing data that we rely on for management guidance.

Ketamine is an injectable anesthetic agent which is mainly used for procedures where skeletal muscle relaxation is not needed, especially short procedures. It is sometimes used off-label for super-refractory SE.[11] Ketamine should only be administered by providers experienced in its use and with rigorous critical care. Further study with this medication is under way, so we should watch for updates.

TABLE 8.3.1 OVERALL OUTCOME OF ANESTHETIC THERAPY

Outcome	Thiopental/ pentobarbital ($n = 192$) (%)	Midazolam ($n = 585$) (%)	Propofol ($n = 143$) (%)
Control	64	78	68
No control ever achieved	5	16	11
Breakthrough seizures	0	3	1
Withdrawal seizures	9	<1	6
Therapy failure because of side effects	3	<1	6
Death during therapy	19	2	8

Fosphenytoin (FOS) is a prodrug of phenytoin and, as such, is in part of the hydatoid family. It is given by IV or intramuscular (IM) injection for SE. Approved uses include SE in adults and children and also nonemergent treatment of tonic-clonic seizures and partial-onset seizures. Fosphenytoin is rapidly metabolized to phenytoin, but does not have some of the infusion adverse effects of IV phenytoin. The effectiveness of fosphenytoin is solely based on phenytoin.

Midazolam is a benzodiazepine used predominately as a preoperative sedative and as an aid to induction of general anesthesia. Midazolam is often used for SE although this is off-label use.[12] It is also used as a nasal spray preparation (Nayzilam) for treatment of prolonged seizures outside of hospital settings.

Lorazepam is a benzodiazepine commonly used for sedation. It is used intravenously for patients with prolonged seizures. It also is a very good rescue medication in that it reduces the risk of recurrent seizures in patients with cluster-type seizures. Lorazepam is the most effective medication for benzodiazepine challenge for patients with possible NCSE when electroencephalogram (EEG) is unavailable or inconclusive.

Propofol is an injected anesthetic used for monitored anesthesia care (a step up from moderate sedation) and for general anesthesia. Propofol is an alternative for benzodiazepine-refractory SE, but this is off-label use.[13] Propofol administration requires comprehensive critical care and controlled airway and continuous monitoring of vital functions.

8.4

Nonmedical Treatment

HASAN H. SONMEZTURK

Partial epilepsies are much more likely than generalized epilepsies to be drug-resistant. These patients are the most likely to benefit from surgical therapy. These treatments include temporal lobectomy, selective amygdalohippocampectomy, lesionectomy, hemispherectomy, multiple subpial transection, and corpus callosotomy.

Patients with generalized epilepsy are usually not candidates for resective (curative) surgical therapy. However, some nonpharmacological treatments can be helpful. Dietary therapy is an effective treatment for patients able to comply with this therapy. Vagal nerve stimulation (VNS) has been used mainly for partial onset seizures, but there is evidence to suggest that VNS can be helpful for idiopathic and symptomatic generalized epilepsies.

NEUROSTIMULATION TECHNIQUES

Vagus Nerve Stimulation

VNS is approved for adjunctive therapy for partial onset seizures in adults and adolescents 12 years of age and older. In addition, there is more recent approval for selected patients with refractory depression. Improvement in seizure control with VNS seems to increase over time. However, less than 10% are seizure-free. Because of the greater chance of seizure freedom with epilepsy surgery, patients are advised to consider it first if they are felt to be good candidates. There are reports of VNS being helpful in patients with refractory generalized epilepsy, although this is not an indication approved by the US Food and Drug Administration (FDA). As with many epilepsy therapies, VNS was tested in and approved for partial-onset seizures, but its clinical utility extends beyond FDA indications.

The electrodes are placed on the left vagus nerve, and the stimulator is usually placed subcutaneously beneath the left clavicle. The stimulator

settings are adjusted as needed based on seizure control and adverse effects. The default stimulation cycle is stimulation for 30 sec followed by 5 min of no stimulation. Adjustment usually involves increasing the current intensity, but other parameters can also be adjusted.

In addition to cyclical stimulation, single VNS stimulation cycles can be generated on demand with magnet activation. The magnet-activated current can be programmed with parameters that differ from the recurrent output current. Patients can initiate on-demand stimulation with the magnet if they experience an aura, or a family member or caregiver can initiate the on-demand stimulation at the beginning of a seizure. Magnet activation is more likely to be helpful at the onset of a seizure and less likely to help after the seizure has progressed. In addition, the magnet can turn the stimulator off by holding it over or tapping it to the stimulator.

Newer VNS models also have an "autostimulation mode" that can detect increases in heart rate as a proxy for seizures and will then initiate an additional VNS cycle similar to a magnet-triggered event.

One VNS side effect to be expected is voice change or hoarseness. This improves over time. Individuals who sing or speak in public may want to turn off the stimulator temporarily during performances (by taping a magnet over it).

Deep Brain Stimulation

Deep brain stimulation (DBS) is used for treatment of patients with medically refractory epilepsy. DBS delivers electrical stimuli to reduce seizure generation. Electrodes are placed in one of a number of structures, with the anterior thalamic nucleus being the most common target. Stimulation is continuous in an open-loop manner, usually with 30 sec on and 3 min off. While the mechanism of action is not completely understood and may be somewhat different for different clinical scenarios, mechanisms implicated include elevating the seizure threshold and/or reducing seizure propagation as a result of desynchronization.[1]

Efficacy with anterior nucleus of the thalamus stimulation was found in one double-blind randomized trial to be 56% mean reduction in seizure frequency.[2]

DBS should only be placed at comprehensive epilepsy centers and managed by providers well-trained in the use and management of the devices.

Responsive Neurostimulation

Responsive neurostimulation (RNS) can be used for patients who do not respond adequately to medical management. Unlike VNS, RNS responds to recorded rhythms, producing a closed-loop brief bursts of electrical stimulation in response to rhythms that the device is programmed to consider potentially epileptogenic. The stimulation produces an interruption in the generation of seizure.[3] The patient is typically unaware of the stimulation.

RNS has been found to reduce seizures up to 75% in 9 years.[4] There is associated improvement in quality of life and improved cognitive functioning with neurostimulation, greater than that seen with DBS or VNS.[5] RNS has a learning curve for both the device and the physician, and its efficacy improves as the detection parameters and stimulation strengths are adjusted to most effective levels.

DIETARY TREATMENT OF EPILEPSY

Dietary therapy, which was popular many years ago, was nearly forgotten during the explosion of newer anti-seizure medications (ASMs), but has regained some interest with the realization that the new ASMs are not the miracle drugs we might have hoped. However, dietary therapy is used more in the pediatric population than in adults and is discussed in Chapter 8.1.

Ketogenic Diet

Ketogenic diet is a high-fat low-carbohydrate diet. This diet has been shown to be effective for a substantial minority of patients, with about 10% seizure-free and a 40–50% or greater reduction in seizure frequency.[6] Young children are more likely to benefit than older children and adults, partly because of better compliance; in addition, the more likely genetic etiologies of their epilepsy may respond better to the ketogenic diet.

The ketogenic diet can be used for patients with refractory seizures of almost any type, especially if there is difficulty with tolerating seizure medications. Particular types of epilepsy that may respond better than others include epilepsy due to glucose transporter deficiency or pyruvate dehydrogenase deficiency, myoclonic-astatic epilepsy, tuberous sclerosis, or infantile spasms. Ketogenic diet should not be used in patients with mitochondrial disorders, pyruvate carboxylase deficiency, and β-oxidation defects.

Difficulty maintaining compliance is the main limitation of the ketogenic diet. Hence it is most useful in individuals for whom compliance is not an issue, for example tube-fed subjects or infants receiving formula. Other diets have been explored to improve compliance with dietary therapy.

Modified Atkins Diet

The modified Atkins diet is a response to the difficulty of tolerating the ketogenic diet. The diet is also low carbohydrate, but with no restriction in proteins, fats, or calories.

This diet has been used for a variety of epilepsies with reported success in children that is not very different from the ketogenic diet.[7] It is better tolerated and has less adverse effects than the ketogenic diet and may be considered as an alternative for select patients, particularly adolescents and adults.

Low Glycemic Index Diet

The low glycemic index diet is another low-carbohydrate diet that is a bit more permissive in that it allows carbohydrates with a low glycemic index (meaning they will not raise blood glucose). It has also shown seizure reduction in children with refractory seizures.[8]

8.5

Surgical Treatment of Epilepsy

HASAN H. SONMEZTURK

HISTORICAL PERSPECTIVE

Early attempts at epilepsy surgery may date back to the Medieval age. However, the modern era of epilepsy surgery began on May 25, 1886, with the first epilepsy surgery performed by Sir Victor Horsley in collaboration with Hughlings Jackson at the National Hospital for Paralyzed and Epileptics in London. By the end of 1886, Horsley had completed nine successful surgeries for epilepsy, thus establishing the efficacy of the procedure. With the advancement of neurosciences, the real advancement was spearheaded by Wilder Penfield an American-Canadian neurosurgeon, and Herbert Jasper, an American neurologist and neurophysiologist, at Montreal Neurological Institute (MNI). Penfield and Jasper were the first to use electroencephalogram (EEG) to localize "psychomotor seizures" to the temporal lobe in 1951. Gibbs and Bailey first reported surgical resection of epileptogenic brain tissue on the basis of EEG findings alone again in 1951. Ever since, temporal lobe resections continue to be the most commonly performed and generally successful surgical treatment for epilepsy.[1]

During the Penfield and Jasper era, seizure focus localization depended on particular attention to auras and early motor phenomena, interictal EEG recordings, and intraoperative spike evaluation with electrocorticography. They also depended heavily on recreating habitual auras and seizures with intraoperative electrical stimulation, mapping the eloquent cortices, and visually identifying injured and scarred cortical regions. These techniques have improved dramatically over the past six or seven decades, particularly when digital long-term video-EEG recordings became possible for both intracranial and scalp recordings with captured habitual seizures.

REFRACTORY (DRUG-RESISTANT) EPILEPSY

Drug-resistant epilepsy is defined as failure of adequate trials of two tolerated, appropriately chosen and dosed anti-seizure medication (ASM) schedules (whether as monotherapies or in combination) to achieve sustained seizure freedom.[2] This definition was based on the findings published by Kwan and Brodie a decade earlier. The rate of seizure freedom with a first-tried ASM was 47%, another 14% became seizure-free during treatment with a second ASM, and only 3% more achieved seizure control with three or more ASMs (Figure 8.5.1). A more recent study in which drug-resistant epilepsy patients were followed prospectively showed that 34.6% of patients will enter seizure remission when followed over the course of 7 years. However, the relapse rate was high, at 71.2%. In general, with the availability of new ASMs and continued trials of different combinations, about 5% of drug-resistant patients per year will enter seizure remission with high risk of recurrence.[3]

FOCAL EPILEPSIES

Focal epilepsies constitute about 66% of all epilepsies; the remaining are generalized epilepsies (23–26%) and unknown epilepsy types. In general, about 36% of focal epilepsy patients develop drug-resistant (refractory) seizures, and this ratio is higher in temporal lobe epilepsy. Despite the discovery or development of multiple new ASMs with different mechanisms of action, this refractory group could not be penetrated over the past four decades. No matter how aggressive the ASM management, only about 3–5% of this group achieves seizure freedom. It is not very well known what determines refractoriness, however, pharmacogenetics is suspected to be the culprit. Surgical options provide higher chances of seizure freedom in this patient population, particularly for those with well-localized seizure foci.

It is estimated that about 1 million (one-third) of all epilepsy patients in the United States have refractory epilepsy. About 10–50% of these patients could benefit from surgical resection

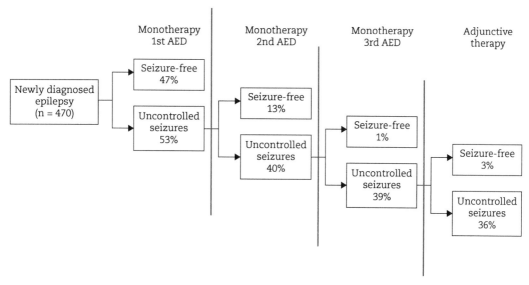

FIGURE 8.5.1 Staged drug response algorithm for epilepsy.

or transection. If only 10% was considered, this number adds up to 100,000 patients. However, only 5% (5,000 patients) are referred for epilepsy surgery, and only 2% (2000 patients) end up having epilepsy surgery. The last published survey in 1990, and more recent data from the National Association of Epilepsy Centers (NAEC) showed that these numbers have not changed, indicating extreme underutilization of epilepsy surgery. A majority of these patients (75–85%) who eventually do have epilepsy surgery undergo a noninvasive (Phase 1) presurgical workup only. About 15–25% require invasive investigation (Phase

2) with intracranial electrodes for seizure focus localization (Figure 8.5.2).[4, 5, 6]

Methods of Epilepsy Surgery

Table 8.5.1 presents some of the modalities for epilepsy surgery. The particular technique used depends on specifics of the case, including etiology, localization, age, concurrent medical condition, and type of seizure.

PATIENT EXAMPLE

A 47-year-old right-handed woman presented to an epilepsy clinic with a history of seizures since

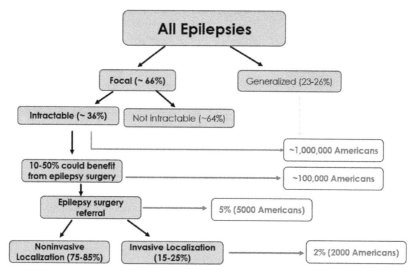

FIGURE 8.5.2 Patient involvement in surgical treatment of epilepsy.

TABLE 8.5.1 MODALITIES OF SURGICAL THERAPY AND THEIR INDICATIONS

Modality	Indication
Lesionectomy	Focal lesion associated with single epileptogenic zone; in some cases, the resection must include surrounding brain tissue (e.g., hemosiderin-stained tissue surrounding a cavernous malformation).
Temporal lobectomy	Well-localized temporal lobe focus, particularly nondominant. This is most appropriate for nonlesional temporal lobe epilepsy when it is not known if the epileptogenic zone is mesial or lateral temporal.
Selective amygdalohippocampectomy	Well-localized mesial temporal focus, particularly if associated with hippocampal sclerosis. This had been reserved for dominant foci, but this is no longer so.
Tailored neocortical resection	Localized neocortical epileptogenic zone.
Multilobar resection	Epileptogenic zone involves more than one lobe in one hemisphere.
Hemispherectomy, hemispherectomy	Well-lateralized widespread epileptogenic zone and severe associated or anticipated motor deficit (e.g., Rasmussen syndrome); if there are no independent finger movements, no significant worsening in motor function will be expected in the long term.
Multiple subpial transections	Neocortical epileptogenic zone well-localized over functional (eloquent) cortex; most often used with motor, sensory, or language cortex. May be combined with resection.
Corpus callosotomy	Palliative surgery that can be useful if the dominant seizure manifestations require rapid spread to the opposite hemisphere (e.g., drop attacks). This surgery does not usually eliminate seizures, but it may eliminate some debilitating manifestations, such as falls.

age 11. She had never been seizure-free and had failed a total of six ASMs. After her first visit to an adult epilepsy clinic, she was referred to an epilepsy monitoring unit (EMU) for seizure classification and focus localization.

The patient's EMU monitoring recorded 11 typical seizures. All were focal impaired awareness seizures with clinical features consisting of freezing, staring, and not responding to examiners. These were followed by lip smacking and right-hand automatisms. Seizures lasted on average 1 min followed by a short 2- to 3-min post-ictal period with minimal confusion. Patient was amnestic to her seizures. Ictal EEG showed focal onset in the left anterior temporal region with a pattern suggesting mesial temporal localization (Figure 8.5.3). The interictal epileptiform discharges were also exclusively in the right anterior infero-mesial temporal region (Figure 8.5.4).

Other noninvasive workup revealed left hippocampal sclerosis on epilepsy protocol brain magnetic resonance imaging (MRI) (Figure 8.5.5), hypometabolism over the left mesial temporal regions on brain positron emission tomography (PET) (>20% compared to right side) (Figure 8.5.5), and diminished verbal memory on neuropsychological testing indicating left temporal localization. The patient also underwent Wada testing that showed right hemispheric dominance for language and memory.

Upon these findings patient underwent left selective amygdalohippocampectomy, as shown in Figure 8.5.6.

After her surgery, the patient became seizure-free and has been free of all seizures for the past 7 years. She used to have 1–3 seizures every week presurgically. Her ASMs were tapered off after an initial 2 years of seizure freedom. The patient has been off medications for the past 5 years. This is just one example demonstrating how life-changing epilepsy surgery can be.

EFFICACY OF EPILEPSY SURGERY

To date, there has only been one randomized controlled trial (RCT) investigating the efficacy of epilepsy surgery. No further studies were done because the benefit of surgical treatment compared to medical management was strikingly and undoubtedly more successful in achieving seizure freedom. The first trial was by Wiebe et al. in 2001, which enrolled 80 patients with an average duration of refractory focal epilepsy for 17 years. Half (40 patients) were randomly assigned to receive presurgical workup and surgery if qualified, and other half (40 patients) were randomly assigned to medical management group. As the randomization was prior to presurgical workup, not all patients in the surgical group qualified for surgical resection. Despite that, 58% of the surgical group became seizure-free compared to only 8% of the medical group, showing a striking and statistically significant difference.[7] The seizure-free rate of those who actually had surgery was 64%.

A second trial by Engel et al. in 2012 was the multicenter Early Randomization Surgical Epilepsy Trial (ERSET).[8] Patients were enrolled within the first 2 years of refractoriness, and they were randomly assigned after presurgical testing

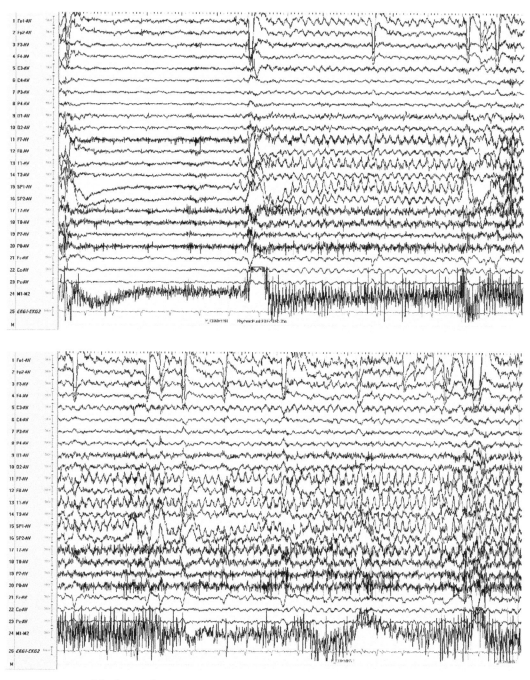

FIGURE 8.5.3 Ictal discharges. (Top, Bottom, and next frame.)

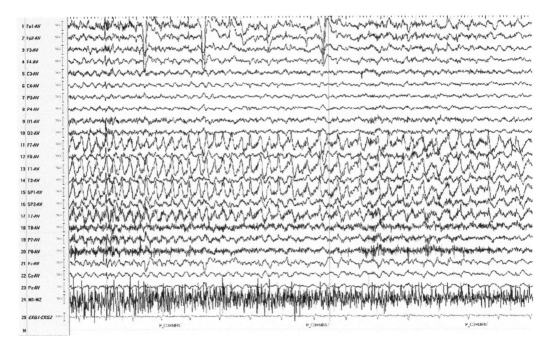

FIGURE 8.5.3 Continued

and confirmation of candidacy for anteromesial temporal resection. Despite 16 US centers contributing, only 38 patients could be randomly assigned in 2 years; therefore, the study was terminated prematurely. During the second year of the study, 85% of the surgical arm were seizure-free and none medical arm was seizure-free.

A meta-analysis by Engel and colleagues (2003) involving 24 non-overlapping surgical series between 1990 and 2000 showed two-thirds of patient remained seizure-free after temporal

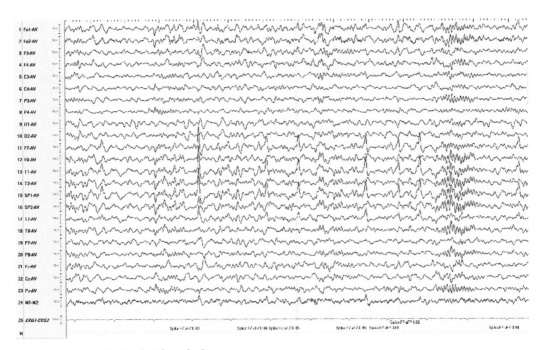

FIGURE 8.5.4 Interictal epileptiform discharges

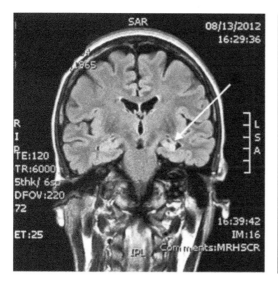

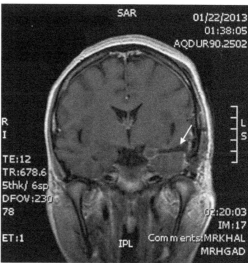

FIGURE 8.5.6 Selective left amygdalohippocampectomy.

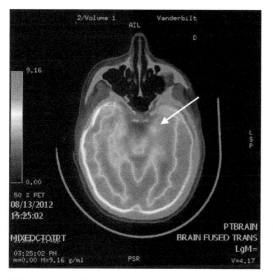

FIGURE 8.5.5 Top: agnetic resonance imaging showing left hippocampal sclerosis, with corresponding positron emission tomography below. Bottom: Positron emission tomography (PET) scan.

resections for temporal lobe epilepsy.[9] These results projected a need-to-treat number for benefit of 2. One of every two patients treated with epilepsy surgery will achieve seizure freedom, yet underutilization of epilepsy surgery is substantial. A more recent population-based retrospective cohort study from a publicly funded universal healthcare system (Ontario, Canada) identified 10,661 patients with refractory epilepsy. Within 2 years of being defined as medically intractable, only 124 (1.2%) had undergone epilepsy surgery. Only 234 (2.2%) of these patients had video-EEG monitoring. This shows

how underutilized EMUs and epilepsy surgery can be.[10]

The mortality of patients treated with focal resection or transections drops dramatically compared to nonsurgical patients. Mortality per 1,000 person-years was 5.2 in patients who had surgery and were seizure-free, 10.4 in patients who had surgery and were not seizure-free, and 25.3 in patients who had no surgery. These data were gathered from 1,110 patients with surgical treatment and 104 nonsurgical patients for a total follow-up of 8,126.62 person-years from 1986 to 2013 (Figure 8.5.7).[11]

Epilepsy Surgery Misconceptions

Why is epilepsy surgery so underutilized? Multiple factors contribute to this fact. Undoubtedly there is inadequate dissemination regarding the safety and efficacy of modern approaches to surgical treatment for epilepsy. There are also misconceptions about surgical management on both sides, patients and physicians. A survey among neurologists questioning their knowledge of and attitudes toward epilepsy surgery discovered more than half of neurologists did not believe lack of seizure freedom would be a reason for epilepsy surgery referral. Nearly half did not realize failing two ASMs constituted drug-resistant epilepsy, and they were not aware of the American Academy of Neurology (AAN) clinical practice guidelines for epilepsy surgery.[12] Better clinical exposure for neurology residents who have relatively few to no didactics focused on the nonpharmacologic treatment of

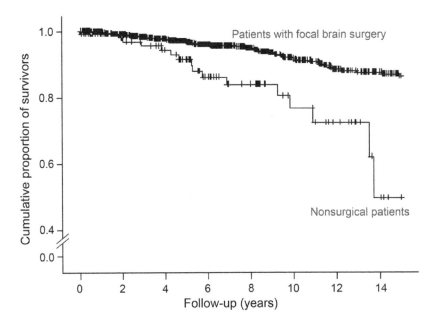

FIGURE 8.5.7 Efficacy of epilepsy surgery.

From Michael R. Sperling et al. *Neurology* 2016;86:1938–1944.

refractory epilepsy and better outreach to non-neurologists could help improve the utilization of epilepsy surgery.

Other misconceptions about surgical candidates are shown in (Figure 8.5.8).

There are misperceptions among patients as well. An ad hoc questionnaire administered to 228 adult patients attending epilepsy clinics revealed widespread fears and misconceptions irrespective of diagnosis, seizure type, and degree of intractability.[13]

Here is what adult epilepsy surgery clinic patients thought about epilepsy surgery:

- 56% said epilepsy surgery is "very dangerous,"
- 47% said paralysis is possible,
- 61% say brain damage is possible,

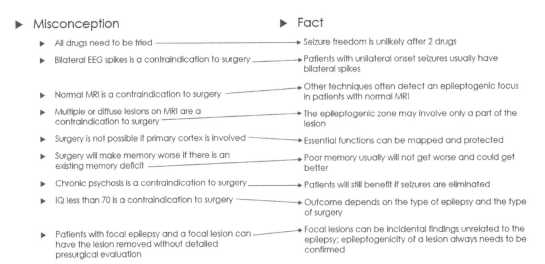

FIGURE 8.5.8 Misconceptions and facts regarding epilepsy surgery.[14]

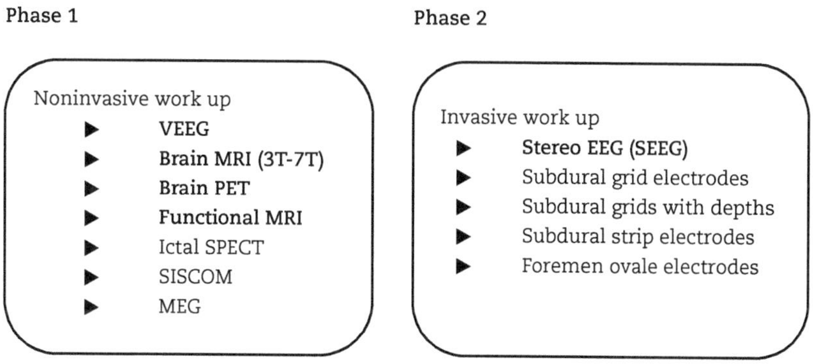

Phase 1

Phase 2

Noninvasive work up
- ▶ **VEEG**
- ▶ **Brain MRI (3T-7T)**
- ▶ **Brain PET**
- ▶ **Functional MRI**
- ▶ Ictal SPECT
- ▶ SISCOM
- ▶ MEG

Invasive work up
- ▶ **Stereo EEG (SEEG)**
- ▶ Subdural grid electrodes
- ▶ Subdural grids with depths
- ▶ Subdural strip electrodes
- ▶ Foremen ovale electrodes

FIGURE 8.5.9 Phases of evaluation for epilepsy surgery.

- 45% reported concern for loss of independence,
- Nearly 30% of patients had preexisting negative attitudes,
- 73% thought surgery should be a last resort,
- 56% would not undergo surgery unless a 100% success rate could be guaranteed.

All these misperceptions about epilepsy surgery exist despite undeniable evidence by one RCT, thousands of additional publications, and more than 20 textbooks on epilepsy surgery. Epilepsy surgery related mortality risk is minimal at less than 1%, and morbidity risk is around 3%. Pharmacoresistent epilepsy has a mortality 5–10 times that of general population. It is known that surgical treatment increases life span. The cost of surgery is considerably less than the cost of lifetime disability, and third-party payers are willing to approve and cover the costs of surgery. Yet still the average delay from onset of epilepsy to surgery is 22 years.

EPILEPSY SURGERY WORKUP

Epilepsy surgery workup consists of two phases. Phase 1 includes noninvasive testing, and the majority of patients can proceed to resective surgery after completing Phase 1 testing alone. Phase 2 consists of invasive workup with intracranial electrodes. Over the past six decades variable methods were used for seizure focus localization, but stereo EEG has been the predominantly used method for the past decade (Figure 8.5.9).

ASM MANAGEMENT AFTER SURGERY

ASM therapy is usually continued for at least 1–2 years after surgery. However, the ASM regimen can be simplified and doses could be reduced in seizure-free patients. However, there is a risk of seizure recurrence after ASM withdrawal. Such recurrence is less common after temporal lobe surgery for mesial temporal lobe epilepsy than surgery for neocortical epilepsy. It is also less common in children than adults. In fact, recurrence is predicted by older age at surgery and longer duration of epilepsy before surgery. Recurrent seizures may be harder to control in patients taken off ASMs after neocortical epilepsy surgery than after mesial temporal lobe epilepsy surgery.

Our recommendation is to go very slowly and be cautious about discontinuation of ASMs after epilepsy surgery.

8.6

Comorbidities

KARL E. MISULIS

Comorbid conditions have become a recent focus of epilepsy evaluation and management.[1] These need to be addressed and managed as part of comprehensive epilepsy management. Here, we discuss some of these conditions.

ANXIETY AND DEPRESSION

Mood disorders including anxiety and depression are more common in patients with epilepsy than in the general population. As clinicians, we should be alert for signs of mood disturbance, and screening is recommended.[2]

MIGRAINE

Migraine and epilepsy are linked in multiple ways.[3] There are undoubtedly pathogenic similarities and genetic links, but more relevant to the individuals are headaches separately and around the time of seizures, whether pre-ictal, ictal, or post-ictal.

Medication selection for patients with both epilepsy and migraine may consider agents that are effective for both, if clinically appropriate. Among the common anti-seizure medications (ASMs) which can be helpful for migraine are topiramate, valproate, and, for some patients, zonisamide, especially in patients who do not tolerate topiramate well.[4]

SUBSTANCE USE AND ABUSE

Substance use complicates epilepsy management by effects of intoxication, withdrawal, and risk of noncompliance or overdose.[5] In addition, the absence of open communication with the providers is a significant barrier to management.

Assessment begins with discussion at a time and venue that is conducive to openness. A non-judgmental attitude is essential. This discussion is best had when there is trust between the patient and provider. We have found that sometimes patients are more open to discussing substance use as well as compliance information with nurses rather than physicians.

CARDIOVASCULAR DISEASE

Epilepsy and cardiovascular disease frequently coexist, with causes being shared risks as well as the effects of one on the other.[6] Patients with epilepsy have a higher incidence of cardiac arrhythmias, some possibly due to common genetic predisposition and some due to effects of the seizures themselves, such as ictal asystole and other arrhythmias.[7]

COGNITIVE DISTURBANCE

Cognitive disturbance can develop in patients with epilepsy for many reasons. There are potentially cognitive manifestations of the genetic and structural disorders which cause the epilepsy, ASMs may affect cognitive function, some surgical procedures for epilepsy can have deleterious cognitive effects, and depression associated with epilepsy can impair cognitive performance.[8,9] Screening for cognitive disturbance should be considered in the course of epilepsy management.[10]

SLEEP DISORDERS

Sleep disorders are more common in patients with epilepsy, particularly sleep apnea, restless legs syndrome, insomnia, and parasomnias.[11] Sleep apnea is predominately obstructive rather than central sleep apnea. Sleep disorders and associated cardiovascular effects may be part of the link between epilepsy and sudden unexpected death in epilepsy (SUDEP).

SOCIAL DIFFICULTIES

Patients with epilepsy have increased risk for difficulties with social function, successful employment, interpersonal relations, and communication.[12] The reasons for this are broad and include the psychological and neurologic manifestations of the disorder and any associated deficits, cognitive difficulties, limitations of societal permissions (e.g., driving, sports), and effects of ASMs.

8.7

Quality of Care Standards and Counseling

BASSEL ABOU-KHALIL

QUALITY OF CARE STANDARDS

The American Academy of Neurology developed standardized quality measures for epilepsy care. The latest quality measurement set includes the following:

- Counseling for women of childbearing potential, at least once a year;
- Comprehensive epilepsy care center referral for discussion for patients with intractable epilepsy;
- Quality-of-life assessment, at least once;
- Quality-of-life outcome, at a visit at least 4 weeks after initial assessment;
- Depression and anxiety screening at every office visit.

The measures were primarily developed for quality improvement projects. Providers were encouraged to identify measures most meaningful for their patients and to implement these measures to drive improvement in practice.

COUNSELING

Counseling for patients with epilepsy is complex, with specific recommendations depending on the specific clinical issue.

Driving and Other Safety Issues

There are specific laws regulating driving in specific states and countries. Those need to be followed. Within the bounds of regulations and laws, we generally practice with the following guidelines:

- If a seizure disorder is an established pattern of purely nocturnal events or if the patient is under complete control neurologically, then they can be allowed to drive.
- If a seizure is due to a provoking incident which is avoidable, then they are allowed to drive after 1 month without further events.

- If a patient has had an accident, especially if an event was implicated, more caution is needed.
- For patients with epilepsy, we recommend not swimming alone. Shower rather than bathe or bathe in a safe depth of water.
- For patients with psychogenic nonepileptic events, there is a restriction but the restriction can be reduced depending on the clinical details at the discretion of the clinician.
- For patients who have recently come off anti-seizure medications (ASMs) after being seizure-free, it is wise to not drive for at least 1 month after cessation of ASM.

Common sense dictates that patients who have seizures, arrhythmia with syncope, and other medical conditions that interfere with mental activities and neurologic functioning should not be driving, working with heavy moving machinery, working at unprotected heights, or performing other risky duties. Driving is only one part of the discussion of safety.

The period of seizure-freedom before a patient can drive varies between states, from 3 months to 1 year. Also, there are differences between states concerning whether the patient must surrender the driver's license or just not drive, and whether the physician must report patients with uncontrolled seizures to the state. Physicians must be familiar with laws in their state. In addition, some businesses have activity restrictions that are more stringent than the state law for driving.

Some states allow exceptions to the driving restriction for people with purely nocturnal seizures, focal aware seizures that do not interfere with ability to drive (e.g., isolated auras), or patients with long auras that allow them time to get off the road before altered awareness. These leniencies are not without risk and merit careful discussion between clinician and patient and total awareness of the laws in their locale. The pattern of purely nocturnal sleep-related seizures or pure focal aware seizures must have been established for at least 6 months in order to remove restrictions.

Inheritance

Many epilepsies have a genetic basis or a genetic component. Genetic tests are available for only a few forms of epilepsy. While there are few instances where epilepsy genetics predict ASM efficacy, obtaining a genetic diagnosis can be very valuable for closure and to avoid unnecessary continued search for an etiology. An underlying genetic etiology is often evident without specific genetic testing. Most commonly, patients are interested to know the risk of epilepsy in their children, or parents may want to know the risk of having another affected child. Most genetic epilepsy syndromes, such as juvenile myoclonic epilepsy, are polygenic and the risk of epilepsy in a child is less than 6–7%. However, epilepsy is monogenic in some families, with higher associated risk in offspring.

8.8

Medications A–Z

BASSEL ABOU-KHALIL AND KARL E. MISULIS

At the time of this writing, we have 27 medications for the management of epilepsy. Note that many of the uses of these medications are not formally approved by the US Food and Drug Administration (FDA). This is not to say that there is not good evidence for efficacy, but, in many circumstances, the applications to change FDA-approved indications and dosing have not been filed. This is especially true for some of the older medications which are available as generics.

Medications discussed in this text are summarized here, with key information for each agent. Because of the possibility of unintentional errors or omissions and the progress of medical science, the reader should consult published prescribing information and current literature for clarifications, corrections, and updates to this information. Readers always should consult the most recent information regarding the use and monitoring of these agents. Sites that we often use include DailyMed from the National Institutes of Health (NIH)[1], and the digital version of the *Physician's Desk Reference* (PDR). Note that the latter includes indications that are not FDA-approved but for which there is evidence of appropriate clinical use.

Abbreviations of medications in common use are frequently used, but because there may be alternative abbreviations, they are not part of the official approved prescribing information. Therefore, when prescribing, use the entire name to avoid potential misunderstanding.

This section focuses on medications which are used for initial and maintenance therapy of epilepsy. Medications used predominately or solely for status epilepticus are discussed in Chapter 8.3.

Anti-seizure medications (ASMs) as a class carry a safety warning on the risk of suicidality, as requested by the FDA. This is based on a meta-analysis of placebo-controlled clinical trials of 11 ASMs that showed that suicidality was twice as high among patients who received the active ASM

as among patients who received placebo (~4 per 1,000 versus 2 per 1,000 patients). The FDA decision to issue a class warning has been criticized. The prescribing information for all these medications also warns against abrupt discontinuation except in the instance of serious adverse event.

BRIVARACETAM (BRIVIACT)

Brivaracetam (BRV) is a levetiracetam analog which is approved for treatment of focal-onset seizures age 4 years to adult. However, there is evidence that it is effective against generalized-onset seizures as well. Its mechanism of action, like that of levetiracetam, involves altering neurotransmitter release by binding to synaptic vesicle protein SV2A. However, it is thought to be more selective in its action. It seems to have less behavioral adverse effects than levetiracetam, and, when substituted to levetiracetam in patients experiencing irritability and other behavioral adverse effects, most reported improvement in these adverse effects. BRV is not effective when used in combination with levetiracetam.

There are intravenous (IV) as well as oral (PO) formulations.

CANNABIDIOL (EPIDIOLEX)

Cannabidiol (CBD) is an oral cannabinoid approved for treatment of seizures associated with Lennox-Gastaut syndrome (LGS), Dravet syndrome, or tuberous sclerosis complex. This includes children 2 years and older and adults. There is some evidence that CBD has a broad spectrum of efficacy, including for focal-onset seizures. Its mechanism of action includes enhancing gamma-aminobutyric acid (GABA) activity and modulating intracellular calcium.

Adverse effects include somnolence, diarrhea, fatigue, rash, insomnia, sleep disturbance, and transaminase elevation. Hepatic enzyme monitoring is recommended. Risk of hepatic complications is increased in patients who are also treated with valproate or clobazam and in patients who have baseline elevation in transaminases. It has potential for interactions. CBD concomitant use with clobazam or everolimus (and the related tacrolimus and sirolimus) can increase levels of these medications.

CARBAMAZEPINE (TEGRETOL, TEGRETOL XR, EQUETRO, EPITOL, CARBATROL)

Carbamazepine (CBZ) is a tricyclic ASM with approved use for focal-onset and generalized tonic-clonic seizures. It is not effective against absence or myoclonic seizures and may in fact worsen the seizure types. Its mechanism of action is through blocking sodium channels.

CBZ has always been available as an oral medication, but an IV formulation was recently approved for replacement therapy when the oral route is not available. An extended-release preparation is available and has proven tolerability as well as suggestion of better efficacy than the immediate-release formulation.

Adverse effects include the potential for serious dermatologic reactions which are particularly increased in patients of Asian descent who carry the HLA-B*1502 allele. Although it had the best balance of efficacy and tolerability among first-generation ASMs, its use has declined because of its potent induction of liver enzymes and considerable interactions.

In addition to its epilepsy indication, it is indicated for trigeminal neuralgia, and one of the extended-release formulations is indicated for bipolar disorder.

CENOBAMATE (XCOPRI)

Cenobamate is a carbamate and, as such, is chemically related to felbamate. It is approved for focal-onset seizures in adults. Its mechanism of action is through enhancement of GABA activity as well as by blocking sodium channels. In adjunctive therapy clinical trials it had an unusually high seizure-free rate. There are limited data on monotherapy use.

Adverse reactions include dose-related somnolence, dizziness, and fatigue. It has interactions mainly due to inhibition of CYP 2C19 so that doses of some baseline seizure medications have to be reduced. The list includes phenobarbital, phenytoin, and clobazam.

CLOBAZAM (ONFI)

Clobazam (CLB) is a benzodiazepine which is approved for use as adjunctive therapy for patients

with LGS, age 2 years or older. However, clobazam appears to have a broad spectrum of efficacy against focal and generalized seizure types.[2] Adverse effects include those commonly associated with benzodiazepines, mainly somnolence. However, it is less sedating and less habituating than other benzodiazepines. It has an active metabolite with long half-life, likely responsible for much of its efficacy. The active metabolite can accumulate when clobazam is used with cannabidiol or cenobamate.

CLONAZEPAM (KLONOPIN)

Clonazepam (CLZ) is a benzodiazepine which is approved for use alone or as adjunctive therapy for patients with LGS and akinetic and myoclonic seizures. There is evidence of a broad spectrum of efficacy.

Adverse effects include sedation and development of tolerance, with waning efficacy over time. It is sometimes used for a limited time as bridge therapy when changing doses of other ASMs or reinstituting long-term ASM therapy after a gap in care.

ESLICARBAZEPINE ACETATE (APTIOM)

Eslicarbazepine acetate (ESL) is the newest agent in the dibenzazepine carboxamide family that includes carbamazepine and oxcarbazepine. It is rapidly converted to S-licarbazepine, the active S-enantiomer of licarbazepine, which is the active metabolite of oxcarbazepine. A major advantage over oxcarbazepine is absence of cerebrospinal fluid (CSF) peak concentration and longer CSF half-life allowing once-daily dosing. Like other agents in the family, it works through blocking sodium channels.

Eslicarbazepine is approved for treatment of focal-onset seizures in patients age 4 years and older. It can be considered a first-line treatment, although cost could be a limitation.

ETHOSUXIMIDE (ZARONTIN)

Ethosuximide (ESM) is a succinimide in the same class as methsuximide. Its mechanism of action is blocking T-type calcium currents. It is FDA-approved for treatment of absence seizures. It is not effective against any other seizure type. It is the drug of choice for patients with generalized absence seizures. However, in patients with both absence and generalized tonic-clonic seizures, an alternative or adjunctive medication with efficacy against generalized tonic-clonic seizures has to be used.

Ethosuximide's adverse effects are mainly gastrointestinal (GI)-related and require 2–3 times daily dosing despite its long half-life.

FELBAMATE (FELBATOL)

Felbamate (FBM) is approved for use in patients with epilepsy which has not responded to other medications with better safety profiles. Its use should be carefully considered only when the potential benefits outweigh the potential risks. Felbamate has a black-box warning for aplastic anemia and hepatic failure. Approved indications are for treatment of focal-onset seizures in adults and for seizures with LGS in children age 2–14 years. There is evidence that felbamate has a broad spectrum of efficacy for focal and generalized seizures.

Felbamate appears to have multiple mechanisms of action, including modulation of GABA$_A$ receptors, blocking N-methyl-D-aspartate (NMDA) receptors, and blocking sodium channels.

The most common felbamate adverse experiences are GI-related, requiring three times daily dosing and administration with food. It has the potential for interactions due to inhibition of metabolism of phenytoin, phenobarbital, valproate, carbamazepine epoxide, and the active clobazam metabolite.

FENFLURAMINE (FINTEPLA)

Fenfluramine is indicated for the treatment of seizures associated with Dravet syndrome in patients 2 years of age and older. The most common adverse effects are decreased appetite and sedation.

GABAPENTIN (NEURONTIN)

Gabapentin (GBP) is chemically related to GABA yet does not appear to interact with the GABA receptor. Its mechanism of action is through binding the alpha-2-delta subunit of voltage-gated calcium channels, reducing influx of calcium and neurotransmitter release. It is approved for adjunctive therapy for focal-onset seizures in adults and children age 3 years and older. It is not effective against generalized seizure types and may even exacerbate generalized myoclonic and generalized absence seizures. GBP is also approved for management of postherpetic neuralgia, but has a wider general off-label use for neuropathic pain especially in diabetic neuropathy, headache, and insomnia, and there is post-marketing evidence of efficacy in these realms.[3]

There are extended-release formulations of gabapentin that are approved for restless leg syndrome and postherpetic neuralgia, but not for seizures (Gralise and Horizant).

GBP absorption is limited due to saturable active transport system. GBP is not metabolized and is excreted unchanged in the urine. Its short half-life requires twice daily or 3 times daily dosing.

GBP most common adverse effects are sedation and dizziness.

LACOSAMIDE (VIMPAT)

Lacosamide (LCM) is a modified amino acid which exerts its anti-seizure effect by enhancement of the slow inactivation of voltage-gated sodium channels. It is approved for treatment of focal-onset seizures in patients 4 years of age and older, as well as adjunctive treatment of generalized-onset tonic-clonic seizures. It is available in multiple formulations, including injection, when oral administration is not possible. LCM can be used as first-line treatment for focal seizures in certain situations, but cost may be a limiting factor.

Use for status epilepticus is not approved but is in widespread use. There is good evidence for efficacy[4] and even for relative safety of IV-push administration.[5]

LCM's most common adverse effects are dizziness, nausea, fatigue, and sedation, all dose-related and more likely when LCM is used in combination with other sodium channel blockers. LCM may produce a dose-dependent prolongation in the PR interval.

LAMOTRIGINE (LAMICTAL)

Lamotrigine (LTG) is chemically related to dihydrofolate reductase inhibitors but this is not believed to be its mechanism of action. It likely works through blocking voltage-gated sodium channels. It is approved for use for adjunctive therapy of focal-onset seizures, generalized tonic-clonic seizures, and the generalized seizures of LGS. LTG is a common first-line treatment for focal seizures, but it has a broad spectrum of efficacy. It is less effective against generalized absence seizures than ethosuximide or valproate but remains an option for patients who do not respond to or are unable to take these medications.

There is a black-box warning regarding serious rash, including Stevens-Johnson syndrome. This is more likely in children than in adults and tends to occur within the first few weeks of initiation of therapy. The risk is likely increased by coadministration with valproate, initiation of therapy at doses higher than recommended, and escalation of therapy faster than recommended. LTG requires a slow titration as a result of the risk of rash.

LTG is generally well-tolerated and less likely to interfere with cognitive function and alertness than many other medications. The most common adverse effects are dizziness, blurred vision, unsteadiness, and nausea, all dose-related. Peak-related adverse effects are alleviated by the extended-release preparation. Adverse effects are more likely to occur when LTG is used in conjunction with other sodium channel blockers.

LTG has important interactions. Its clearance is increased by coadministration of estrogen, during pregnancy, and when used with enzyme-inducing drugs. On the other hand, its clearance is markedly reduced by coadministration with valproate. It should be noted that the LTG-valproate combination has well-documented synergy.

LEVETIRACETAM (KEPPRA)

Levetiracetam (LEV) is a pyrrolidine derivative whose mechanism of action involves altering neurotransmitter release by binding to synaptic vesicle protein SV2A.[6] It is a broad-spectrum ASM. It is indicated for adjunctive therapy for focal-onset seizures in patients 1 month of age and older, myoclonic seizures in patients 12 years of age and older with juvenile myoclonic epilepsy, and for generalized-onset tonic-clonic seizures in patients 6 years of age and older with idiopathic generalized epilepsy. The IV formulation is available for use in patients unable to take PO. Use of LEV for status epilepticus is off-label but part of common medical practice. Efficacy seems comparable to that of fosphenytoin and valproate for benzodiazepine-refractory status epilepticus.[7]

Levetiracetam is only partially metabolized in the blood and is excreted mostly unchanged in the urine. It has no significant interactions. Its short half-life requires twice-daily dosing, but an extended-release preparation allows once-daily dosing.

The most common adverse effects are sedation, dizziness, and asthenia. Due to its rapid onset of action, its general safety, and its ease of use, LEV has become the most widely prescribed ASM. However, behavioral adverse effects of irritability, hostility, and depression are a limiting factor in its use.

METHSUXIMIDE (CELONTIN)

Methsuximide (MSX) is a succinimide anticonvulsant in the same class as ethosuximide. It is approved for use for absence epilepsy that is refractory to ethosuximide. However, there is evidence that methsuximide is effective against focal epilepsy as well, unlike ethosuximide, which has a very narrow spectrum of efficacy against generalized absence seizures.

Methsuximide is converted to an active metabolite with a long half-life. However, its GI side effects require twice-daily or 3 times daily dosing.

OXCARBAZEPINE (TRILEPTAL)

Oxcarbazepine (OXC) is an analog of carbamazepine but with very different metabolic pathway and pharmacokinetic profile. Although it does have a potential for enzyme induction, this is much more selective and less potent than carbamazepine. Its mechanism of action is similar to that of carbamazepine, through blocking of sodium channels. It is approved for focal-onset seizures in adults as monotherapy or adjunctive therapy and for use as monotherapy for focal-onset seizures in children 4 years and older and adjunctive therapy for focal-onset seizures in children 2 years and older.

OXC is a first-line treatment for focal-onset seizures, largely replacing carbamazepine due to its pharmacokinetic advantages. It has fewer interactions than carbamazepine but may still reduce the efficacy of oral contraceptives at daily doses of 900 mg or more. However, it is more likely than carbamazepine to cause hyponatremia. Hyponatremia had an incidence of about 2.5% in trials and usually developed during the first 3 months of therapy, although it can occur later as well. It is most likely in older individuals and much less likely to be encountered in children. Other adverse experiences typical of most sodium channel blockers include drowsiness, fatigue, dizziness, blurred vision, nausea, and ataxia, all dose-related. Peak adverse effects and relatively short half-life require twice-daily dosing, but an extended-release preparation is available for once-daily dosing.

PERAMPANEL (FYCOMPA)

Perampanel (PER) is indicated for treatment of focal-onset seizures in patients age 4 years and greater and as adjunctive therapy for generalized-onset tonic-clonic seizures in patients age 12 and older. It has a broad spectrum of efficacy with evidence of some efficacy against other generalized seizure types. Its mechanism of action is selective noncompetitive alpha-amino-3-hydroxy-5-methyl-4-isoxazolepropionic acid (AMPA) glutamate receptor antagonism.

It has a long half-life allowing once-daily dosing. Its efficacy is reduced by administration with enzyme-inducing drugs. The most common adverse effects were dizziness, somnolence, fatigue. Behavioral issues including hostility and aggression were observed in a nontrivial proportion of patients, 12–20% at higher doses, but much less frequently at the initial target dose of 4 mg/d.

It is most appropriately used as adjunctive therapy due to limited data on initial monotherapy use. Its long half-life is a major advantage, with less risk of breakthrough seizures due to missed doses.

PHENOBARBITAL (LUMINAL)

Phenobarbital (PHB) is a barbiturate and one of the oldest ASMs; it is effective against focal-onset and generalized tonic-clonic seizures. However it is not effective against generalized absence seizures. It has also been used as a sedative. An IV form can be used for treatment of status epilepticus.

Phenobarbital is a potent liver enzyme inducer. Several inhibitors (including valproate, felbamate, and cenobamate) can result in its accumulation. Its main adverse effects are sedation and decreased concentration. Long-term use is associated with decreased bone density and some connective tissue changes.

The use of phenobarbital in the treatment of epilepsy has declined in developed countries due to its sedative adverse effect and its potent hepatic enzyme induction. However, it remains the only affordable ASM in many countries with limited resources.

PHENYTOIN (DILANTIN)

Phenytoin (PHT) is a hydantoin which supplied in a variety of forms. Mechanism of action is believed to be related to blocking of sodium channels, like carbamazepine. It is indicated for treatment of focal-onset seizures and generalized-onset tonic-clonic seizures. It is also indicated for seizure prophylaxis after neurosurgery. An IV formulation was frequently used for treatment of status epilepticus in adults and children. It has been largely replaced by the water-soluble prodrug Fosphenytoin, which can be administered faster and is less likely to cause local reactions.

PHT is not effective against generalized absence and generalized myoclonic seizures. It may even exacerbate these seizures.

PHT's dose-related adverse effects are typical of sodium channel blockers. They include ataxia, incoordination, and diplopia. Idiosyncratic reactions including rash may occur. There are also long-term adverse effects including gingival hyperplasia and reduced bone density.

PHT is unique among ASMs in its nonlinear kinetics, so that within the therapeutic range small dose increments can produce a disproportionate increase in serum concentration. PHT absorption is also variable and influenced by co-administered agents. As a result, PHT concentrations may be unstable in some individuals.

PHT is a potent enzyme inducer and is subject to many interactions. It was the most frequently used ASM for decades, but its use has declined with the availability of newer medications with more favorable pharmacokinetics.

PREGABALIN (LYRICA)

Pregabalin (PGB) is similar structurally and chemically to gabapentin. It has the same mechanism of action. It is approved for adjunctive therapy of focal-onset seizures in patients 1 month of age or older. It is a narrow-spectrum drug that is not effective against generalized-onset seizures. It can exacerbate generalized absence and generalized myoclonic seizures. In addition to the epilepsy indication, there are nonepileptic indications, including neuropathic pain due to diabetic neuropathy or spinal cord injury, fibromyalgia, and postherpetic neuralgia. It is also used off-label for generalized anxiety disorder, insomnia, and social phobia disorder.

PGB has more reliable absorption than gabapentin, but otherwise has very similar pharmacokinetics with no metabolism, no protein-binding, and excretion in the urine. Its short half-life requires twice-daily or 3 times daily dosing. It has the same adverse effects as gabapentin, including dizziness, somnolence, as well as weight gain and peripheral edema.

Its use in epilepsy is relatively limited and is much less common than for nonepileptic indications.

PRIMIDONE (MYSOLINE)

Primidone (PRM) is a barbiturate analog which is approved for use against focal-onset seizures and generalized-onset tonic-clonic seizures. Its major metabolite is phenobarbital. It is commonly used off-label for treatment of essential tremor.[8]

PRM was less well-tolerated than phenobarbital, phenytoin, or carbamazepine in a large comparative trial. As a result, it is used infrequently. It requires a slow titration to avoid acute toxicity related to the parent drug.

Primidone is a potent enzyme inducer and has the expected pharmacokinetic interactions of its main metabolite, phenobarbital.

RUFINAMIDE (BANZEL)

Rufinamide (RFM) is a triazole derivative (containing a triazole ring: C_2N_3). Mechanism of action may be related to blocking the sodium channel and prolongation of its inactive state. It is approved for adjunctive therapy of seizures associated with LGS in adults and children age 1 year and up. It is occasionally used off-label for adjunctive treatment of refractory focal-onset seizures in adults.[9]

RFM has an important interaction with valproate which reduces its clearance, causing accumulation. Its most common adverse effects are dizziness, fatigue, somnolence, and headache. It may shorten the QT interval.

STIRIPENTOL (DIACOMIT)

Stiripentol is a novel ASM, unrelated chemically to other ASMs. It is approved for use as adjunctive therapy for patients with Dravet syndrome age 2 years and older taking clobazam (Onfi).

Since it is typically used with clobazam, a benzodiazepine, worsening somnolence is a potential adverse effect, and, to reduce this risk, the dose of clobazam may be reduced by 25% with institution of stiripentol therapy.

Mechanism of action is thought to be mediated directly via binding to the $GABA_A$ receptor and indirectly by reducing metabolism of clobazam and its active metabolite.

TIAGABINE (GABITRIL)

Tiagabine (TGB) inhibits GABA reuptake at the synapse, resulting in increased GABA concentration. It is indicated as adjunctive therapy in adults and children 12 years and older in the treatment of focal-onset seizures. It is a narrow-spectrum drug that is ineffective against generalized-onset seizures and may exacerbate generalized absence and myoclonic seizures. It is also used off-label in treatment of spasticity and addiction and to increase the proportion of deep sleep.

TGB has a short half-life requiring 3 times daily dosing. Its clearance is increased by enzyme-inducing drugs. It requires a slow titration for tolerability. The most common adverse effect is dizziness. TGB may be associated with those related episodes of encephalopathy or nonconvulsive status epilepticus that may occur even in people who do not have epilepsy. Its use is markedly limited due to this.

TOPIRAMATE (TOPAMAX)

Topiramate (TPM) is an ASM with weak carbonic anhydrase inhibitor properties. It has multiple mechanisms of action, most importantly AMPA/kainate receptor antagonism, augmentation of GABA activity, and blocking of voltage-gated sodium channels. Approved indications include monotherapy and adjunctive therapy for focal-onset and generalized-onset tonic-clonic seizures in patients age 2 years and older. It is also approved for adjunctive therapy of seizures in patients with LGS age 2 years and older. Thus, TPM is a broad-spectrum drug. However, it does not seem to be effective against generalized absence seizures. TPM is sometimes used for super-refractory status epilepticus with some evidence of benefit.[10]

In addition to epilepsy indications, it is approved for migraine prophylaxis in patients age 12 and older; because of this co-indication, topiramate is used commonly in patients with both epilepsy and migraine. It is also indicated for weight loss in a combination that includes phentermine.

Topiramate has tolerability issues, mainly due to cognitive adverse effects. Kidney stones may appear in about 1.5% of patients. Decreased appetite and weight loss are usually welcome, but could be problematic in some individuals. Paresthesias may occur due to the carbonic anhydrase inhibition.

While pharmacokinetic interactions are minimal, topiramate may reduce the efficacy of the oral contraceptive at greater than 200 mg/d.

VALPROATE (DEPAKOTE, DEPAKENE, DEPACON)

Valproate (VPA) is a small molecule which is a weak organic acid. Approved indications are for monotherapy or adjunctive treatment of focal-onset seizures in adults and children age 10 years and older and of generalized absence seizures. Although not explicitly indicated for other generalized seizure types, there is ample evidence that valproate is a broad-spectrum medication effective against all seizure types, including generalized-onset tonic-clonic and generalized myoclonic seizures. Valproate IV formulation is often prescribed for patients with refractory status epilepticus, but this is an off-label use.[11]

VPA is also indicated for treatment of manic episodes associated with bipolar disorder and to prevent migraine headaches.

VPA has multiple mechanisms of action, including potentiation of GABA, blocking of T-type calcium channels, and blocking of sodium channels.

VPA is extensively metabolized, and its clearance is increased by enzyme inducers. In addition, it is an enzyme inhibitor, reducing the clearance of several medications, including phenobarbital, lamotrigine, rufinamide, and carbamazepine epoxide, thus causing accumulation of these agents.

Adverse effects include gastric irritation, fatigue, drowsiness, tremor, weight gain, hair loss, and peripheral edema. GI adverse effects are less common with the divalproex sodium extended-release preparation. A boxed warning concerns potential hepatic failure, which appears to be more likely in children younger than 2 years, in patients on multiple anticonvulsants, and in patients with mitochondrial disease. The warning also includes fetal risk of major congenital malformations and risk of pancreatitis in children and adults.

VIGABATRIN (SABRIL)

Vigabatrin (VGB) was designed to inhibit GABA-transaminase thereby increasing GABA levels in the brain. Approved use includes monotherapy for treatment of infantile spasms in children age 1 month to 2 years of age and for refractory focal-onset seizures in adults and children age 10 years and older. It is not effective against generalized-onset seizures and may exacerbate generalized absence and myoclonic seizures.

VGB is not metabolized and is excreted unchanged in the urine. It has minimal interactions.

VGB has a boxed warning of risk of peripheral visual loss resulting in progressive and irreversible visual field constriction. Because of this, periodic visual assessment is recommended at baseline and every 3 months. Treatment should only be continued if the observed benefit justifies the risk.

ZONISAMIDE (ZONEGRAN)

Zonisamide (ZNS) is a sulfonamide ASM approved for adjunctive therapy of adults with focal-onset seizures. However, there is evidence that it is a broad-spectrum drug effective against generalized-onset as well as focal-onset seizures. ZNS is sometimes used off-label for migraine prevention.[12]

ZNS's mechanisms of action include blocking T-type calcium channels, blocking sodium channels, and weak inhibition of carbonic anhydrase activity.

ZNS has minimal interactions. Its long half-life justifies once-daily dosing, even though the official indication is for twice-daily dosing based on clinical trials.

Adverse effects include sedation, ataxia, dizziness, nausea, fatigue, irritability, decreased appetite, and weight loss. Cognitive dysfunction may occur with higher doses, but it is less pronounced than that seen with topiramate. Kidney stones may occur.

Although zonisamide is acceptable as a first-line treatment, it is rarely the first choice due to its cognitive adverse effects.

PART 9

Samples and Case Discussions

9.1

Teaching Case Discussions with Dr. Abou-Khalil

BASSEL ABOU-KHALIL

CASE 1

A 36-year-old right-handed woman presented with recurrent convulsive seizures. She worked as a special education teacher. The first attack was 1 month before presentation. She felt odd, then turned her head to the left, became stiff, and started having generalized jerking. She was transported to the emergency room and had another similar episode there. She turned her head to the left, as if following something, stiffened all over, and had generalized jerking. Her dose of pregabalin, previously prescribed for fibromyalgia, was increased. Five days later, she had two more convulsive events. Her mother, who witnessed the last event, insisted that she saw extreme head turning to the right before the generalized jerking. She was then started on levetiracetam 750 mg twice daily. There was no recurrence of attacks, but she felt anxious and experienced insomnia. Pyridoxine 100 mg/d was added to help reduce the anxiety. A 2-hour electroencephalogram (EEG) was normal in waking drowsiness and sleep. Brain magnetic resonance imaging (MRI) was normal.

She had no recurrence of convulsive events for 1.5 years, then they recurred, initially after missing 2 days of her levetiracetam, but later without clear trigger, every 2–6 months. She also developed what she called "partial seizures" in which she would go into a dream state. She said that she could hear people talking but could not tell what they were saying. She estimated 2–3 such episodes per month. They were brought on by stress. They continued, even after her dose of levetiracetam was increased to 1,000 mg in the morning and 1,500 mg in the evening.

She was admitted to the epilepsy monitoring unit (EMU). Levetiracetam was stopped on the day of admission. A cluster of small events (Figure 9.1.1), as well as two major convulsive events were recorded.

The video-EEG study recorded two bilateral tonic-clonic seizures, both of which started with head deviation to the left followed by generalized tonic then clonic activity.

Does head turning at ictal onset indicate that we are dealing with focal epilepsy? The corresponding EEG started with generalized bifrontally predominant mixed 12 Hz rhythmic sharp activity and 4–4.5 Hz spike-and-wave activity. This was associated with staring. Attenuation with higher frequency rhythmic activity marked the transition to the tonic-clonic phase.

Could we truly be dealing with generalized epilepsy when the onset was at age 36 years? The patient was diagnosed with adult-onset idiopathic generalized epilepsy with generalized absence and generalized tonic-clonic seizures. At the end of the EMU study, levetiracetam was resumed at 1,000 mg twice daily and lamotrigine was titrated up to 200 mg twice daily. She has been seizure-free for 9 years. She did not wish to take any risks with medication withdrawal.

This case illustrates several points.

- Head deviation at onset of tonic-clonic activity is contralateral to the epileptogenic zone in focal epilepsy. Can this presumably focal sign be seen with generalized epilepsy?

Head deviation to one side is common in primary generalized seizures. It may occur in up to 60% of seizures.[1, 2] The head turning may be in opposite directions in different seizures, which should be considered a clue favoring primary generalized tonic-clonic seizures.

- Idiopathic generalized epilepsy usually starts in the first two decades of life. Can it start in adulthood?

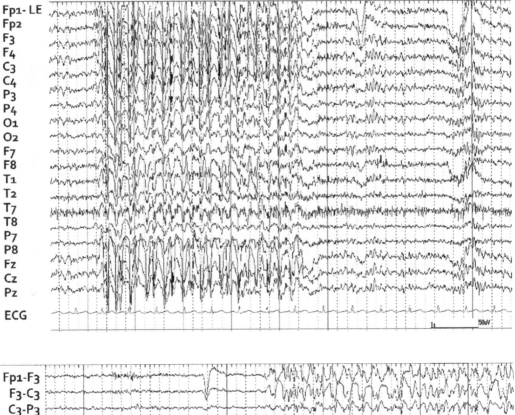

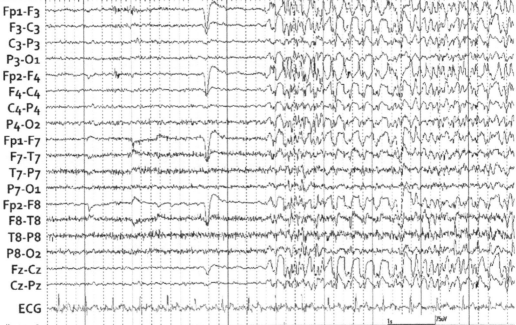

FIGURE 9.1.1 Case 1. Electroencephalogram (EEG) associated with a brief behavioral arrest and staring. This is a series of 11 frames. There was a cluster of these episodes. The EEG showed generalized 4 Hz spike-and-wave activity. Next frame: EEG discharge in association with a tonic-clonic seizure.

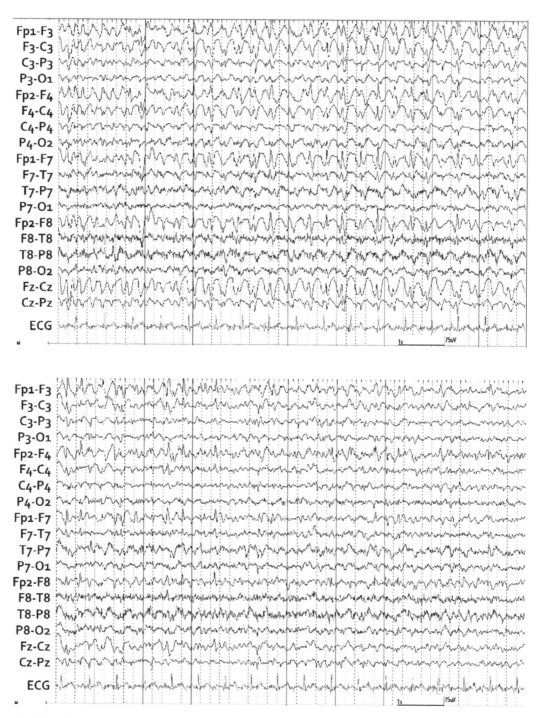

FIGURE 9.1.1 Continued

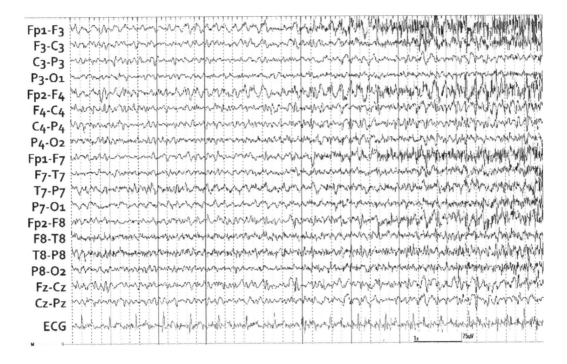

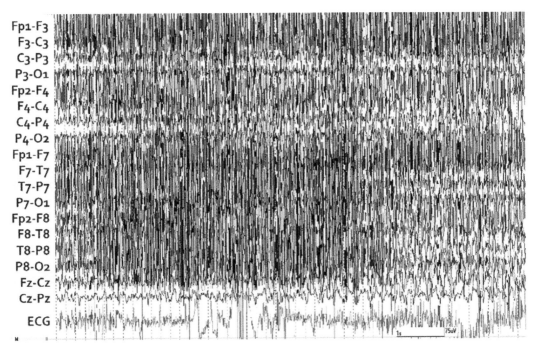

FIGURE 9.1.1 Continued

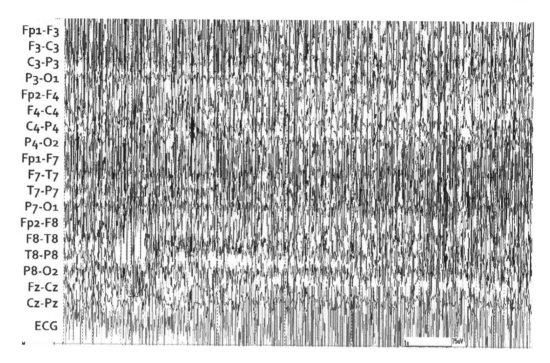

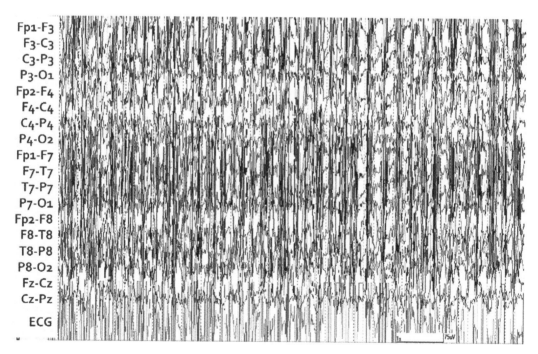

FIGURE 9.1.1 Continued

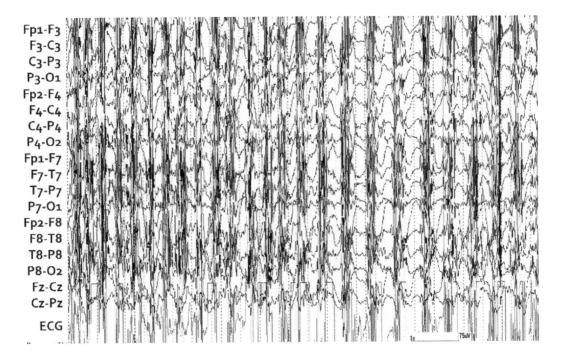

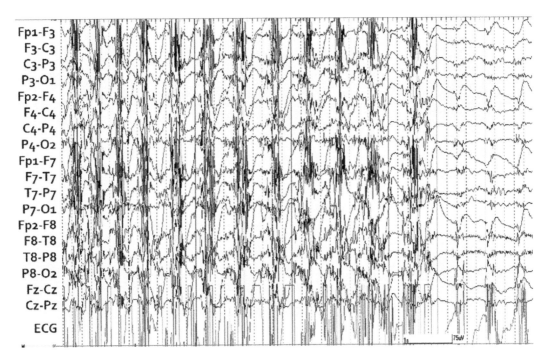

FIGURE 9.1.1 Continued

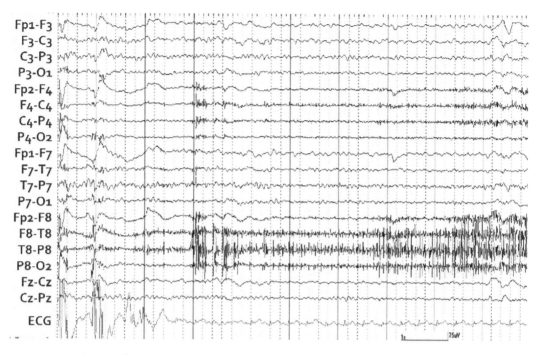

FIGURE 9.1.1 Continued

Idiopathic generalized epilepsy may start in adulthood. Onset after age 20 is reported in up to 28% of patients.[3,4,5,6,7] , It is possible that subtle absence seizures or myoclonic seizures may have been present but not recognized until tonic-clonic seizures occur.

- The EEG showed that the tonic-clonic seizure evolved from absence. Can this happen?

Generalized absence seizures may evolve into generalized tonic-clonic seizures,[8,9] just as they may evolve from myoclonic seizures. The latter are recognized in the new seizure classification as generalized myoclonic-tonic-clonic seizures and commonly occur in patients with juvenile myoclonic epilepsy.

- What about the 12 Hz rhythmic activity intermixed with spike-and-wave activity? Is this compatible with absence?

Generalized absence seizures may include fast 10–15 Hz rhythms intermixed with typical spike-and-wave activity.[10] This activity does not have any negative prognostic implication. It is of unknown clinical significance.

CASE 2

A 70-year-old woman presented for management of seizures starting at age 62. With the first event, her coworker noticed that her head turned to the right, after which she was unresponsive for approximately 30 sec. An EEG showed left temporal sharp waves. MRI showed only scattered foci of increased white matter T2 signal. She was started on oxcarbazepine 300 mg twice a day. However, seizures continued to recur once a month. They were characterized by staring, lip twitching, inability to talk, and unresponsiveness. She thought that she was awake, but she was unable to respond. She complained that oxcarbazepine caused excessive tiredness and cognitive dysfunction.

She was switched to lamotrigine. She had increased seizure frequency as oxcarbazepine was tapered, but after the lamotrigine dose was increased to 200 mg twice a day she had a remission for more than a year. The remission ended when she developed recurrent passing out episodes that were different from her prior seizures. She would slump over with no warning. A neurologist who witnessed one of her episodes in church concluded that it was a syncopal event rather than a seizure. She also developed recurrence of her habitual seizures with staring and unresponsiveness followed by confusion and disorientation. When the dose of lamotrigine was increased she developed diplopia and disequilibrium. These adverse effects improved with switching to extended-release lamotrigine. However, the passing out episodes continued every few months, along with her habitual seizures. A tilt table test was positive, so she was advised to increase her salt intake. She also reduced her extended-release lamotrigine dose from 500 to 400 mg/d based on the diagnosis of syncope. She increased the dose back to 500 mg/d after an increase in frequency of both her habitual seizures and the passing out and slumping episodes. Passing out episodes that recurred despite the addition of fludrocortisone. She felt as if she was standing. At times there was associated vomiting. A 48-hour ambulatory EEG study was negative and did not record any events. She was admitted to the EMU for continuous video-EEG monitoring. Lamotrigine was stopped for the purpose of the study. Five seizures were recorded. The ictal onset was bitemporal independent (three right temporal and two left temporal), and interictal epileptiform discharges were also bitemporal independent. One of the attacks with left temporal onset was associated with slumping. The electrocardiogram (EKG) showed ictal bradycardia then asystole for 9 sec preceding the slumping (Figure 9.1.2).

- What is the connection between the left temporal seizure and the bradycardia/asystole?

The bradycardia started approximately 8 sec after the ictal discharge was first noted. The patient had bradycardia with 4 of 5 seizures recorded and asystole in 3. It was clear that the seizure discharge was a precursor. This represents ictal bradycardia and ictal asystole.

She had a pacemaker implanted. Levetiracetam was also added to her regimen at a dose of 500 mg twice a day. She had no recurrence of syncope over 9 years of follow-up.

- Ictal bradycardia-asystole is a rare event, estimated to occur in about 0.27–0.4% of patients undergoing video-EEG monitoring.[11]
- It is most common in temporal or frontal lobe seizures.[12]
- The incidence may be higher in select patients with drug-resistant epilepsy and an implanted loop recorder.

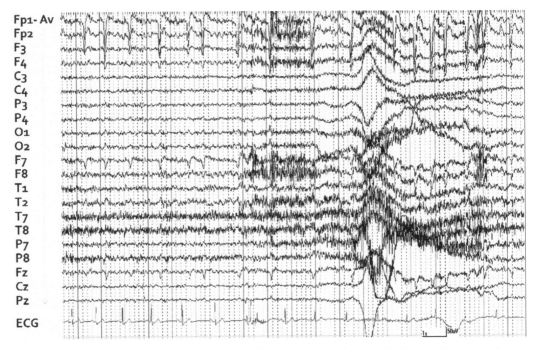

FIGURE 9.1.2 Case 2. Electroencephalogram (EEG) demonstrating a left temporal seizure with associated bradycardia and asystole. Average reference montage. This is a series of 6 frames from the same patient.

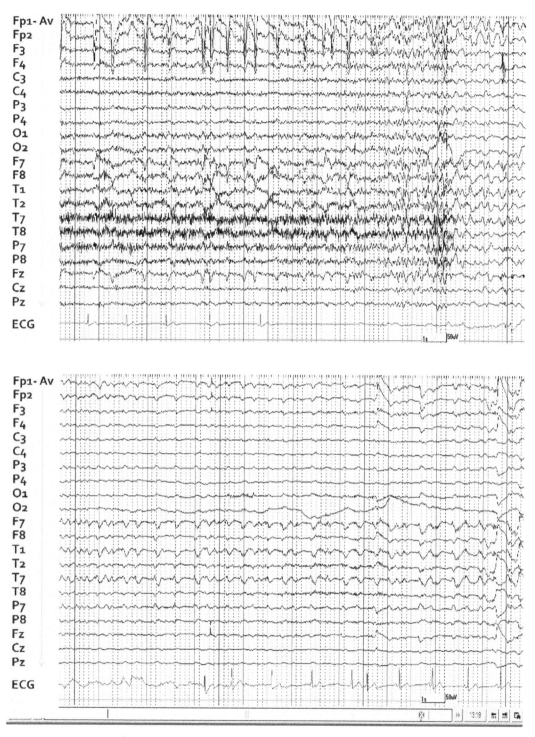

FIGURE 9.1.2 Continued

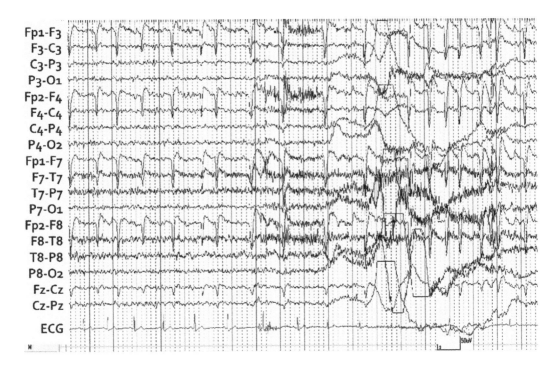

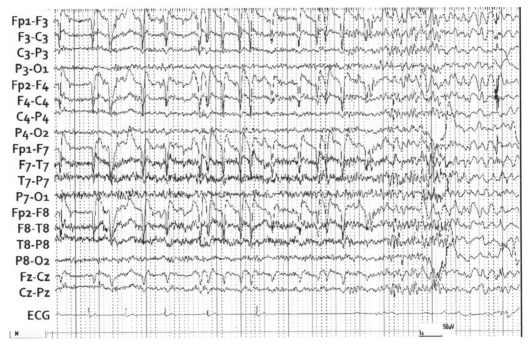

FIGURE 9.1.2 Continued

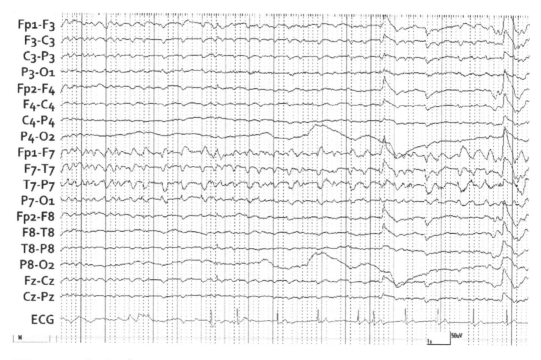

FIGURE 9.1.2 Continued

- Syncope occurs after about 6 sec of asystole.[13]
- Although it is concerning and the syncope can be associated with injury, it is usually self-limited and not related to sudden unexpected death in epilepsy (SUDEP).

CASE 3

A 13-year-old right-handed boy has had seizures since age 5, as well as developmental delay. Seizures are characterized by sudden contraction of all extremities and trunk for a few seconds, then staring and unresponsiveness for up to 30 sec. A typical seizure was recorded on video-EEG (Figure 9.1.3).

- What is this seizure?

The initial EEG change was with low-voltage fast activity, associated with increased muscle artifact, consistent with a tonic seizure. However, after 8 sec, the EEG has evolved to 1.5–2 Hz generalized spike-and-wave activity, consistent with atypical generalized absence seizure.

This uncommon seizure type has been called *tonic-absence seizure*.[14] One study reported 29 seizures of this pattern in eight patients; 26 of 29 seizures demonstrated generalized activity 14–30 Hz, lasting 2–8 sec followed by generalized 1–2 Hz spike-and-wave for 3–50 seconds. The predominant clinical correlate was bilateral tonic activity followed by a period of inattentiveness. These seizures were differentiated from typical tonic seizures by prolonged impaired attention/responsiveness after the end of the tonic contraction. This prolonged inattention could initially appear to be post-ictal in the absence of an EEG, which confirms its ictal nature.

CASE 4

A 51-year-old man with type 2 diabetes mellitus was found by hospital security in the parking lot leaning on the hood of his car, not responding appropriately. In the emergency room, he was found to have a rightward gaze deviation, and he was minimally responsive, intermittently. Blood glucose was 542. He was given insulin and admitted to the hospital. On examination, he was awake but nonverbal. He followed commands inconsistently. He had an episode of right arm jerking and was given lorazepam. The next morning he was back to baseline except for visual symptoms. He was able to relay that he started feeling funny after he left a clinic appointment; had visual difficulties,

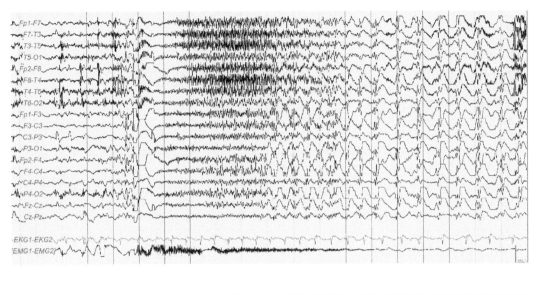

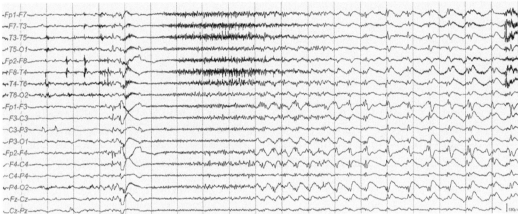

FIGURE 9.1.3 Case 3. Top: Longitudinal bipolar montage. Bottom: Longitudinal bipolar montage.

particularly trouble with estimating distances; had a hard time finding his car; and could not get into his car. He lost memory after that. On examination, he had a right homonymous hemianopia. Brain MRI did not show any infarct or clearly abnormal contrast enhancement.

An EEG was performed. Figure 9.1.4 shows the sequential pages.

- What is the nature of the activity in Figure 9.1.4?

We are seeing recurrent left occipital ictal discharges. Quantitative EEG analysis (discussed later) shows recurrent ictal discharges with 19 discharges in the span of 2 hours. EEG changes with seizures show up best on the left hemisphere rhythmicity spectrogram (increased rhythmicity with every ictal discharge), asymmetry spectrogram (increased left

power in blue with a color display, with every ictal discharge, but showing dark on these figures), and amplitude-integrated EEG (aEEG), with a peak corresponding to every ictal discharge.

After correction of hyperglycemia, EEG ictal discharges resolved without anti-seizure medications (ASMs), and the hemianopia resolved over several days.

- Are the ictal discharges connected to the hemianopia?

Occipital lobe seizures that remain localized to the occipital lobe most often manifest with positive symptoms, such as elementary visual hallucinations, but negative symptoms such as hemianopia or even blindness may occur. Hemianopia may also be a post-ictal manifestation, particularly with frequent recurrent ictal discharges.

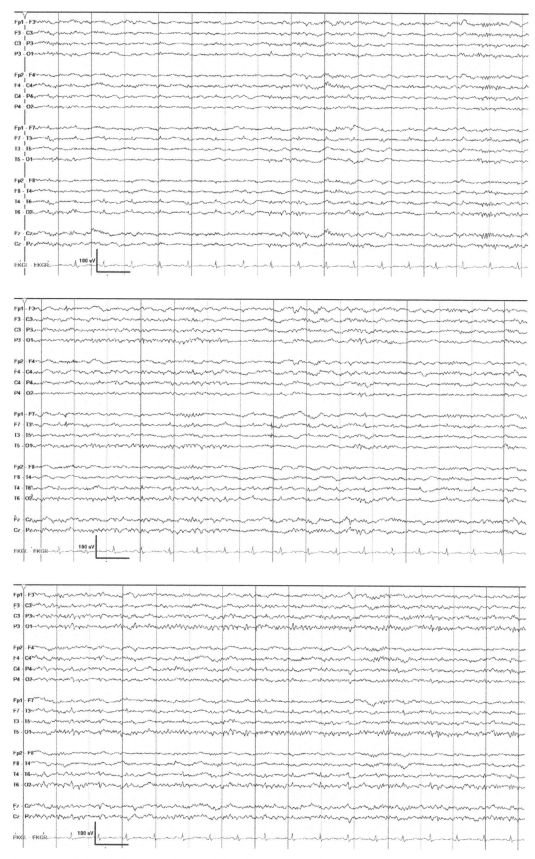

FIGURE 9.1.4 Case 4. Five sequential pages followed by two pages of quantitative EEG analysis. Longitudinal bipolar montage.

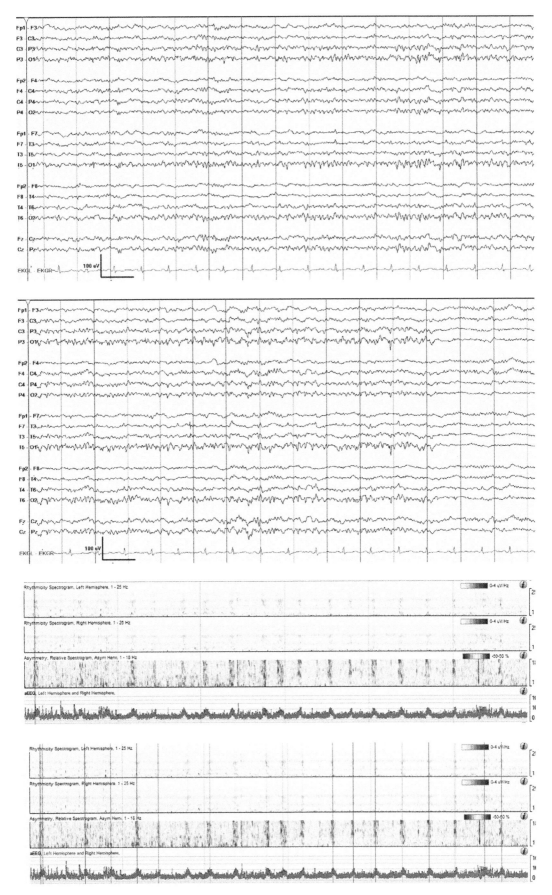

FIGURE 9.1.4 Continued

- Are the seizures and hemianopia connected to the hyperglycemia?

Indeed, nonketotic hyperglycemia is associated with focal seizures. In particular, hemianopia has been described as a transient manifestation,[15] demonstrated secondary to occipital ictal activity.[16]

CASE 5

This case presents a 21-year-old man with seizures starting at age 13. Seizures consisted of upper extremity twitching, and he also developed convulsions. Over time, the convulsions increased to monthly. They were most often in the early morning, often preceded by a cluster of jerks. Single or clustered jerks involved the upper extremities, caused him to drop items, and affected his writing. Their frequency varied from daily to weekly.

EEG revealed frontally dominant generalized 3.5–4 Hz spike-and-wave and polyspike-and-wave discharges as well as a photoparoxysmal response. There were also rare right occipital spikes. He was diagnosed with juvenile myoclonic epilepsy and initially treated with phenytoin and levetiracetam. Major seizures came under control for about 1 year, then they recurred with increasing frequency. The myoclonic jerks increased to daily and the tonic-clonic seizures to weekly. Addition

of topiramate resulted in transient remission of tonic-clonic seizures. He was then weaned off phenytoin, which was replaced with lamotrigine. A vagus nerve stimulator was implanted, then valproate was added. These changes resulted in another transient remission of tonic-clonic seizures and improvement in myoclonic seizures. However, he developed concentration difficulty, postural tremor and asterixis on examination, and was found to have elevated ammonia. Valproate had to be removed, but hyperammonemia did not resolve until topiramate was discontinued. Seizures were very frequent, with two clusters of convulsive seizures per week plus daily jerks. He was admitted to the EMU for medication management. On admission he had been trialed on 15 ASMs. He was started on valproate again and his regimen of five ASMs that he took prior to admission was simplified.

The EMU study recorded (1) 16 ictal discharges associated with clusters of myoclonic jerking, in five instances evolving to clonic seizures; these ictal discharges started with irregular generalized 4–6 Hz spike-and-wave activity; (2) abundant generalized, bifrontal predominant, 4–6 Hz spike-and-wave discharges, often in clusters usually lasting 1–2 sec, but up to 4–9 secs; at times there were associated myoclonic jerks; And (3) generalized slow activity (Figure 9.1.5).

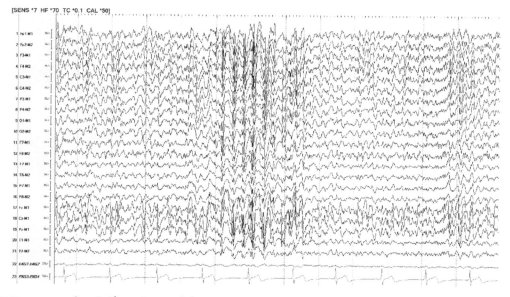

FIGURE 9.1.5 Case 5. Above: Interictal electroencephalogram (EEG). Ipsilateral ear reference. Following 10 frames in sequence: Case 5. Ictal EEG with a cluster of generalized myoclonic seizures evolving to a generalized clonic seizure. Longitudinal bipolar reference.

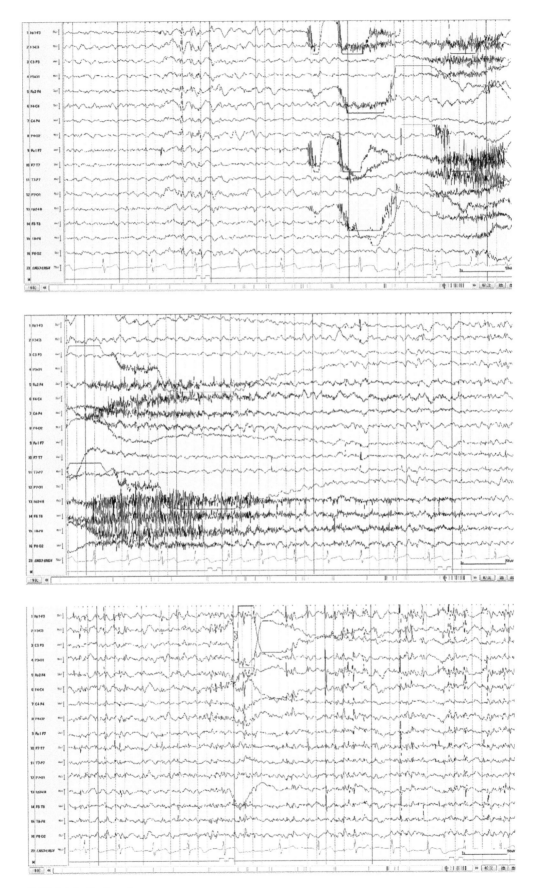

FIGURE 9.1.5 Continued

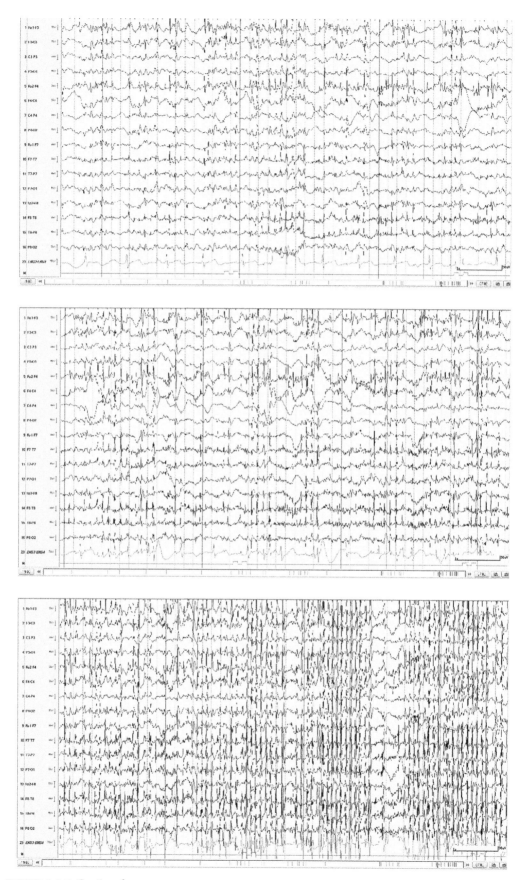

FIGURE 9.1.5 Continued

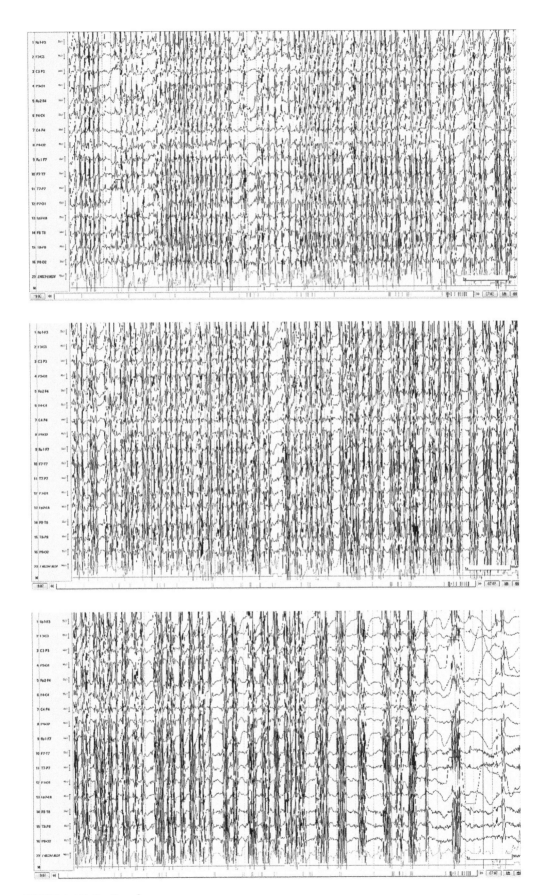

FIGURE 9.1.5 Continued

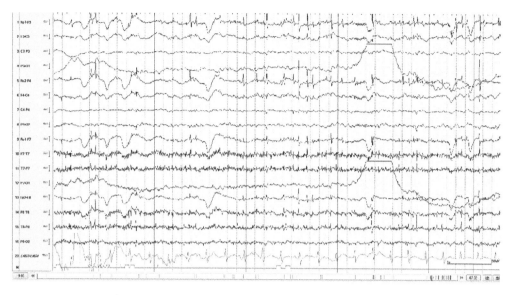

FIGURE 9.1.5 Continued

The activity noted on EEG is a combination of cerebral EEG activity and artifact.

- Are the clinical and EEG features consistent with juvenile myoclonic epilepsy?

Several features are atypical for juvenile myoclonic epilepsy and raised the possibility of progressive myoclonic epilepsy.[17]

- The very high seizure frequency,
- The resistance to several appropriate drugs,
- The apparent progressive nature of the condition,
- The recording of clonic seizures, which are unusual for juvenile myoclonic epilepsy and more common with progressive myoclonic epilepsy,
- The increased slow activity in the background.

Genetic testing was performed. It was positive for a mutation of cystatin B, diagnostic of Unverricht Lundborg disease.[18]

He was started on perampanel, in addition to levetiracetam, zonisamide, valproate, clobazam. The addition of perampanel produced marked improvement in myoclonus and only rare convulsive seizures persisted, every 3–6 months.

Perampanel appears to be particularly helpful in Unverricht-Lundborg disease.[19,20]

CASE 6

A 24-year-old man presented after a motor vehicle accident while unrestrained by a seatbelt. Head CT demonstrated left-sided subdural hematoma, evolving hemorrhagic left hemisphere contusions, and 7 mm of midline shift. On examination, he was unresponsive to verbal stimulation but withdrew to painful stimulation. He was intubated and hyperventilated. An intracranial pressure (ICP) monitor was placed, and his elevated ICP was treated with mannitol, then an external ventricular drain, then a pentobarbital coma. An EEG showed a burst suppression pattern. The bursts did not include any epileptiform discharges (Figure 9.1.6).

As pentobarbital was weaned, a pattern of generalized, frontally dominant periodic discharges recurring at 3/sec was recorded, concerning for nonconvulsive status epilepticus (Figure 9.1.6). There was no observable motor accompaniment.

- Does the above represent nonconvulsive status epilepticus?

Generalized periodic discharges (GPDs) may be a transient pattern during withdrawal of pentobarbital and propofol.[21] This pattern has been called GPDs related to anesthetic withdrawal (GRAW). The pattern will resolve spontaneously without treatment. Electroclinical features that may identify GRAWs include

- New-onset GPDs after anesthetic withdrawal, especially after drug-induced burst-suppression;
- No GPDs prior to anesthetic use;
- GPDs differ from pre-anesthetic EEG pattern (e.g., pre-anesthetic EEG with focal ictal discharges);
- Spontaneous electrographic and clinical improvement without treatment;
- Recurrence of pattern with repeated anesthetic withdrawal;
- Absence of confounding conditions (e.g., generalized convulsive status epilepticus, prion disease, anoxic brain injury, or diffuse toxic/metabolic processes);
- Absence of clinical ictal signs other than coma.

In this patient, the GPDs resolved spontaneously after 9 hours, as seen in frames 5 and 6 of Figure 9.1.6.

The patient was eventually discharged 25 days after admission. He was alert and oriented to time and place, but had significant deficits in attention, working memory, insight, and mental control.

CASE 7

A 21-year-old woman developed passing out events at age 20. Passing out events occurred without warning. She would be out for a few seconds,

then, upon regaining consciousness, she felt foggy and slow. Events gradually increased in frequency to weekly. She also started to have some warning symptoms, including numbness and tingling in the fingers and throbbing headaches. Cardiac and autonomic evaluations were negative. A routine EEG by her local neurologist was interpreted as abnormal due to paroxysmal bursts, possibly consistent with generalized epilepsy. She was referred for video-EEG monitoring.

On examination in the EMU, the only findings were give-way weakness on the left side and inconsistency in sensory perception on the left side. There were no objective abnormalities.

The interictal EEG recorded generalized sharply contoured alpha theta bursts during drowsiness (first frame of Figure 9.1.7).

- Are these bursts abnormal?

The bursts recorded can occur normally in drowsiness. In one study, 10% of normal subjects had bursts of irregular, frontocentral, large-amplitude, sharp theta/delta activity lasting less than 1 sec during the waking–drowsy transition. Occasional normal subjects had bursts of generalized, fronto-central predominant, large-amplitude, 2.5–7.5 Hz, irregular sharp activity lasting up to 4 sec.[22] These sharp bursts are sometimes misinterpreted as an abnormal finding suggestive of generalized epilepsy.

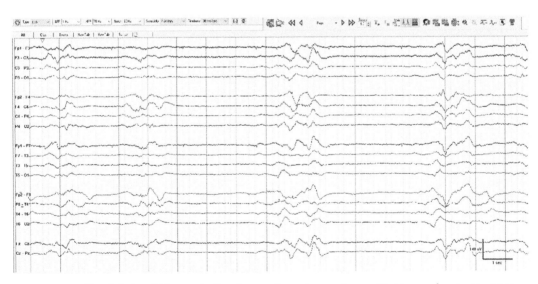

FIGURE 9.1.6 Case 6. Series of 6 frames starting above and on subsequent pages. First two are burst suppression pattern with increasing interburst interval in conjunction with deepening coma (LB montage). Next two are generalized 3/sec periodic discharges noted after pentobarbital was stopped (LB and linked ear). The last two are 9 and 17 hours after anesthetic withdrawal (LB).

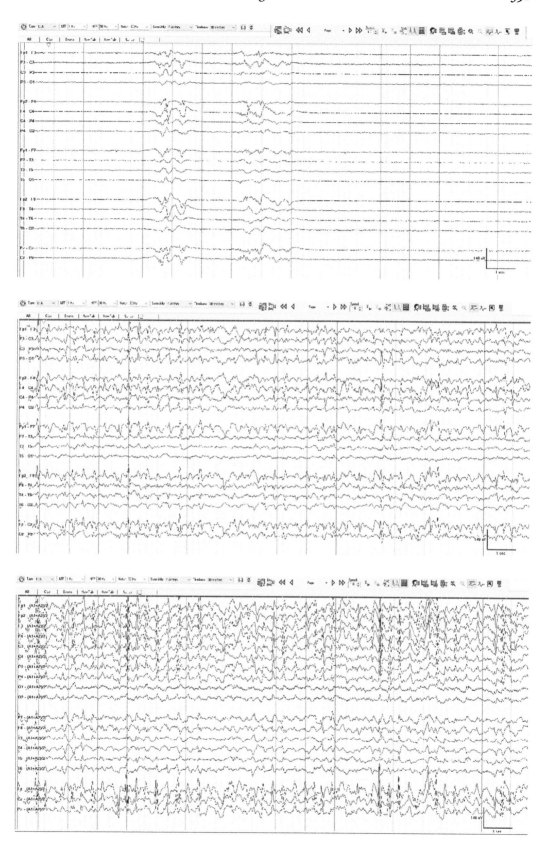

FIGURE 9.1.6 Continued

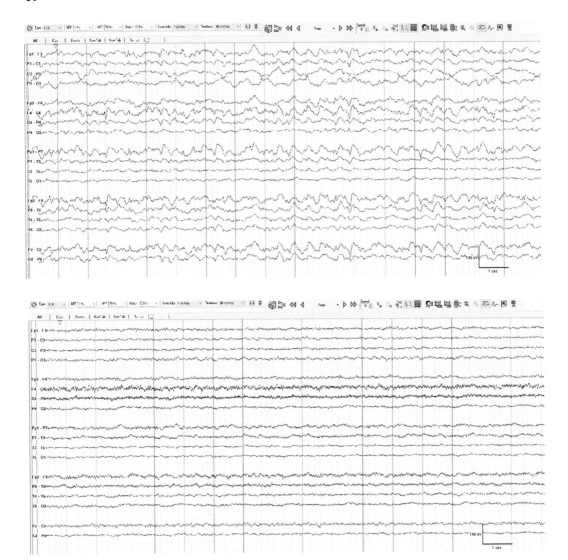

FIGURE 9.1.6 Continued

The video-EEG study of this patient recorded two typical events characterized by dropping her head to the left for 5–10 sec, with associated unresponsiveness. Upon recovery, she reported left arm numbness and headache. There were no associated EEG changes. By both EEG and clinical criteria, these spells were nonepileptic, most probably psychogenic in nature. In addition, there were no definite interictal EEG abnormalities, so the study failed to provide support for co-existent epilepsy.

CASE 8

A 48-year-old woman reported seizures starting at age 30. Her main risk factor for epilepsy was pneumococcal meningitis at 8 months, with recurrent convulsions for 5 days. Initial seizures were characterized by behavior arrest and staring. Seizures came under control for 4 years on carbamazepine, then they recurred, and, over time, seizure manifestations became more complex. She reported no aura; she would rub her hands, then began rowing arm motions that became unilateral on the right, with the left arm relatively immobile and she would have lip-smacking. She continued to speak at times during some seizures and had no word-finding difficulty post-ictally. She reported 1–2 seizures monthly despite trials of several ASM regimens. She expressed interest in epilepsy surgery and was admitted to the EMU to record seizures on video-EEG.

Figure 9.1.8 is an EEG example representative of four recorded seizure events.

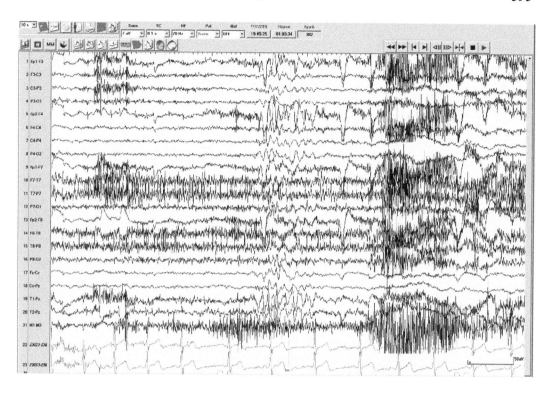

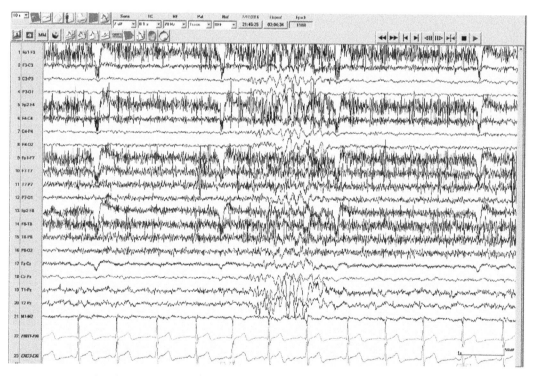

FIGURE 9.1.7 High-voltage generalized alpha theta bursts during drowsiness. Three frames starting above; first and second are LB montage, and third is ipsilateral ear reference montage.

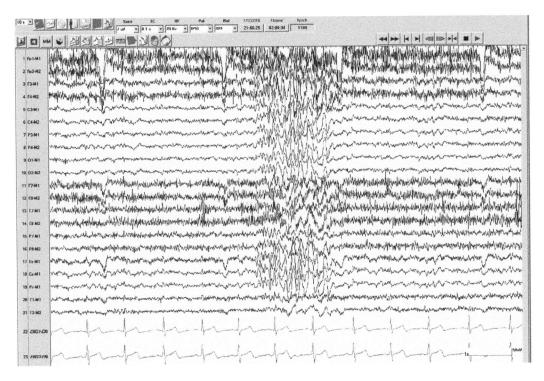

FIGURE 9.1.7 Continued

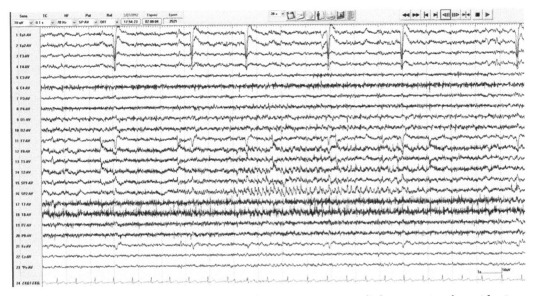

FIGURE 9.1.8 Focal 6 Hz rhythmic activity at Sp2>T2 lasting 8 sec. Sequence of 3 frames starting above. After 8 sec of what appeared to be normal interictal electroencephalogram (EEG), there was widespread rhythmic 5 Hz activity with right frontotemporal predominance. The third segment shows the 8 sec gap between the initial train of focal rhythmic theta activity and the more widespread rhythmic ictal discharge. Average reference montage.

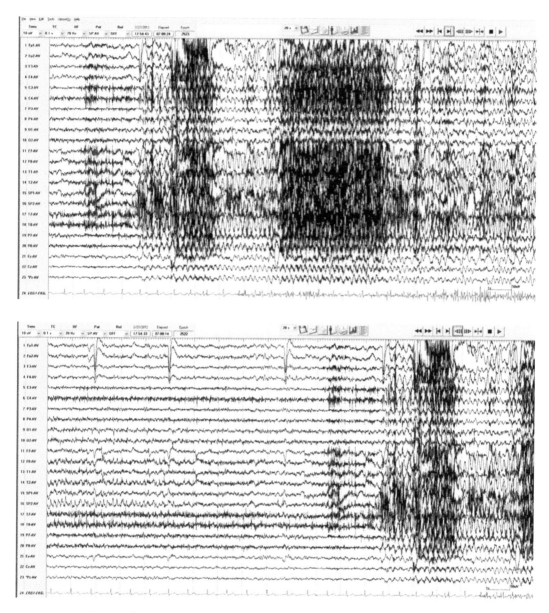

FIGURE 9.1.8 Continued

It is clear that the widespread rhythmic activity was an ictal discharge associated with a clinical seizure.

- What about the initial focal 8-second train?

The initial rhythmic activity was in fact the focal right inferomesial temporal ictal onset of the same seizure. The following attenuation may reflect transient seizure propagation away from the surface. This represents the start-stop-start phenomenon.[23] The first "start," which is typically more focal, corresponds to the ictal onset zone. The second "start" tends to have a wider field and less clear localization.

The EMU study recorded 10 ictal discharges of right inferomesial temporal origin, four of which were associated with a start-stop-start phenomenon. There were also frequent sharp waves in the right inferomesial-anterior temporal region, frequent right inferomesial-anterior-midtemporal intermittent rhythmic delta activity (TIRDA), and irregular delta activity. The main clinical features of the seizures were bilateral proximal and distal automatisms involving the upper extremities, including folding hands, rubbing hands, and sweeping both arms backward in a semicircular fashion repetitively (resembling breaststroke swimming), dystonic posturing of the left arm in some seizures, staring, and well-formed speech in some seizures.

The MRI showed bilateral hippocampal atrophy, more on the left, but with increased signal on the right. The patient had a right temporal lobectomy, which rendered her seizure-free. She remained in remission off seizure medications.

CASE 9

A 26-year-old man reported facial twitching, more on the right side, triggered by reading. He would typically stop reading temporarily when he experienced these, except for one instance when he continued reading: the episode evolved to loss of consciousness and generalized jerking.

He had an EEG study during which he read to trigger one of his events. Figure 9.1.9 is an EEG sample corresponding to subtle facial twitches not appreciated on video review.

- Is there a relation between the single spike-and-wave discharges and the jaw jerks?

The discharges are typical of that seen in association with jaw jerks in reading epilepsy. Reading epilepsy is a rare form of reflex epilepsy.[24] The EEG correlate of jaw jerks is single brief spike-and-wave discharges or sharp theta wave discharges that may be generalized, bi-frontocentrotemporal with left predominance, or lateralized to the left hemisphere.[25]

CASE 10

A 38-year-old man presented with seizures since 5 years of age. Clinically, seizures started with speech arrest, looking around, hand fidgeting, lip-smacking and post-ictal aphasia. Seizures rarely evolved to bilateral tonic-clonic activity, with versive head and eye deviation to the right.

He was admitted to the EMU to be evaluated for epilepsy surgery. Figure 9.1.10 is a recording of interictal epileptiform discharges followed by ictal onset.

- Is the seizure frontal or temporal?

F7 is physically overlying inferior frontal cortex but is most often recording anterior temporal activity. To determine whether the discharge is recording inferior frontal or anterior temporal

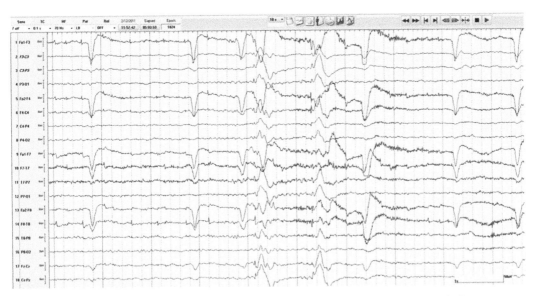

FIGURE 9.1.9 Two spike-and-wave discharges better appreciated on the ear reference montage. The first is generalized with left frontocentrotemporal predominance, and the second is focal left frontocentral. Above is longitudinal bipolar montage and Below is same epoch with linked ear reference montage.

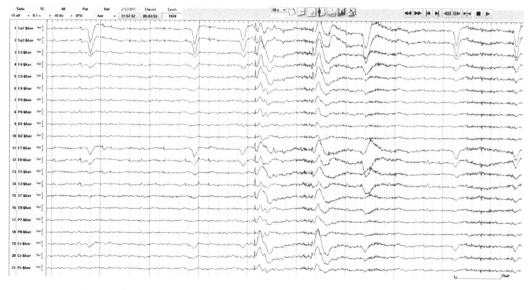

FIGURE 9.1.9 Continued

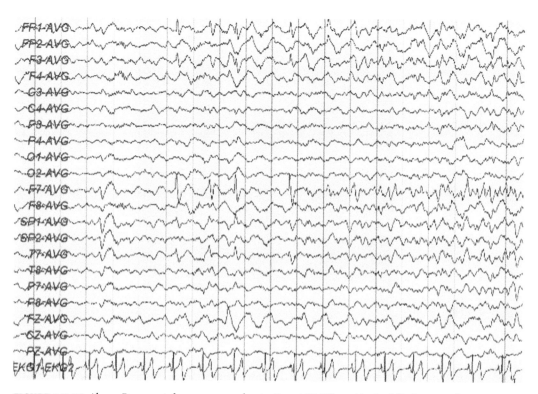

FIGURE 9.1.10 Above: Recurrent sharp waves predominating at F7, followed by ictal discharge predominant at F7 as well. Average reference montage. Next page top: The second segment shows bilateral propagation of the ictal discharge with frontotemporal predominance. Next page MRi image: Fluid-attenuated inversion recovery (FLAIR) magnetic resonance imaging (MRI) sequence demonstrating left inferior frontal cortical lesion with increased T2 signal.

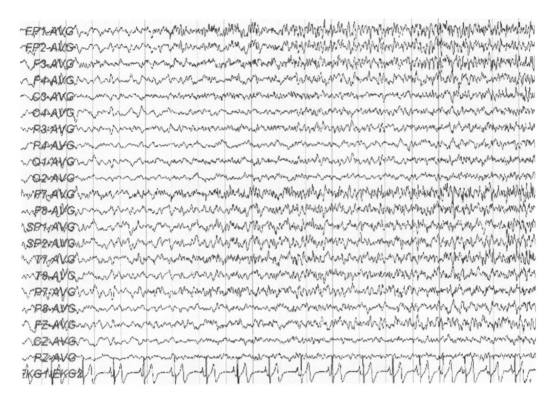

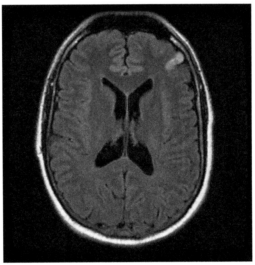

FIGURE 9.1.10 Continued

activity, one has to examine the field of the discharge. Looking at the field of the sharp waves preceding the ictal onset, there is usually greater involvement of Fp1 and F3 than temporal electrodes Sp1 and T7. This favors an inferior frontal origin. Indeed, the MRI showed a left inferior frontal cortical lesion (Figure 9.1.10).

The lesion was resected. The pathology was a dysembryoplastic neuroepithelial tumor (DNET) tumor. The patient is in medication-free remission.

9.2

Pediatric Teaching Case Discussions with Dr. Ess

KEVIN C. ESS

PEDIATRIC EPILEPSY CASE 1

Patient is a 38-month-old girl who began having seizures around 6 weeks of life. Her seizures began with intermittent eye deviation and head turning to the right. Duration of each seizure was several seconds, and frequency would increase when tired. She developed a left-hand preference by 1 year of age though her development was otherwise normal, including expressive and receptive language. She was treated with levetiracetam at 2 months of life. This was initially effective, but around 1 year of age she began to have breakthrough seizures and oxcarbazepine was added. This also provided good control for about 1 year, then seizures became more frequent and longer. Further evaluations for epilepsy surgery were then initiated. Language at age 2 years was delayed, using only 1–2 word phrases. Receptive language seemed intact. Interictal electroencephalogram (EEG) (Figure 9.2.1) shows very frequent, quasi-rhythmic sharp waves and slowing in the left frontal region, greatest around F3 and Fp1 but also involving F7.

EEG at ictal onset is characterized by fast and diffuse left frontal/central discharges that stands out from the interictal discharges, becoming more organized and rhythmic. The EEG onset always preceded the clinical onset, and at times

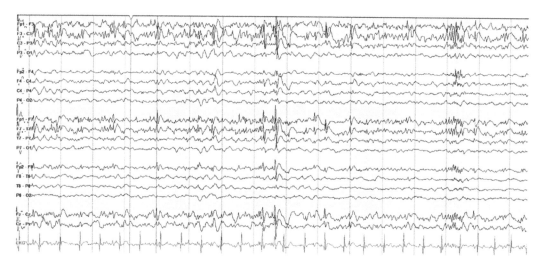

FIGURE 9.2.1 Case 1. Above: Frequent interictal discharges involving the left frontal lobe. Longitudinal bipolar montage. Next page top: Frequent interictal discharges involving the left frontal lobe, maximal in Fp1, F3, and F7 electrodes. Average montage. Next page middle: Ictal onset of typical seizure. Electroencephalogram (EEG) discharges become more rhythmic and organized, maximal at the F3 and C3 electrodes (within blue box). The family noted clinical onset of right eye deviation and altered mental status about 10 sec after the electrographic onset. Next page bottom: left panel, T2 brain magnetic resonance imaging (MRI) coronal view reveals extensive cortical dysplasia in the left frontal lobe within the black box. Right panel, fluorodeoxyglucose (FDG)-positron emission tomography (PET). The role of this procedure is to detect metabolically active. Coronal image showing increased uptake of the radioligand in the left frontal region corresponding to the region of dysplasia.

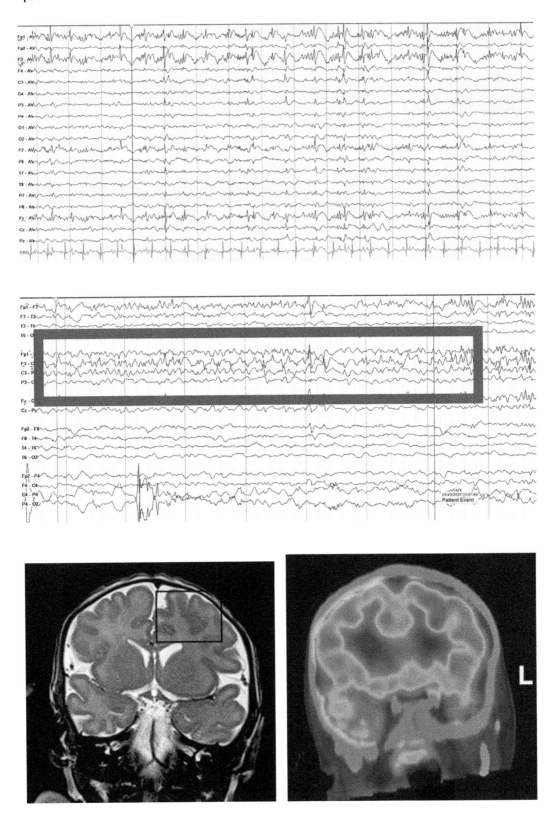

FIGURE 9.2.1 Continued

similar discharges were seen with no clinical accompaniment.

Brain magnetic resonance imaging (MRI) (Figure 9.2.1, left image) showed likely extensive region of cortical dysplasia involving the left frontal lobe. A fluorodeoxyglucose-positron emission tomography (FDG-PET) scan was also done (Figure 9.2.1, right image) and showed increased FDG uptake.

This was interpreted as an ictal PET scan given the almost constant left frontal activity seen in all prior EEGs, including during injection of the FDG-PET ligand.

Multiple stereo-EEG electrodes were placed in the left frontal lobe, and the ictal onset of her seizure onset was defined. The region of seizure generation was readily identified and found to be almost constantly having rhythmic discharges with intermittent spread to other electrodes. Cortical mapping was done to define the primary motor cortex; mapping for expressive language was also done. No eloquent cortex was immediately adjacent to the region of seizure onset.

A focal resection of the left frontal lobe was then done at around the age of 28 months. Pathological evaluation confirmed cortical dysplasia Type 2A with disorganized cortical layers and enlarged neurons. The patient remained seizure-free after surgery and did not have any motor deficits or worsening of language. In fact, her language began to improve rapidly over the next 12 months. Levetiracetam was weaned off after 1 year of seizure freedom, and she remains on oxcarbazepine monotherapy.

PEDIATRIC EPILEPSY CASE 2

This is a 4-year-old boy with tuberous sclerosis complex (TSC). He presented before birth with referral of his mother to a maternal–fetal clinic for evaluation of cardiac rhabdomyomas identified by screening obstetric ultrasound. After an uneventful birth, a neonatal brain MRI confirmed TSC with findings of cortical tubers and subependymal nodules.

Genetic testing was positive for a pathogenic mutation in the *TSC2* gene. The patient began to have seizures around 4 months of age; they were characterized as multifocal and initially treated with levetiracetam. These focal seizures at first were under reasonable control although the semiology evolved over 3 months to epileptic (infantile) spasms. Vigabatrin was then initiated and spasms rapidly resolved. Vigabatrin was weaned off after 6 months of therapy, and the patient did well on levetiracetam monotherapy until 2 years of age. He then began to again have focal seizures with a suspected right central onset on EEG (Figure 9.2.2), with seizures characterized by abrupt facial grimace upon waking or stopping activity, frequently associated with grabbing his left arm with his right hand and head drops. He failed appropriate medication trials with oxcarbazepine, zonisamide, and everolimus.

Brain MRI and alpha methyl tryptophan (AMT) PET were done and revealed an area of increased uptake adjacent to a prominent tuber.

He ultimately had stereo-EEG placement covering the right frontal and central regions as well as the perituberal region and right temporal lobe.

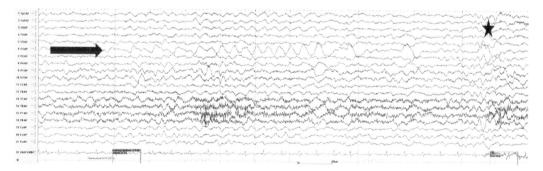

FIGURE 9.2.2 Case 2. Above: Focal seizure in 4-year-old with tuberous sclerosis complex (TSC). Clinical onset was preceded by rhythmic discharge maximal at the right central (C4) electrode (*arrow*). About 12 sec after electrographic seizure onset, the patient was noted to have head drop (*star*).

Next page top: Brain fluid-attenuated inversion recovery (FLAIR) magnetic resonance imaging (MRI) sequence from 4-year-old with TSC. Tuber for seizure onset within the right frontal lobe marked by red arrow. Next page subsequent frame: Alpha methyl tryptophan positron emission tomography (AMT-PET) scan in same patient showing focal increased uptake in the right frontal lobe.

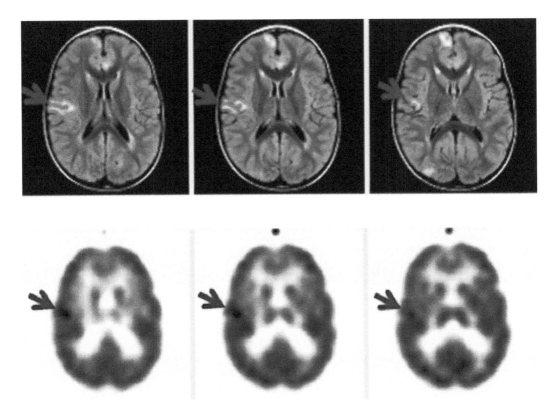

FIGURE 9.2.2 Continued

Focal seizure onset was confirmed from the right perituberal region with rapid secondary spread to the right temporal lobe. A right frontal lobe resection was then done around age 3 years; there were no motor deficits following surgery.

Neuropathological analyses confirmed extensive dysplasia and giant cells consistent with TSC.

The patient had a greater than 90% reduction in seizures following surgery and also had dramatic improvement in cognitive development as well as social interactions.

PEDIATRIC EPILEPSY CASE 3

This is a 16-year-old girl with Lennox-Gastaut syndrome. The etiology was initially unknown but later genetic testing revealed a de novo loss of function mutation in the *STXBP1* gene.

Her initial seizures at age 8 months were generalized tonic-clonic and tonic. She later developed atonic and atypical absence seizures. Her development was delayed in all domains, but she is able to say several words and ambulate independently.

EEG patterns showed frequent slow spike-and-wave discharges as well as multifocal and generalized discharges (Figure 9.2.3 (Top)).

Seizures were difficult to control with medications; she had trials of levetiracetam, oxcarbazepine, zonisamide, lamotrigine, and rufinamide. Her best seizure control was at age 2 years with the initiation of the ketogenic diet. She then had, on average, monthly generalized tonic-clonic and atonic seizures that were exacerbated when febrile. She started to refuse any form of the diet around 5 years of age. Additional medication trials included clobazam, topiramate, and cannabidiol.

She underwent further evaluations for palliative epilepsy surgery. Her seizures then were atonic and tonic with secondary head and face trauma (Figure 9.2.3 (Bottom)).

Given the intractability of these seizures to multiple medications, consideration was given to

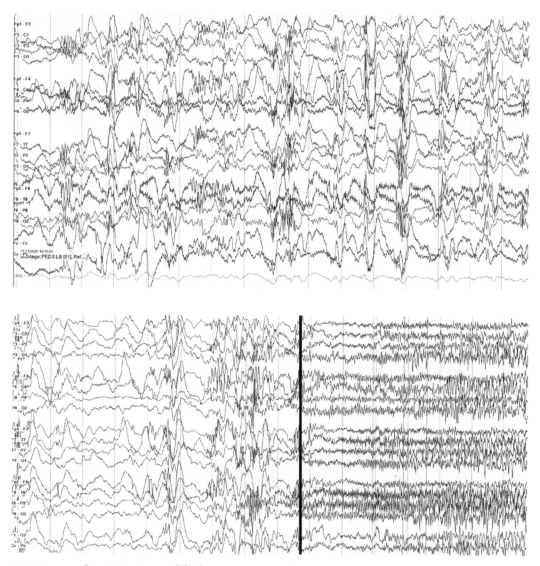

FIGURE 9.2.3 Case 3. Top: Interictal discharges in patient with *STXBP1* mutation. Frequent multifocal as well as generalized high-voltage discharges were seen. Bottom: Tonic seizure in patient with *STXBP1* mutation. The frequent high-voltage interictal discharges were replaced (*vertical black line*) by low-amplitude generalized fast activity admixed with muscle artifact. This correlated clinically with whole-body tonic stiffening that, if patient was standing, usually results in falling and injury.

implantation of a vagal nerve stimulator or a corpus callosotomy. Ultimately, a two-thirds anterior corpus callosotomy was done at age 14 years.

She had mild bilateral leg weakness postsurgery which resolved over several weeks. Language was unchanged. Atonic and tonic seizures were essentially abolished although monthly generalized tonic-clonic seizures and weekly staring seizures remained.

9.3

Teaching Case Discussions with Dr. Sonmezturk

HASAN H. SONMEZTURK

CASE 1

Our patient is a 76-year-old woman who was referred to an epilepsy clinic for recurring seizures for the past 1 year. She initially had memory difficulties which led to a brain magnetic resonance imaging (MRI), which found a right parietal meningioma (2.5 cm in diameter) causing mild cortical mass effect and edema. The meningioma was removed, and, few months after that, she had her first event which started with a left upper extremity (LUE) weakness followed by generalized shaking. She started having these frequently, and she was given tissue plasminogen activator (tPA) twice during her repeated emergency room (ER) visits due to suspected strokes. Patient was eventually started on levetiracetam, however, her events continued with variable features and increasing frequency. Lacosamide was also added and titrated to a dose of 150–200 mg/d.

Event description per family members:

Most of the patient's events would manifest with sudden-onset flaccid left arm weakness followed by loss of ability to use her left-sided extremities. She would be confused and unable to walk right. Patient would often be taken to ER during these events where she would start having very violent shaking of her head (extension + flexion) and violent asynchronous flailing movements of her upper extremities. These events would last as long as an hour or more. During some of these events and violent shaking patient would be fully awake and asking "why am I shaking?" Patient never had tongue-biting or loss of bowel or bladder control with these events.

- What is your diagnosis?
- Are these seizures?
- If they are seizures, what type of seizures are they?

- If they are not seizures, what is the differential diagnosis?
- What would you do next?

The clinic attending's most likely diagnosis was events of unknown nature most likely nonepileptic and psychogenic. Levetiracetam was tapered off and lacosamide was continued at the same dose. A follow up phone-call with patient's daughter revealed that the patient's events were decreased by about 75% after levetiracetam discontinuation. However, patient would still have sporadic LUE weakness followed by shaking.

- What would you do next?

An epilepsy monitoring unit (EMU) admission was requested. Patient had 10 typical events during the 5-day admission, during which her lacosamide was stopped. Her events consisted of subjective feeling of ringing in her ears, subjective feeling of LUE weakness, left leg and hand shaking followed by tremors in both upper extremities. She had retained awareness and would cry and hyperventilate during these events. Her electroencephalogram (EEG) was normal throughout the admission. She was diagnosed with psychogenic nonepileptic spells (PNES) and discharged to home off anti-seizure medications (ASMs). However, her ride did not show up, and she had to stay one more night in the EMU, until the next day. That night she restarted having recurring LUE flaccid weakness episodes. The events were initially dismissed as nonepileptic by the on-call house-staff. However, the nursing staff were concerned enough to call a code stroke alert. Patient was then taken to radiology for stroke protocol brain MRI and cranial computed tomography (CT) perfusion. While on the MRI table patient had three generalized (bilateral) tonic-clonic seizures and went into convulsive status epilepticus. The review of the video-EEG of her LUE weakness events confirmed "inhibitory seizures" with right parietal onset (P8, P4 > T8, C4) focal ictal discharges manifesting with flaccid LUE paralysis (Figure 9.3.1).

Clinical seizures most often cause excitatory and positive symptoms such as jerking, shaking, or increased distorted sensations, sounds, or visual phenomena. Inhibitory or negative symptoms as a result of a seizure are very rare. Inhibitory seizures can however rarely occur, particularly with

posterior quadrant seizures. This patient had both epilepsy and coexisting PNES. It is critical to keep an open mind while evaluating patients with frank PNES events in the EMU. If this patient had left a day earlier, she would probably have had these seizures at her home and they would be dismissed as nonepileptic. In one extensive review, Chen-Block et al.[1] showed that 5.2% of 1,567 adult EMU admissions had both epilepsy and PNES. When only patients with epilepsy were analyzed, 12.3% were found to have coexisting PNES, and when PNES-only patients were analyzed, 14.8%

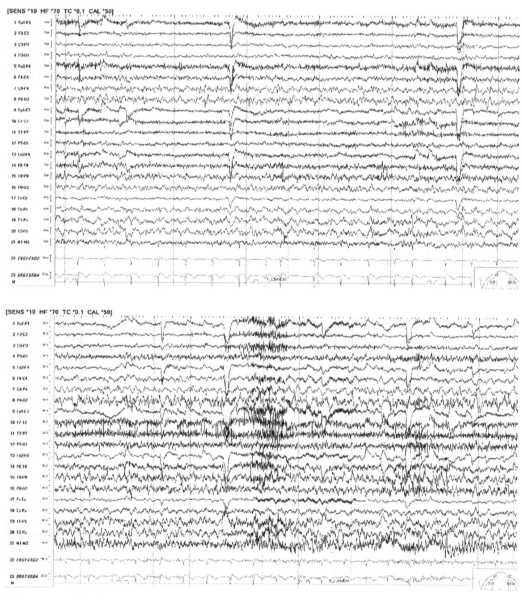

FIGURE 9.3.1 Case 1.

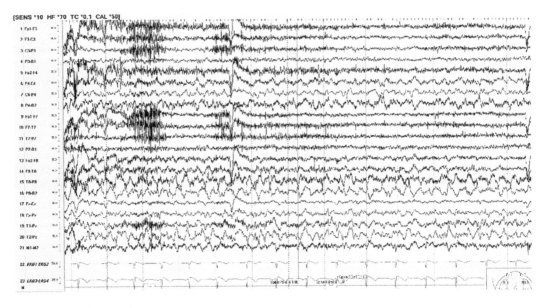

FIGURE 9.3.1 Continued

were found to have coexisting epilepsy. Please also note that the approximately 75% decrease in event frequency after levetiracetam discontinuation was because levetiracetam is known to worsen and increase the number of PNES events.

CASE 2

This patient is a 51-year-old man with long-standing right spastic hemiplegia and epilepsy due to a left hemispheric large arteriovenous malformation (AVM). He used to live alone with minimal assistance from his sister and has never been on ASMs by choice. He always refused to use them. One day the patient was found down at his home by his neighbors and taken to a local hospital where he had altered mental status with a creatine phosphokinase (CPK) level of 6,689 and a reported fever of 101.5°F. He was then transferred to a tertiary care center where he was afebrile. Seizures were thought to be the most likely cause of his presentation, and a video-EEG was done emergently.

Preliminary review of the EEG reported no seizures. However, patient had a convulsive event that night, and he was loaded with levetiracetam and maintained on 1,000 mg IV q12h (Figure 9.3.1 First frame). The next day, patient became less responsive and had two more convulsive events resulting in an additional load of levetiracetam and a dose increase to 1,500 mg IV q12h. The events were described as generalized stiffening and shaking (Figure 9.3.1 Second frame). Patient became comatose and unresponsive to noxious stimuli

with a burst attenuation pattern on his EEG (Figure 9.3.2 Third frame). His CK was normalized, and a complete blood count (CBC) and comprehensive metabolic panel (CMP) were also normal.

- What is your most likely diagnosis?
- What is causing this patient's comatose state?
- Is the recorded event a seizure, considering the EEG finding in Figure 9.3.2 Second frame?

Epilepsy consultation confirmed that the patient's events were not epileptic in nature and were instead spasm attacks with motion artifact on EEG. The events were often initiated by a cough followed by repeated torso thrusting and generalized stiffening which was followed by trembling in all extremities before ending. The events lasted 15–25 sec each. Patient's cranial imaging showed a very large left hemispheric AVM (Figure 9.3.2 Fourth frame).

After this finding, the epilepsy consult service considered the possibility that levetiracetam may have been causing the comatose state due to the baseline paucity of neuronal reserves. A recommendation was made to decrease the dose to 250 mg IV q12h. The patient woke up 24 hours later, and he was cooperative and clear mentally. He was quickly extubated and returned to his baseline. It is important to note that even though levetiracetam is considered to be a nonsedating ASM, in patients with limited neuronal reserves it can cause severe sedation or coma-like state.

CASE 3

This is a 19-year-old man who presented with recurrent episodes of behavioral arrest followed by weird behavior and confusion state suggestive of focal impaired awareness seizures. He reportedly had several generalized tonic-clonic seizures after his presentation to an outside hospital. His radiologic and metabolic workup was unrevealing. He was then referred to a tertiary care center where he was found to be lethargic and mildly encephalopathic but able to follow commands. He had intermittent left facial focal motor seizures manifesting with left-sided lip and facial twitching. His brain MRI was normal, and a cerebrospinal fluid (CSF) exam showed 61 white cells (75% lymphocytes). Protein and glucose were normal. Polymerase chain reaction (PCR) tests for multiple viral agents and oligoclonal bands were negative, with a normal IgG index level. Patient's initial video-EEG showed 3–5/hour focal ictal discharges in the right frontal region (Fp2 > F8 > F4) each lasting 40–70 sec.

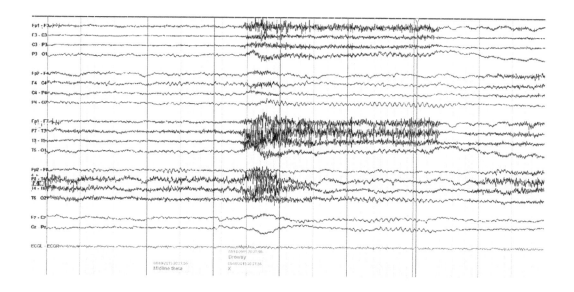

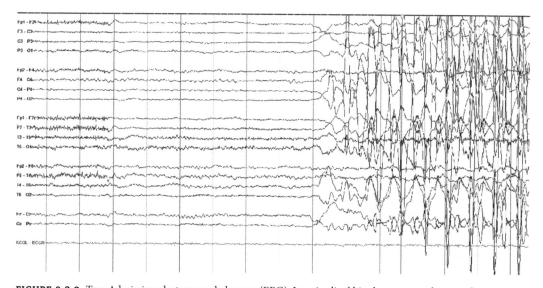

FIGURE 9.3.2 Top: Admission electroencephalogram (EEG). Longitudinal bipolar montage showing clear posterior dominant rhythm (PDR). Bottom: The EEG showing the beginning of convulsive event. Next page top: EEG after levetiracetam administration, showing burst attenuation pattern with no PDR. Next page lower: Head computed tomography (CT) images showing a very large arteriovenous malformation (AVM) covering entire left hemisphere.

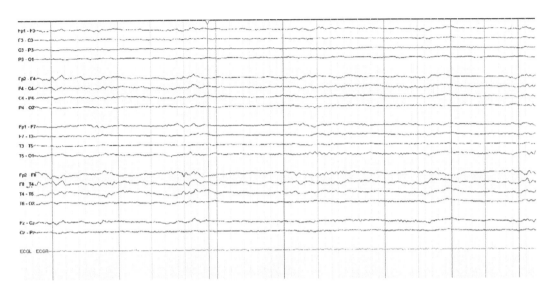

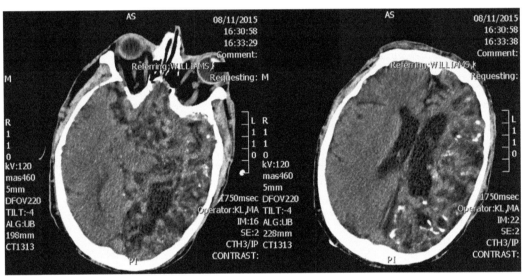

FIGURE 9.3.2 Continued

Interictally, EEG showed continuous lateralized periodic discharges (LPDs) plus a fast pattern in the same region. Patient's seizures became more intense, causing altered awareness intermittently and an EEG showing seizures spreading to the right temporal region then to left frontal and then to left temporal region (Figure 9.3.3). Patient was not responding to nonsedating ASMs. He was intubated for third-line sedative agent administration for seizure control. Over the next 42 days, the patient failed seven drug-induced (propofol, midazolam, and pentobarbital) deep coma sessions, the shortest lasting 24 hours and longest lasting 7 days. He also failed eight different ASMs managed, in addition to drug-induced

coma (levetiracetam, oxcarbazepine, valproic acid, topiramate, lacosamide, phenobarbital, clobazam, fosphenytoin), at maximum doses. Recurrent multifocal seizures, both with clear motor phenomena and no visible motor phenomena, continued nonstop. Seizures with motor activity often started with left facial twitching and then progressed to bifacial and bilateral upper extremity jerking, as depicted on seizure detection trendograph and on ictal brain positron emission tomography (PET) scan.

- What is your diagnosis?
- If your answer was status epilepticus, what type of status epilepticus can you classify?

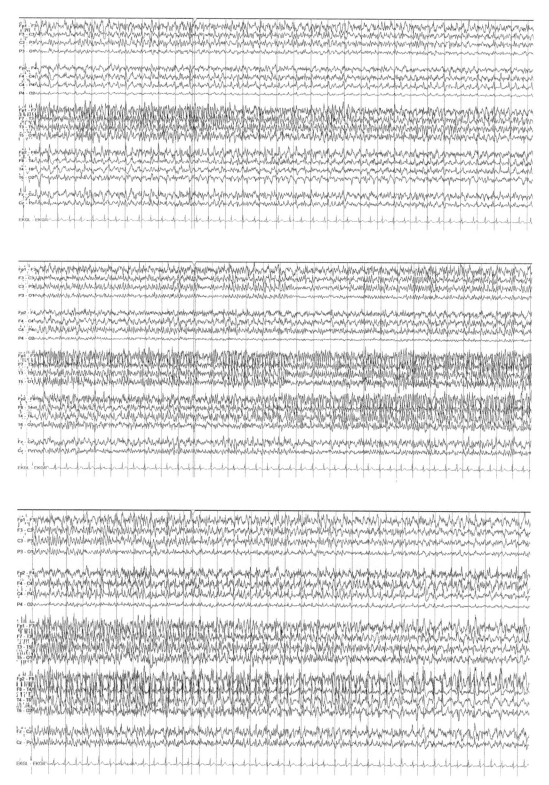

FIGURE 9.3.3 Sequence of 3 frames above. Seizure onset and propagation of a seizure with no clinical correlate. Next page, top 2 frames: Seizure detection software showing recurrent seizures with motor phenomena (Next page Upper frame) and no motor phenomena (Next page Lower frame). Next page Bottom frame: Brain positron emission tomography (PET) showing multifocal increased brain metabolism corresponding to the multifocal seizures detected on electroencephalogram (EEG).

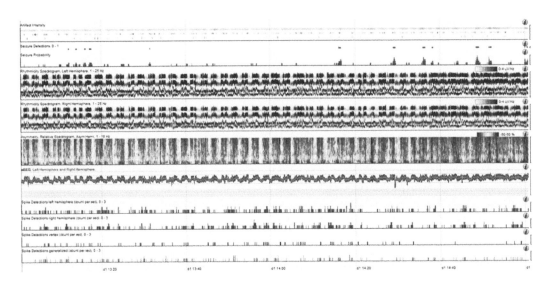

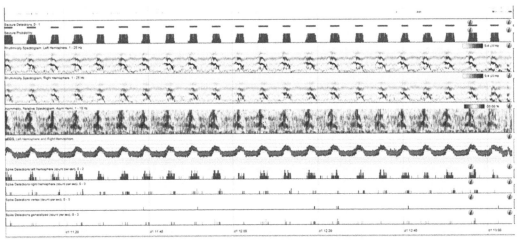

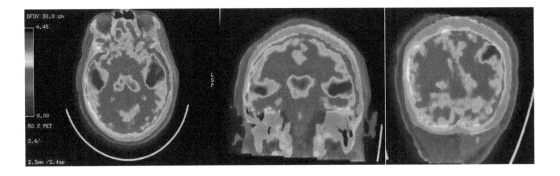

FIGURE 9.3.3 Continued

- After classification according to the International League Against Epilepsy (ILAE) Task Force's SE classification scheme, can you further subcategorize with a more specific name for this type of status epilepticus?
- What would be your next step in the management of this patient?

The diagnosis is clearly status epilepticus. To classify this status epilepticus, we need to take a staged approach. The patient presented with recurrent discrete simple motor (left facial twitching) seizures without loss of awareness, thus qualifying for "focal motor status epilepticus" with repeated focal motor seizures. These then progressed to more intense seizures with impairment of awareness, thus qualifying for "focal motor status epilepticus" evolving to "focal nonconvulsive status epilepticus with impaired consciousness." When the frequency reached 12–15 seizures per hour, without recovery between them and involving bilateral facial and bilateral upper extremities with synchronous jerking, at that moment this would be classified as "convulsive status epilepticus with focal onset evolving into bilateral convulsive status epilepticus." This is the formal classification according to semiologic findings proposed by the ILAE Task Force. However, if we consider the constellation of findings, such as age of the patient, lack of prior history of seizures, type of seizures, his refractoriness to medical management, and lack of etiologic findings (normal brain MRI and bland CSF findings except mildly elevated white cells which could be secondary to recurrent seizures), one specific status epilepticus type comes to mind and that is *new-onset refractory status epilepticus* (NORSE).

- What would be the next step?

After 42 days of recurrent drug-induced coma sessions and failed multiple ASM at maximum doses, when is it time to give up? In a 19-year-old man with no comorbidities and absent brain MRI abnormalities (brain MRI repeated three times during his 42-day course), the answer is "never." One should never give up trying to stop seizures in this clinical scenario. However, due to weekly changing primary teams, both the attendings and house-staff on multiple services (neurology, neuro ICU, anesthesiology), it is not uncommon to contemplate withdrawal of care in these patients. It is critical to remember

that these patients are in coma mostly because of the strong and long-acting sedatives we use. We will not know if they can sustain an awake state until all sedating drugs clear from their systems. Pentobarbital may need up to 72–96 hours to drop to nonsedating blood levels. Withdrawing care prior to sedative washout would risk unintentional euthanasia. In this patient, withdrawal of care was contemplated but stopped when the epilepsy team on board asked for one last trial of a different approach. All IV sedation was stopped with continued ventilator support. This approach allowed a real-time assessment of treatment response to aggressive nonsedating ASM therapy while the multifocal convulsive and nonconvulsive seizures were ongoing as long as the ictal discharges were not bihemispheric, bisynchronous, or generalized. It also eliminated potentially fatal IV anesthetic-induced complications and prevented anesthetic withdrawal seizures. The next medication used was perampanel, which was given through a nasogastric tube at a loading dose of 24 mg followed by 12 mg through the tube twice daily. Perampanel stopped all clinical seizures within 12 hours; however, the patient's subclinical multifocal ictal discharges continued (Figure 9.3.3 Second frame). Perampanel use made sense at the cellular and molecular levels as it is a selective noncompetitive antagonist of α-amino-3-hydroxy-5-methyl-4-isoxazolepropionic acid (AMPA) receptors, the major subtype of ionotropic glutamate receptors that become externalized/potentiated with prolonged refractory seizures. Opposite to that, gamma-aminobutyric acid (GABA) receptors become internalized with prolonged seizures, rendering GABAergic drugs ineffective. Nonconvulsive multifocal ictal discharges continued despite very high doses of perampanel and phenobarbital. The nonconvulsive seizures eventually stopped when lidocaine was given at a 100 mg loading dose followed by a 1.5 mg/min IV infusion for 24 hours.

Two to three days after cessation of all seizures, a gradual taper of phenobarbital and other ASMs was initiated. Over the following days and weeks, the patient was able to speak, eat independently, and walk on his own. He was discharged to inpatient rehab on hospital day 70 and seen back in clinic 92 days after his initial presentation. He had no neurologic deficits beyond subtle ataxia and slower speech patterns which resolved after phenytoin was tapered off. This case was published as a case report by the authors. Please refer to the case report for further details.[2]

9.4

EEG Examples

BASSEL ABOU-KHALIL AND KEVIN C. ESS

PERIODIC DISCHARGES WITH ANOXIA

Figure 9.4.1 shows the electroencephalogram (EEG) of a 56-year-old with witnessed tonic-clonic jerking after cardiac arrest. The EEG showed a continuously evolving pattern and frequency, with abrupt termination of rhythmic EEG activity with attenuation followed by periodic activity. The evolution is consistent with an ictal pattern. However, the anoxic etiology implies a poor prognosis.

HSV ENCEPHALITIS

Figure 9.4.2 shows a 94-year-old woman with HSV encephalitis. She had been having episodes of eye twitching, which in retrospect may have been small seizures, for several days. Then she had a decline in level of activity progressing to a nonverbal state. She was in stupor at the time of the EEG, which shows a disorganized and slow background with left temporal periodic discharges. Magnetic resonance imaging (MRI) showed a T2 hyperintense lesion of the left anterior and lateral-medial temporal lobe. She had a positive cerebrospinal fluid (CSF) test for herpes simplex virus-1 (HSV-1).

WICKET SPIKES

Figure 9.4.3 shows a 75-year-old woman with spells that were determined to be nonepileptic when evaluated with inpatient video-EEG monitoring. Her EEG was previously interpreted by a general neurologist as showing right and left midtemporal spikes and an electrographic seizure from the left temporal area. The EEG recording in Figure 9.4.3 shows wicket patterns from both temporal regions, but predominant on the left. The higher voltage sharply contoured waves are components of a monorhythmic activity that waxes and wanes in its voltage, but does not evolve in frequency.

BREACH RHYTHM

A 77-year-old man with altered mental status is seen in Figure 9.4.4. He had old right thalamic stroke. The EEG showed increased beta activity and fragments of mu rhythm at C3, suggesting breach rhythm. The computed tomography (CT) scan confirmed the presence of a skull defect. There had been no mention of craniotomy in his hospital notes, but a search of the records determined that he had had craniotomy for placement of a cortical stimulating electrode to relieve thalamic pain syndrome.

CREUTZFELDT-JAKOB DISEASE

Figure 9.4.5 shows a 74-year-old man with rapidly progressive dementia. The EEG showed intermittent left hemisphere periodic discharges activated with arousal and stimulation. The MRI shows typical increased left posterior and right frontal cortical ribbon signal on diffusion MRI images. The finding is absent in the FLAIR MRI. The autopsy confirmed the diagnosis of prion disease with the characteristics of sporadic Creutzfeldt-Jakob disease.

COUGH SYNCOPE

Figure 9.4.6 shows a 48-year-old man with obesity and spells of unclear nature that were determined to be nonepileptic. He had an episode of brief multifocal myoclonus and altered responsiveness after persistent cough in the setting of hyperventilation. The EEG showed generalized slow activity then generalized attenuation, followed by slow activity then recovery of normal EEG rhythms. The findings represent an episode of cough syncope.

PENTOBARBITAL COMA

A 24-year-old man with severe traumatic brain injury from a motorcycle accident is shown in Figure 9.4.7. CT showed right frontal

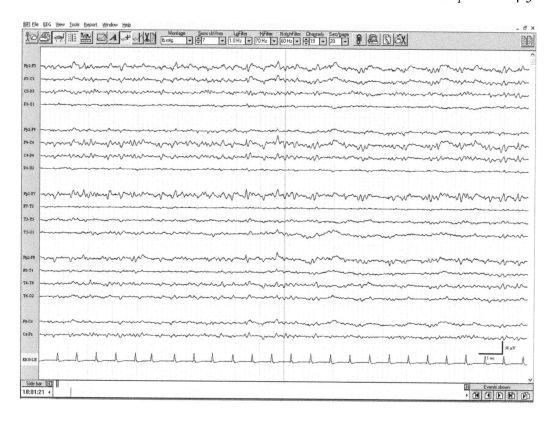

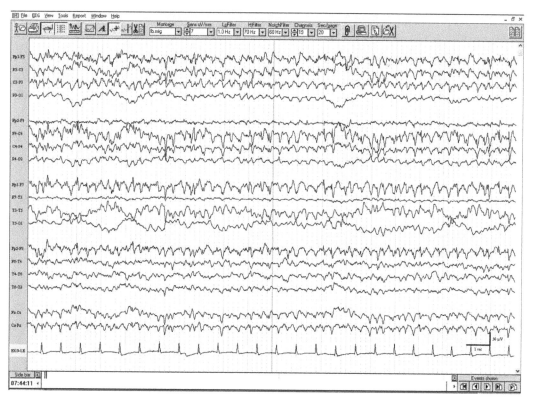

FIGURE 9.4.1 Anoxic encephalopathy. Series of 4 frames. Longitudinal bipolar montage.

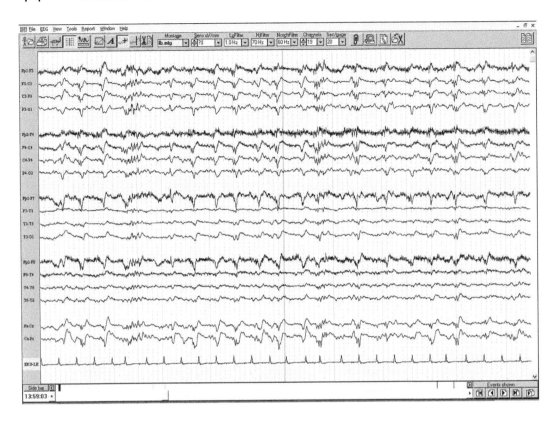

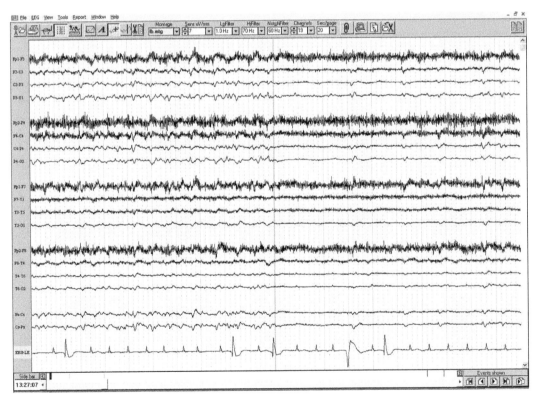

FIGURE 9.4.1 Continued

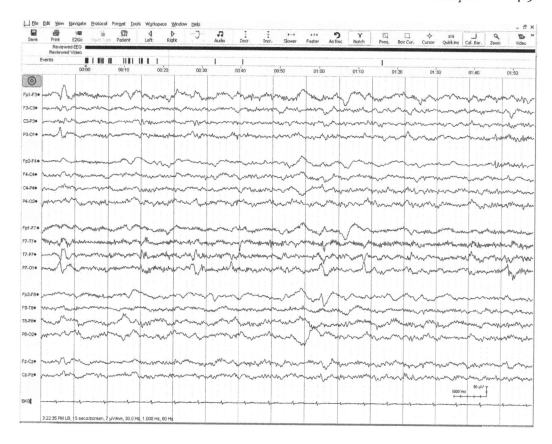

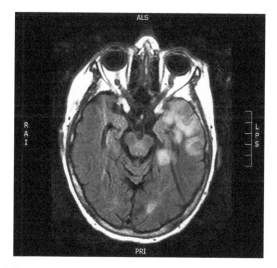

FIGURE 9.4.2 HSV encephalitis. Top: Longitudinal bipolar montage. Bottom: MRI brain.

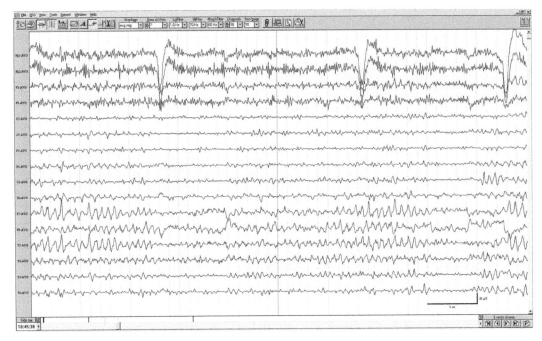

FIGURE 9.4.3 Wicket spikes. Average reference montage.

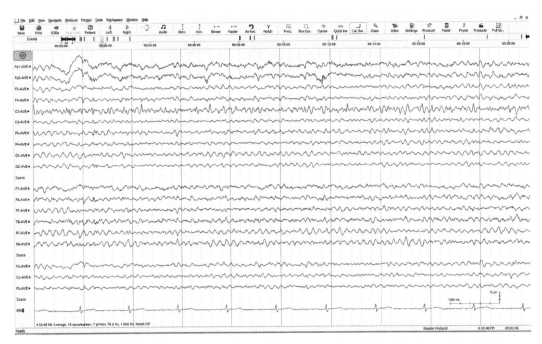

FIGURE 9.4.4 Breath rhythm. Above: Average reference. Next page top: Longitudinal bipolar montage. Next page bottom CT brain.

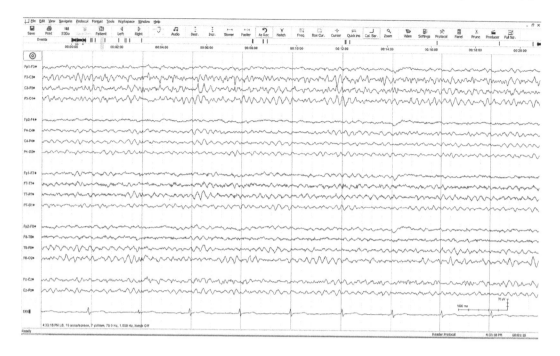

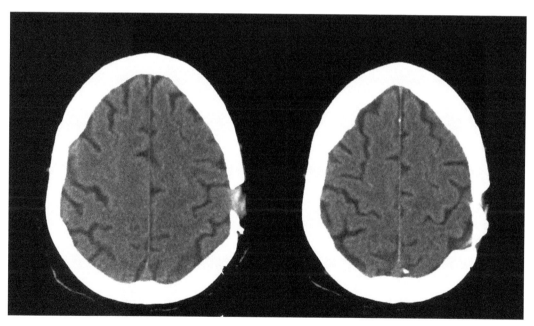

FIGURE 9.4.4 Continued

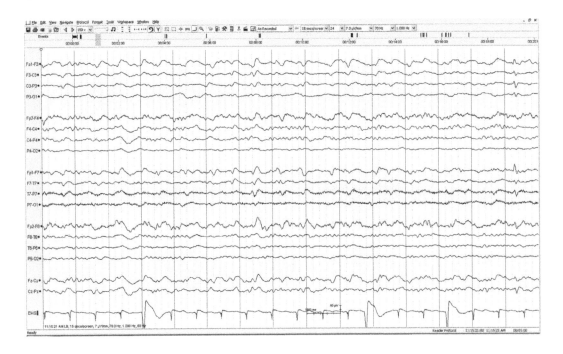

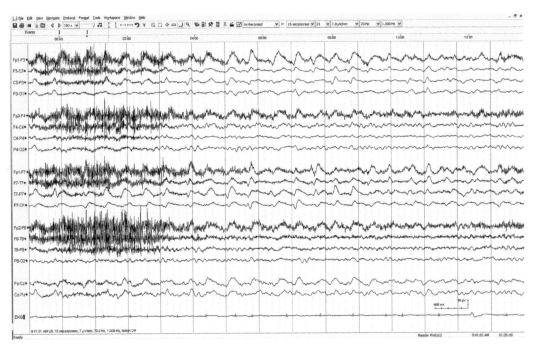

FIGURE 9.4.5 Creutzfeldt-Jakob disease. Top is earlier in disease. Bottom is later. Top of next page is MRI. Longitudinal bipolar montage.

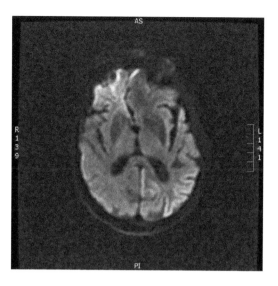

FIGURE 9.4.5 Continued

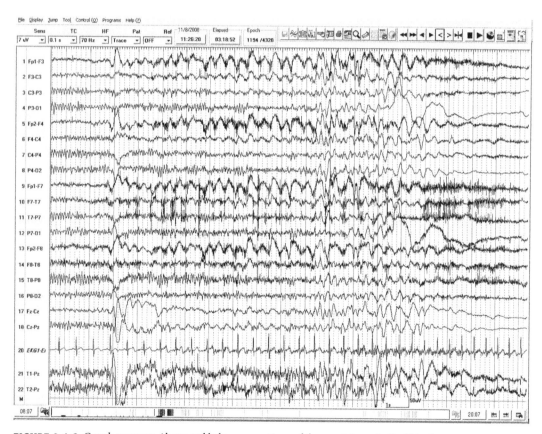

FIGURE 9.4.6 Cough syncope. Above and below are portions of the event. Longitudinal bipolar montage.

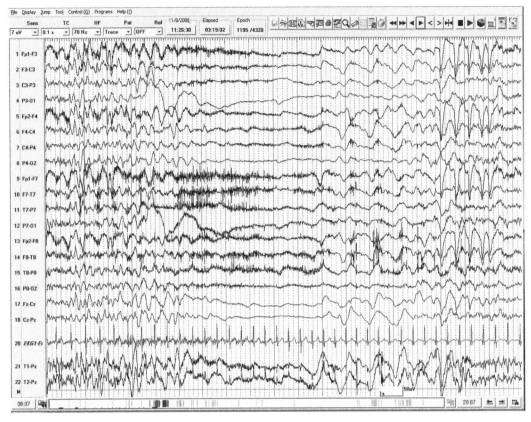

FIGURE 9.4.6 Continued

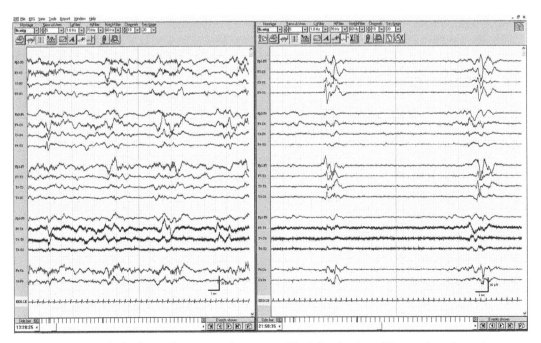

FIGURE 9.4.7 Pentobarbital coma for traumatic brain injury. Top left and right and Bottom show deepening induced coma.

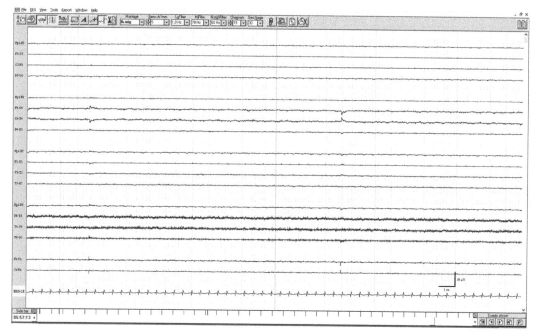

FIGURE 9.4.7 Continued

intraparenchymal hemorrhage, diffuse subarachnoid hemorrhage, subdural hematoma along the
falx, extensive intraventricular hemorrhage predominantly on the left, right to left midline shift,
and uncal herniation. He was placed in pentobarbital coma for treatment of increased intracranial
pressure. The EEG segments show the effect of
deepening pentobarbital coma, with increasing
duration of interburst intervals, until complete
suppression.

PARKINSONISM WITH
TREMOR

An 84-year-old man with advanced Parkinson's
disease complicated by anxiety and dementia is
shown in Figure 9.4.8. Examination showed bilateral resting and postural tremor, worse with stress-
ful discussions. He also had a mild head tremor
and chin tremor. EEG was obtained because of
episodes of unresponsiveness. The EEG shows
tremor artifact in the left posterior head region.

ATTENUATION WITH
SUBDURAL HEMATOMA

A patient with subdural hematoma with signs on
CT of acute and chronic blood is shown in Figure
9.4.9. The EEG shows attenuation over the left
hemisphere. The loss of faster frequencies is evident on this side.

FOCAL ATTENUATION IN
A PATIENT WITH RIGHT
HEMISPHERE STROKE

The patient shown in Figure 9.4.10 has had a
large right hemisphere infarction and subsequently had seizures. EEG shows signs of the
focal damage while the MRI shows typical signs
of acute-subacute infarction. Review of the EEG
shows frontal activity that is attenuated over the
right hemisphere. However, it would be easy to
assume that the left side with the higher amplitude slowing is the more abnormal side.

HYPSARRHYTHMIA

Figure 9.4.11 shows a 9-month-old boy with
prematurity and 1 month of epileptic spasms.
His MRI was normal. The study recorded three
clusters of infantile spasms. The associated
EEG changes were high-voltage slow waves
with superimposed fast activity followed by
1–2 sec of generalized attenuation. The interictal EEG showed multifocal epileptiform discharges, most often right parietal, and a chaotic
high-amplitude disorganized slow background

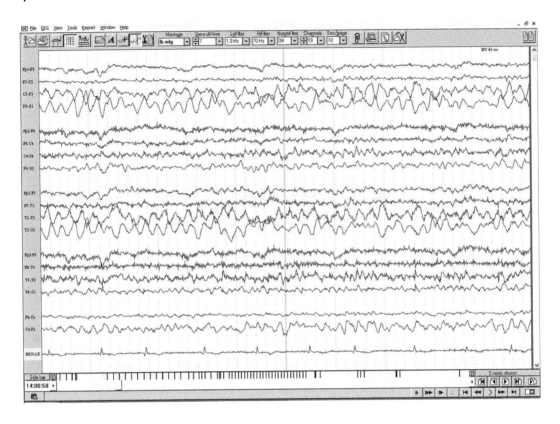

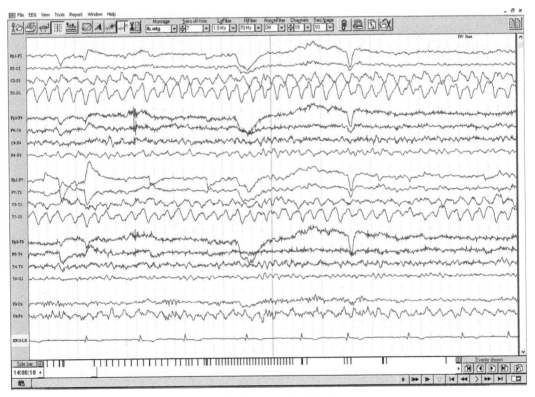

FIGURE 9.4.8 Tremor artifact. Top and Bottom both Longitudinal bipolar montage.

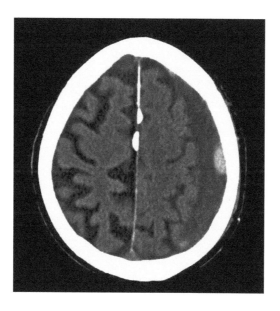

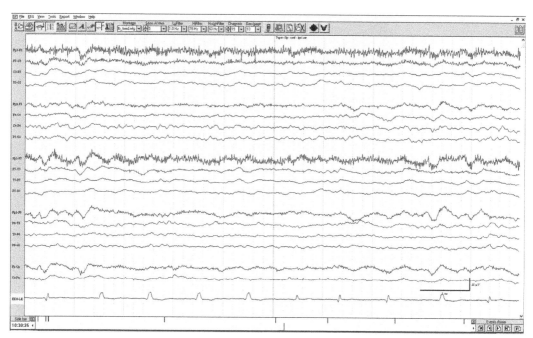

FIGURE 9.4.9 Subdural hematoma. Top: CT brain. Bottom: EEG. Longitudinal bipolar montage.

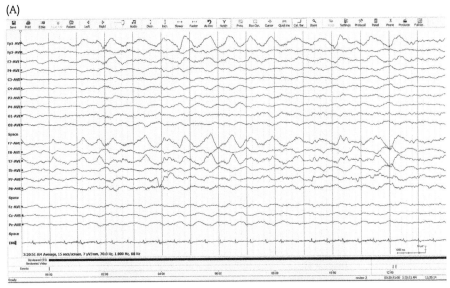

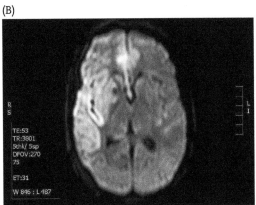

FIGURE 9.4.10 A: Focal attenuation in a patient with right hemisphere stroke. Average reference montage. B: MRI showing right hemisphere infarction.

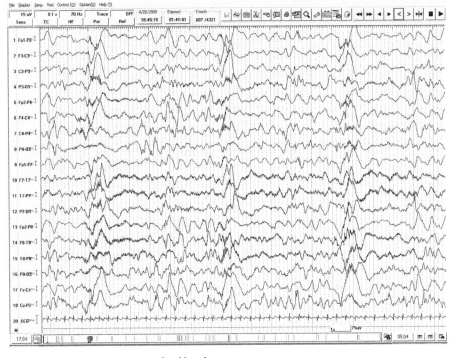

FIGURE 9.4.11 Hypsarrhythmia. Longitudinal bipolar montage.

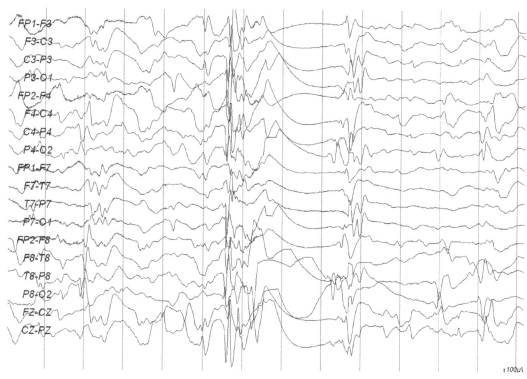

FIGURE 9.4.12 Hypsarrhythmia. Longitudinal bipolar montage.

with no posterior rhythm, consistent with hypsarrhythmia.

HYPSARRHYTHMIA

A 3-year-old boy is being evaluated for seizures and developmental delay (Figure 9.4.12). The EEG background is disorganized and there are high-voltage, polymorphic discharges. This is characteristic of hypsarrhythmia. Patients with hypsarrhythmia are more likely to have seizures, including infantile spasms. West syndrome is the triad of infantile spasms, hypsarrhythmia, and mental retardation, although not all three of the triad have to be present for diagnosis.

PART 10

Appendix

10.1

Abbreviations

ABPE	atypical benign partial epilepsy	ESUS	electrical status epilepticus during sleep
ACNS	American Clinical Neurophysiology Society	FAR	frontal arousal rhythm
AE	adverse effects (of a treatment)	FAS	focal aware seizure
AED	anti-epileptic drug, not termed ASM, anti-seizure medication	FBM	felbamate
		FDG-PET	fluorodeoxyglucose (FDG)-positron emission tomography
AS	active sleep		
ASM	anti-seizure medication	FIAS	focal impaired awareness seizure
BAEP	brainstem auditory evoked potentials	FIRDA	frontal intermittent rhythmic delta activity
BECTS	benign epilepsy with centrotemporal spikes	FOS	fosphenytoin
BETS	benign epileptiform transients of sleep	GABA	gamma-aminobutyric acid
		GBM	glioblastoma multiforme
BiPDs	bilateral independent periodic discharges	GBP	gabapentin
		GCSE	generalized convulsive status epilepticus
BRV	Brivaracetam		
BSSS	benign sporadic sleep spikes	GEFS+	genetic epilepsy with febrile seizures+
CA	conceptional age		
CAE	childhood absence epilepsy	GPD	generalized periodic discharge
CBD	cannabidiol	GPFA	generalized paroxysmal fast activity
CBZ	carbamazepine		
CJD	Creutzfeldt-Jakob disease	GRDA	generalized rhythmic delta activity
CLB	clobazam		
CLZ	clonazepam	GTC	generalized tonic-clonic (seizure)
CNS	central nervous system		
CPR	cardiopulmonary resuscitation	HFF	high frequency filter
CSWS	continuous spike-and-wave during sleep	HIE	hypoxic-ischemic encephalopathy
CT	computed tomography	HV	hyperventilation
ECI	electrocerebral inactivity	ICU	intensive care unit
ECoG	electrocorticography	IFCN	International Federation of Clinical Neurophysiology
EEG	electroencephalogram		
EIEE	early infantile epileptic encephalopathy	ILAE	International League Against Epilepsy
EKG	electrocardiogram	IOM or IONM	intraoperative neuro-monitoring
EMG	electromyogram		
EMU	epilepsy monitoring unit	IPSP	inhibitory postsynaptic potential
EPC	epilepsy partialis continua		
EPSP	excitatory postsynaptic potential	IRDA	intermittent rhythmic delta activity
ES	epileptic spasms (formerly IS: infantile spasms)		
		IS	infantile spasms (now called epileptic spasms [ES])
ESL	eslicarbazepine		
ESM	ethosuximide	JAE	juvenile absence epilepsy

JME	juvenile myoclonic epilepsy	RED	rhythmic epileptiform discharges
LCM	lacosamide		
LEV	levetiracetam	REM	rapid eye movement (sleep)
LFF	Low-frequency filter	RFM	rufinamide
LGS	Lennox-Gastaut syndrome	RMTD	rhythmic mid-temporal theta of drowsiness
LKS	Landau-Kleffner syndrome		
LPD	lateralized periodic discharge	SE	status epilepticus
LRDA	lateralized rhythmic delta activity	SEP or SSEP	somatosensory evoked potentials
LTG	lamotrigine	SIRPID	stimulus-induced rhythmic, periodic, or ictal discharges
MRI	magnetic resonance imaging		
MSX	methsuximide	SMEI	severe myoclonic epilepsy of infancy
NCSE	nonconvulsive status epilepticus		
		SPECT	Single photon emission computed tomography
NEE	nonepileptic event; can be psychogenic or physiologic	SREDA	subclinical rhythmic electrographic discharge of adults
NORSE	new-onset refractory status epilepticus		
		SSPE	subacute sclerosing panencephalitis
OIRDA	occipital intermittent rhythmic delta activity		
		SSS	small sharp spikes
OXC	oxcarbazepine	SSW	slow spine wave
PACS	picture archive and communication system	SUDEP	sudden unexplained death in epilepsy
PDA	polymorphic delta activity	TCeMEP	transcranial electric motor evoked potentials
PDR	posterior dominant rhythm		
PDS	paroxysmal depolarization shift	TD	trace discontinu
		TGA	transient global amnesia
PER	perampanel	TGB	tiagabine
PET	positron emission tomography	TIA	transient ischemic attack
PGB	pregabalin	TIRDA	temporal intermittent rhythmic delta activity
PHB	phenobarbital		
PHT	phenytoin	TLE	temporal lobe epilepsy
PNES	psychogenic nonepileptic seizure, a term retired in favor of nonepileptic events (NEE)	TPM	topiramate
		VEP	visual evoked potential
		VER	visual evoked response
POSTS	positive occipital sharp transients of sleep	VGB	vigabatrin
		VPA	valproate
PRM	primidone	ZNS	zonisamide
QS	quiet sleep		

NOTES

Chapter 1.1

1. Fisher RS, van Emde Boas W, Blume W, et al. Epileptic seizures and epilepsy: Definitions proposed by the International League Against Epilepsy (ILAE) and the International Bureau for Epilepsy (IBE). *Epilepsia*. 2005;46(4):470–472. PMID: 15816939.

2. Fisher RS, Acevedo C, Arzimanoglou A, et al. ILAE official report: A practical clinical definition of epilepsy. *Epilepsia*. 2014;55(4):475–482. PMID: 24730690.

3. Fisher RS, et al. Epileptic seizures and epilepsy.

4. Proposal for revised clinical and electroencephalographic classification of epileptic seizures. From the Commission on Classification and Terminology of the International League Against Epilepsy. Epilepsia. 1981;22(4):489–501. PMID: 6790275.

5. Fisher RS, Cross JH, French JA, et al. Operational classification of seizure types by the International League Against Epilepsy: Position Paper of the ILAE Commission for Classification and Terminology. *Epilepsia*. 2017;58(4):522–530. PMID: 28276060.

6. Scheffer IE, Berkovic S, Capovilla G, et al. ILAE classification of the epilepsies: Position paper of the ILAE Commission for Classification and Terminology. *Epilepsia*. 2017;58(4):512–521. PMID: 28276062.

7. Ibid.

Chapter 1.2

1. McGinty RN, Costello DJ, Kinirons P, McNamara B. Diagnostic yield of routine EEG in adults with active epilepsy. *Ir Med J*. 2019, Jan 15;112(1):851. PMID: 30718615.

2. Mahuwala Z, Ahmadi S, Bozoky Z, Hays R, Agostini M, Ding K. Diagnostic yield of 2-hour EEG is similar with 30-minute EEG in patients with a normal 30-minute EEG. *J Clin Neurophysiol*. 2019;36(3):204–208. PMID: 30845074.

3. Baumgartner C, Pirker S. Video-EEG. *Handb Clin Neurol*. 2019;160:171–183.

4. Fujimoto A, Okanishi T, Kanai S, Sato K, Nishimura M, Enoki H. Real-time three-dimensional (3D) visualization of fusion image for accurate subdural electrodes placement of epilepsy surgery. *J Clin Neurosci*. 2017;44:330–334. PMID: 28694041.

5. Iida K, Otsubo H. Stereoelectroencephalography: Indication and efficacy. *Neurol Med Chir (Tokyo)*. 2017;57(8):375–385. PMID: 28637943.

6. Valentín A, Hernando-Quintana N, Moles-Herbera J, et al. Depth versus subdural temporal electrodes revisited: Impact on surgical outcome after resective surgery for epilepsy. *Clin Neurophysiol*. 2017;128(3):418–423. PMID: 28160747.

7. Joswig H, Steven DA, Parrent AG, et al. Intracranial electroencephalographic monitoring: From subdural to depth electrodes. *Can J Neurol Sci*. 2018;45(3):336–338. PMID: 29644947.

8. Sprengers M, Vonck K, Carrette E, Marson AG, Boon P. Deep brain and cortical stimulation for epilepsy. *Cochrane Database Syst Rev*. 2017 Jul 18;7(7):CD008497. PMID: 28718878.

Chapter 2.1

1. Purves D, Augustine GJ, Fitzpatrick D, et al. *Neuroscience*. New York: Sinauer Associates, Oxford University Press; 2017.

Chapter 2.2

1. The terminology can be confusing since, in a diode configuration, the P-type semiconductor develops a negative charge and the N-type semiconductor develops a positive charge.

2. The terms "high-pass" and "low-pass" imply that they do not allow frequencies above or below those set points to pass, which is incorrect; those frequencies are attenuated in a frequency-dependent manner but not blocked.

Chapter 2.3

1. Halgren M, Ulbert I, Bastuji H, et al. The generation and propagation of the human alpha rhythm. *Proc Natl Acad Sci U S A*. 2019;116(47):23772–23782.

2. Lüthi A. Sleep spindles: Where they come from, what they do. *Neuroscientist*. 2014;20(3):243–256. PMID: 23981852.

3. Diekelmann S, Born J. The memory function of sleep. *Nat Rev Neurosci*. 2010;11(2):114–126. PMID: 20046194.

4. Stern JM, Caporro M, Haneef Z, et al. Functional imaging of sleep vertex sharp transients. *Clin Neurophysiol*. 2011;122(7):1382–1386. PMID: 21310653.

5. Pineda JA. The functional significance of mu rhythms: Translating "seeing" and "hearing" into "doing." *Brain Res Brain Res Rev*. 2005;50(1):57–68. PMID: 15925412.

6. Kane N, Acharya J, Benickzy S, et al. A revised glossary of terms most commonly used by clinical electroencephalographers and updated proposal for the report format of the EEG findings. Revision 2017. *Clin Neurophysiol Pract*. 2017 Aug 4;2:170–185. doi: 10.1016/j.cnp.2017.07.002. Erratum in: *Clin Neurophysiol Pract*. 2019 Jun 15;4:133. PMID: 30214992; PMCID: PMC6123891.

7. Tao JX, Ray A, Hawes-Ebersole S, Ebersole JS. Intracranial EEG substrates of scalp EEG interictal spikes. Epilepsia. 2005;46(5):669–676. PMID: 15857432.

Chapter 3.1

1. Fisher RS, van Emde Boas W, Blume W, et al. Epileptic seizures and epilepsy: Definitions proposed by the International League Against Epilepsy (ILAE) and the International Bureau for Epilepsy (IBE). *Epilepsia*. 2005;46(4):470–472. PMID: 15816939.

2. Fisher RS, Acevedo C, Arzimanoglou A, et al. ILAE official report: A practical clinical definition of epilepsy. *Epilepsia*. 2014;55(4):475–482. PMID: 24730690

Chapter 3.2

1. Bleasel A, Lüders HO. Tonic seizures. In Lüders HO, Noachtar S, eds. *Epileptic Seizures-Pathophysiology and Clinical Semiology*. Philadelphia: Churchill Livingstone; 2000: 389–411.

2. Blume WT, Lüders HO, Mizrahi E, Tassinari C, van Emde Boas W, Engel J Jr. Glossary of descriptive terminology for ictal semiology: Report of the ILAE task force on classification and terminology. *Epilepsia*. 2001;42(9):1212–1218. PMID: 11580774.

Chapter 3.3

1. Proposal for revised clinical and electroencephalographic classification of epileptic seizures. From the Commission on Classification and Terminology of the International League Against Epilepsy. *Epilepsia*. 1981;22(4):489–501.

2. Fisher RS, Cross JH, French JA, et al. Operational classification of seizure types by the International League Against Epilepsy: Position Paper of the ILAE Commission for Classification and Terminology. *Epilepsia*. 2017;58(4):522–530. PMID: 28276060.

Chapter 3.4

1. Williamson PD, Spencer DD, Spencer SS, Novelly RA, Mattson RH. Complex partial seizures of frontal lobe origin. *Ann Neurol*. 1985;18(4):497–504. PMID: 4073842

2. Kotagal P, Bleasel A, Geller E, Kankirawatana P, Moorjani BI, Rybicki L. Lateralizing value of asymmetric tonic limb posturing observed in secondarily generalized tonic-clonic seizures. *Epilepsia*. 2000;41(4):457–462. PMID: 10756413

3. Williamson PD, Engel J Jr. Anatomic classification of focal epilepsies. In Engel JJ, Pedley TA, eds. *Epilepsy: A Comprehensive Textbook*. Philadelphia: Lippincott Williams & Wilkins; 2008: 2465–2477.

4. Striano P, Gambardella A, Coppola A, et al. Familial mesial temporal lobe epilepsy (FMTLE): A clinical and genetic study of 15 Italian families. *J Neurol*. 2008;255(1):16–23. PMID: 18004642.

5. Quevedo-Diaz M, Campo AT, Vila-Vidal M, Principe A, Ley M, Rocamora R. Ictal spitting in nondominant temporal lobe epilepsy: An anatomo-electrophysiological correlation. *Epileptic Disord*. 2018 Apr 1;20(2):139–145. PMID: 29620007

6. Ebner A, Dinner DS, Noachtar S, Lüders H. Automatisms with preserved responsiveness: A lateralizing sign in psychomotor seizures. *Neurology*. 1995 Jan;45(1):61–64. PMID: 7824137.

7. Park HR, Seong MJ, Shon YM, Joo EY, Seo DW, Hong SB. SPECT perfusion changes during ictal automatisms with preserved responsiveness in patients with right temporal lobe epilepsy. *Epilepsy Behav*. 2018 Mar;80:11–14. PMID: 29396356.

8. Kotagal P, Lüders H, Morris HH, et al. Dystonic posturing in complex partial seizures of temporal lobe onset: A new lateralizing sign. *Neurology*. 1989;39(2 Pt 1):196–201. PMID: 2915789.

9. Lee GR, Arain A, Lim N, Lagrange A, Singh P, Abou-Khalil B. Rhythmic ictal nonclonic hand (RINCH) motions: A distinct contralateral sign in temporal lobe epilepsy. *Epilepsia*. 2006;47(12):2189–2192. PMID: 17201723.

10. Kelemen A, Fogarasi A, Borbély C, et al. Nonmanipulative proximal upper extremity automatisms lateralize contralaterally in temporal lobe epilepsy. *Epilepsia*. 2010;51(2):214–220. PMID: 19780800.

11. Foldvary N, Lee N, Thwaites G, et al. Clinical and electrographic manifestations of lesional

neocortical temporal lobe epilepsy. *Neurology.* 1997;49(3):757–763. PMID: 9305337.

12. Zaher N, Haas K, Sonmezturk H, Arain A, Abou-Khalil B. Rhythmic ictal nonclonic hand (RINCH) motions in general EMU patients with focal epilepsy. *Epilepsy Behav.* 2020 Feb;103(Pt A):106666. doi:10.1016/j.yebeh.2019.106666. Epub 2019 Dec 14. PMID: 31848102.

13. Wang L, Mathews GC, Whetsell WO, Abou-Khalil B. Hypermotor seizures in patients with temporal pole lesions. *Epilepsy Res.* 2008;82(1):93–98. PMID: 18760904.

14. Vaugier L, Aubert S, McGonigal A, et al. Neural networks underlying hyperkinetic seizures of "temporal lobe" origin. *Epilepsy Res.* 2009;86(2–3):200–208. PMID: 19619985.

15. Yu HY, Yiu CH, Yen DJ, et al. Lateralizing value of early head turning and ictal dystonia in temporal lobe seizures: A video-EEG study. *Seizure.* 2001 Sep;10(6):428–432. PMID: 11700997.

16. Mercan M, Yıldırım İ, Akdemir Ö, Bilir E. Ictal body turning in focal epilepsy. *Epilepsy Behav.* 2015 Mar;44:253–257. PMID: 25769674.

17. Asadi-Pooya AA, Asadollahi M, Bujarski K, et al. Ictal verbal help-seeking: Occurrence and the underlying etiology. *Epilepsy Behav.* 2016 Nov;64(Pt A):15–17. Epub 2016 Oct 8 PMID: 27723496.

18. Privitera MD, Morris GL, Gilliam F. Post-ictal language assessment and lateralization of complex partial seizures. *Ann Neurol.* 1991 Sep;30(3):391–396. PMID: 1952827.

19. Privitera M, Kohler C, Cahill W, Yeh HS. Post-ictal language dysfunction in patients with right or bilateral hemispheric language localization. *Epilepsia.* 1996 Oct;37(10):936–941. PMID: 8822691.

20. Dupont S, Semah F, Boon P, et al. Association of ipsilateral motor automatisms and contralateral dystonic posturing: A clinical feature differentiating medial from neocortical temporal lobe epilepsy. *Arch Neurol.* 1999;56(8):927–932. PMID: 10448797.

21. Fakhoury T, Abou-Khalil B. Association of ipsilateral head turning and dystonia in temporal lobe seizures. *Epilepsia.* 1995;36(11):1065–1070. PMID: 7588449.

22. Jobst BC, Siegel AM, Thadani VM, Roberts DW, Rhodes HC, Williamson PD. Intractable seizures of frontal lobe origin: Clinical characteristics, localizing signs, and results of surgery. *Epilepsia.* 2000;41(9):1139–1152. PMID: 10999553.

23. Leung H, Schindler K, Clusmann H, et al. Mesial frontal epilepsy and ictal body turning along the horizontal body axis. *Arch Neurol.* 2008;65(1):71–77. PMID: 18195141

24. Souirti Z, Landré E, Mellerio C, Devaux B, Chassoux F. Neural network underlying ictal pouting ("chapeau de gendarme") in frontal lobe epilepsy. *Epilepsy Behav.* 2014 Aug;37:249–257. PMID: 25108117.

25. Munari C, Kahane P, Francione S, et al. Role of the hypothalamic hamartoma in the genesis of gelastic fits (a video-stereo-EEG study). *Electroencephalogr Clin Neurophysiol.* 1995;95(3):154–160. PMID: 7555906.

26. Abou-Khalil B, Fakhoury T, Jennings M, Moots P, Warner J, Kessler RM. Inhibitory motor seizures: Correlation with centroparietal structural and functional abnormalities. *Acta Neurol Scand.* 1995;91(2):103–108. PMID: 7785419

27. Jobst BC, Williamson PD, Thadani VM, et al. Intractable occipital lobe epilepsy: Clinical characteristics and surgical treatment. *Epilepsia.* 2010;51(11):2334–2337. PMID: 20662891.

28. Isnard J, Guénot M, Sindou M, Mauguière F. Clinical manifestations of insular lobe seizures: A stereo-electroencephalographic study. *Epilepsia.* 2004;45(9):1079–1090. PMID: 15329073.

29. Kuznieckky R, Guthrie B, Mountz J, et al. Intrinsic epileptogenesis of hypothalamic hamartomas in gelastic epilepsy. *Ann Neurol.* 1997;42(1):60–67. PMID: 9225686.

30. Chae JH, Kim SK, Wang KC, Kim KJ, Hwang YS, Cho BK. Hemifacial seizure of cerebellar ganglioglioma origin: Seizure control by tumor resection. *Epilepsia.* 2001;42(9):1204–1207. PMID: 11580771.

31. Hirsch E, Panayiotopoulos CP. Childhood absence epilepsy and related syndromes. In Roger J, Bureau M, Dravet C, et al, eds. *Epileptic Syndromes in Infancy, Childhood and Adolescence.* Montrouge: John Libbey Eurotext; 2005: 315–335.

32. Caraballo RH, Fontana E, Darra F, et al. A study of 63 cases with eyelid myoclonia with or without absences: Type of seizure or an epileptic syndrome? *Seizure.* 2009;18(6):440–445. PMID: 19419888.

33. Chin PS, Miller JW. Ictal head version in generalized epilepsy. *Neurology.* 2004;63(2):370–372. PMID: 15277642.

34. Niaz FE, Abou-Khalil B, Fakhoury T. The generalized tonic-clonic seizure in partial versus generalized epilepsy: Semiologic differences. *Epilepsia.* 1999;40(11):1664–1666. PMID: 10565598.

35. Shih TT, Hirsch LJ. Tonic-absence seizures: An underrecognized seizure type. *Epilepsia.* 2003;44(3):461–465. PMID: 12614405.

36. Goldstein J, Slomski J. Epileptic spasms: A variety of etiologies and associated syndromes. *J Child Neurol.* 2008;23(4):407–414. PMID: 18192648.

37. Ramgopal S, Shah A, Zarowski M, et al. Diurnal and sleep/wake patterns of epileptic spasms in different age groups. *Epilepsia.* 2012;53(7):1170–1177. PMID: 22578060.

38. Linane A, Lagrange AH, Fu C, Abou-Khalil B. Generalized onset seizures with focal evolution

(GOFE): A unique seizure type in the setting of generalized epilepsy. *Epilepsy Behav*. 2016 Jan;54:20–29. PMID: 26619379.

39. Williamson R, Hanif S, Mathews GC, Lagrange AH, Abou-Khalil B. Generalized-onset seizures with secondary focal evolution. *Epilepsia*. 2009;50(7):1827–1832. PMID: 19260942.

Chapter 5.2

1. Formerly known as the American EEG Society.

2. Seeck M, Koessler L, Bast T, Leijten F, Michel C, Baumgartner C, He B, Beniczky S. The standardized EEG electrode array of the IFCN. *Clin Neurophysiol*. 2017 Oct;128(10):2070–2077. PMID: 28778476.

3. Beniczky S, Rosenzweig I, Scherg M, et al. Ictal EEG source imaging in presurgical evaluation: High agreement between analysis methods. *Seizure*. 2016;43:1–5. PMID: 27764709

4. Baumgartner C, et al. The standardized EEG electrode array of the IFCN. *Clinical Neurophysiol*. 2017;128:2070–2077.

5. Beniczky S, Conradsen I, Moldovan M, Jennum P, Fabricius M, Benedek K, et al. Automated differentiation between epileptic and nonepileptic convulsive seizures. *Ann Neurol*. 2015;77:348–351. PMID: 25545895.

6. Kasteleijn-Nolst Trenite D, Rubboli G, Hirsch E, Martins da Silva A, Seri S, Wilkins A, et al. Methodology of photic stimulation revisited: Updated European algorithm for visual stimulation in the EEG laboratory. *Epilepsia*. 2012;53:16–24. PMID: 22091642.

7. Acharya JN, Hani AJ, Thirumala PD, Tsuchida TN. American Clinical Neurophysiology Society Guideline 3: A proposal for standard montages to be used in clinical EEG. *J Clin Neurophysiol*. 2016 Aug;33(4):312–316. PMID: 27482795.

8. American Clinical Neurophysiology Society. *J Clin Neurophysiol*. 2006, multiple articles.

9. Privitera MD, Morris GL, Gilliam F. Postictal language assessment and lateralization of complex partial seizures. *Ann Neurol*. 1991 Sep;30(3):391–396. PMID: 1952827.

10. Elmali AD, Bebek N, Baykan B. Let's talk SUDEP. *Noro Psikiyatr Ars*. 2019 Sep 5;56(4):292–301. PMID: 31903040.

11. Mesraoua B, Deleu D, Hassan AH, et al. Dramatic outcomes in epilepsy: Depression, suicide, injuries, and mortality. *Curr Med Res Opin*. 2020 Sep;36(9):1473–1480. PMID: 32476500.

12. Maguire MJ, Jackson CF, Marson AG, Nolan SJ. Treatments for the prevention of Sudden Unexpected Death in Epilepsy (SUDEP). *Cochrane Database Syst Rev*. 2016;7(7):CD011792. Published 2016 Jul 19. PMID: 27434597.

13. Noe KH, Drazkowski JF. Safety of long-term video-electroencephalographic monitoring for evaluation of epilepsy. *Mayo Clin Proc*. 2009;84(6):495–500. PMID: 1948316.

14. Schuele SU, Bermeo AC, Alexopoulos AV, Locatelli ER, Burgess RC, Dinner DS, Foldvary-Schaefer N. Video-electrographic and clinical features in patients with ictal asystole. *Neurology*. 2007;69:434–441. PMID: 17664402.

15. Marynissen T, Govers N, Vydt T. Ictal asystole: Case report with review of literature. *Acta Cardiol*. 2012 Aug;67(4):461–464. PMID: 22998002.

16. Agostini SD, Aniles E, Sirven J, Drazkowski JF. The importance of cardiac monitoring in the epilepsy monitoring unit: A case presentation of ictal asystole. *Neurodiagn J*. 2012 Sep;52(3):250–260. PMID: 23019762..

17. Bestawros M, Darbar D, Arain A, Abou-Khalil B, Plummer WD, Dupont WD, Raj SR. Ictal asystole and ictal syncope: Insights into clinical management. *Circulation Arrhythmia Electrophysiol*. 2015;8:159–164. PMID: 25391254.

18. Herskovitz M, Schiller Y. Atrial fibrillation associated with epileptic seizures. *Arch Neurol*. 2012 Sep;69(9):1197–1199. PMID: 22637287..

19. Monami M, Mannucci E, Breschi A, Marchionni N. Seizures as the only clinical manifestation of reactive hypoglycemia: A case report. *J Endocrinol Invest*. 2005;28(10):940–941. PMID: 16419498.

Chapter 5.3

1. Drury I. 14-and-6 Hz positive bursts in childhood encephalopathies. *Electroencephalogr Clin Neurophysiol*. 1989 Jun;72(6):479–485. PMID: 2471616.

Chapter 5.4

1. Bhatt AB, Popescu A, Waterhouse EJ, Abou-Khalil BW. De novo generalized periodic discharges related to anesthetic withdrawal resolve spontaneously. *J Clin Neurophysiol*. 2014 Jun;31(3):194–198. PMID: 24887600.

2. Beniczky S, Hirsch LJ, Kaplan PW, Pressler R, Bauer G, Aurlien H, Brøgger JC, Trinka E. Unified EEG terminology and criteria for nonconvulsive status epilepticus. *Epilepsia*. 2013 Sep;54 Suppl 6:28–29. PMID: 24001066.

3. Hirsch LJ, LaRoche SM, Gaspard N, et al. American Clinical Neurophysiology Society's Standardized Critical Care EEG Terminology: 2012 version. *J Clin Neurophysiol*. 2013;30(1):1–27. PMID: 23377439.

Chapter 5.6

1. Lv RJ, Wang Q, Cui T, Zhu F, Shao XQ. Status epilepticus-related etiology, incidence and

mortality: A meta-analysis. *Epilepsy Res.* 2017 Oct;136:12–17. PMID: 28734267.

2. Leitinger M, Trinka E, Giovannini G, et al. Epidemiology of status epilepticus in adults: A population-based study on incidence, causes, and outcomes. *Epilepsia.* 2019 Jan;60(1):53–62. doi: 10.1111/epi.14607. PMID: 30478910..

3. DeLorenzo RJ, Pellock JM, Towne AR, Boggs JG. Epidemiology of status epilepticus. *J Clin Neurophysiol.* 1995 Jul;12(4):316–325. PMID: 7560020..

4. Treiman DM. Importance of early recognition and treatment of generalised convulsive status epilepticus. *Lancet Neurol.* 2008 Aug;7(8):667–668. PMID: 18602344..

5. Treiman DM, Meyers PD, Walton NY, et al. A comparison of four treatments for generalized convulsive status epilepticus. *Veterans Affairs Status Epilepticus Cooperative Study Group. N Engl J Med.* 1998 Sep 17;339(12):792–798. PMID: 9738086.

6. Trinka E, Cock H, Hesdorffer D, et al. A definition and classification of status epilepticus: Report of the ILAE Task Force on Classification of Status Epilepticus. *Epilepsia.* 2015;56(10):1515–1523. doi:10.1111/epi.13121. PMID: 26336950.

7. Ibid.

8. Lowenstein DH, Bleck T, Macdonald RL. It's time to revise the definition of status epilepticus. *Epilepsia.* 1999 Jan;40(1):120–122. PMID: 9924914..

9. Trinka et al. A definition and classification of status epilepticus.

10. Leitinger et al. Epidemiology of status epilepticus in adults.

11. Trinka et al. A definition and classification of status epilepticus.

12. Beniczky S, Hirsch LJ, Kaplan PW, Pressler R, Bauer G, Aurlien H, Brøgger JC, Trinka E. Unified EEG terminology and criteria for nonconvulsive status epilepticus. *Epilepsia.* 2013 Sep;54 Suppl 6:28–29. doi:10.1111/epi.12270. PMID: 24001066..

Chapter 5.7

1. Nielsen N, Wetterslev J, Cronberg T, et al. Targeted temperature management at 33°C versus 36°C after cardiac arrest. *N Engl J Med.* 2013;369(23):2197–2206. doi:10.1056/NEJMoa1310519 PMID: 24237006.

2. Makker P, Kanei Y, Misra D. Clinical effect of rebound hyperthermia after cooling postcardiac arrest: A meta-analysis. *Ther Hypothermia Temp Manag.* 2017;7(4):206–209. PMID: 28731840.

3. Lascarrou JB, Merdji H, Le Gouge A, et al. Targeted temperature management for cardiac arrest with nonshockable rhythm. *N Engl J Med.* 2019;381(24):2327–2337. PMID: 3157739.

4. Kawai M, Thapalia U, Verma A. Outcome from therapeutic hypothermia and EEG. *J Clin Neurophysiol.* 2011;28(5):483–488. PMID: 21946362.

5. Rundgren M, Westhall E, Cronberg T, Rosén I, Friberg H. Continuous amplitude-integrated electroencephalogram predicts outcome in hypothermia-treated cardiac arrest patients. *Crit Care Med.* 2010 Sep; 38(9):1838–1844. PMID: 20562694.

6. Granfeldt A, Holmberg MJ, Donnino MW, Andersen LW; CARES Surveillance Group. 2015 guidelines for cardiopulmonary resuscitation and survival after adult and pediatric out-of-hospital cardiac arrest. *Eur Heart J Qual Care Clin Outcomes.* 2020;qcaa027. PMID: 32232441.

7. Iacobone E, Bailly-Salin J, Polito A, Friedman D, Stevens RD, Sharshar T. Sepsis-associated encephalopathy and its differential diagnosis. *Crit Care Med.* 2009;37(10 Suppl):S331–S336. PMID: 20046118.

8. Kaplan PW, Rossetti AO. EEG patterns and imaging correlations in encephalopathy: Encephalopathy part II. *J Clin Neurophysiol.* 2011;28(3):233–251. PMID: 21633250.

9. Sutter R, Kaplan PW, Valença M, De Marchis GM. EEG for diagnosis and prognosis of acute non-hypoxic encephalopathy: History and current evidence. *J Clin Neurophysiol.* 2015;32(6):456–464. PMID: 26629755.

10. Kinney MO, Craig JJ, Kaplan PW. Non-convulsive status epilepticus: Mimics and chameleons. *Pract Neurol.* 2018;18(4):291–305. PMID: 29650639.

Chapter 6.1

1. Thoresen M, Henriksen O, Wannag E, Laegreid L. Does a sedative dose of chloral hydrate modify the EEG of children with epilepsy? *Electroencephalogr Clin Neurophysiol.* 1997 Feb;102(2):152–157. PMID: 9060867.

Chapter 6.2

1. Dan B, Boyd SG. Stimulus-sensitive burst-spiking in burst-suppression in children: Implications for management of refractory status epilepticus. *Epileptic Disord.* 2006;8(2):143–150. PMID: 16793576.

2. Khan S, Al Baradie R. Epileptic encephalopathies: An overview. *Epilepsy Res Treat.* 2012;2012:403592. PMID: 23213494.

Chapter 6.3

1. Glass HC, Shellhaas RA, Tsuchida TN, et al. Seizures in preterm neonates: A multicenter observational cohort study. *Pediatr Neurol.* 2017;72:19–24. PMID: 28558955.

2. Spagnoli C, Falsaperla R, Deolmi M, Corsello G, Pisani F. Symptomatic seizures in preterm

newborns: A review on clinical features and prognosis. *Ital J Pediatr.* 2018;44(1):115. Published 2018 Nov 1. PMID: 30382869.

3. Pavone P, Striano P, Falsaperla R, Pavone L, Ruggieri M. Infantile spasms syndrome, West syndrome and related phenotypes: What we know in 2013. *Brain Dev.* 2014;36(9):739–751. PMID: 24268986.

4. Asadi-Pooya AA. Lennox-Gastaut syndrome: A comprehensive review. *Neurol Sci.* 2018;39(3):403–414. PMID: 29124439.

5. Mastrangelo M. Lennox-Gastaut syndrome: A state of the art review. *Neuropediatrics.* 2017;48(3):143–151. PMID: 28346953..

6. Varadkar S, Bien CG, Kruse CA, et al. Rasmussen's encephalitis: Clinical features, pathobiology, and treatment advances. *Lancet Neurol.* 2014;13(2):195–205. PMID: 24457189.

7. Wirrell EC, Laux L, Donner E, et al. Optimizing the diagnosis and management of Dravet syndrome: Recommendations from a North American consensus panel. *Pediatr Neurol.* 2017;68:18–34.e3. PMID: 28284397.

8. Baykan B, Wolf P. Juvenile myoclonic epilepsy as a spectrum disorder: A focused review. *Seizure.* 2017;49:36–41. PMID: 28544889.

9. Adcock JE, Panayiotopoulos CP. Occipital lobe seizures and epilepsies. *J Clin Neurophysiol.* 2012;29(5):397–407. PMID: 23027097.

10. Caraballo RH, Cejas N, Chamorro N, Kaltenmeier MC, Fortini S, Soprano AM. Landau-Kleffner syndrome: A study of 29 patients. *Seizure.* 2014;23(2):98–104. PMID: 24315829.

11. Duran MH, Guimarães CA, Medeiros LL, Guerreiro MM. Landau-Kleffner syndrome: Long-term follow-up. *Brain Dev.* 2009;31(1):58–63. PMID: 18930363.

12. Veggiotti P, Pera MC, Teutonico F, Brazzo D, Balottin U, Tassinari CA. Therapy of encephalopathy with status epilepticus during sleep (ESES/CSWS syndrome): An update. *Epileptic Disord.* 2012;14(1):1–11. PMID: 22426353.

13. Allen NM, Conroy J, Deonna T, et al. Atypical benign partial epilepsy of childhood with acquired neurocognitive, lexical semantic, and autistic spectrum disorder. *Epilepsy Behav Case Rep.* 2016;6:42–48. Published 2016 Apr 23. PMID: 27504264.

14. Gupta A. Febrile seizures. *Continuum (Minneap Minn).* 2016;22(1 Epilepsy):51–59. PMID: 26844730.

15. Patel AD, Vidaurre J. Complex febrile seizures: A practical guide to evaluation and treatment. *J Child Neurol.* 2013 Jun;28(6):762–7. doi: 10.1177/0883073813483569. Epub 2013 Apr 10. PMID: 23576415..

16. de Lange IM, Gunning B, Sonsma ACM, et al. Outcomes and comorbidities of SCN1A-related

seizure disorders. *Epilepsy Behav.* 2019 Jan;90:252–259 PMID: 30527252..

17. Steel D, Symonds JD, Zuberi SM, Brunklaus A. Dravet syndrome and its mimics: Beyond SCN1A. *Epilepsia.* 2017 Nov;58(11):1807–1816. PMID: 28880996..

Chapter 7.2

1. Baslet G. Psychogenic non-epileptic seizures: A model of their pathogenic mechanism. *Seizure.* 2011 Jan;20(1):1–13. PMID: 21106406.

2. Martin R, Burneo JG, Prasad A, et al. Frequency of epilepsy in patients with psychogenic seizures monitored by video-EEG. *Neurology.* 2003 Dec 23;61(12):1791–2. PMID: 14694050.

3. Benbadis SR, Agrawal V, Tatum WO 4th. How many patients with psychogenic nonepileptic seizures also have epilepsy? *Neurology.* 2001 Sep 11;57(5):915–7. PMID: 11552032.

4. Gröppel G, Kapitany T, Baumgartner C. Cluster analysis of clinical seizure semiology of psychogenic nonepileptic seizures. *Epilepsia.* 2000 May;41(5):610–4. PMID: 10802768.

5. Selwa LM, Geyer J, Nikakhtar N, Brown MB, Schuh LA, Drury I. Nonepileptic seizure outcome varies by type of spell and duration of illness. *Epilepsia.* 2000 Oct;41(10):1330–4. PMID: 11051130.

6. Szabó L, Siegler Z, Zubek L, Liptai Z, Körhegyi I, Bánsági B, Fogarasi A. A detailed semiologic analysis of childhood psychogenic nonepileptic seizures. *Epilepsia.* 2012 Mar;53(3):565–70. PMID: 22332748.

7. DeToledo JC, Ramsay RE. Patterns of involvement of facial muscles during epileptic and nonepileptic events: Review of 654 events. *Neurology.* 1996 Sep;47(3):621–5. PMID: 8797454.

8. Avbersek A, Sisodiya S. Does the primary literature provide support for clinical signs used to distinguish psychogenic nonepileptic seizures from epileptic seizures? *J Neurol Neurosurg Psychiatry.* 2010 Jul;81(7):719–25. PMID: 20581136.

9. Chung SS, Gerber P, Kirlin KA. Ictal eye closure is a reliable indicator for psychogenic nonepileptic seizures. *Neurology.* 2006 Jun 13;66(11):1730–1. PMID: 16769949.

10. Azar NJ, Tayah TF, Wang L, Song Y, Abou-Khalil BW. Postictal breathing pattern distinguishes epileptic from nonepileptic convulsive seizures. *Epilepsia.* 2008 Jan;49(1):132–7. PMID: 17651411.

11. Arain AM, Song Y, Bangalore-Vittal N, Ali S, Jabeen S, Azar NJ. Long term video/EEG prevents unnecessary vagus nerve stimulator implantation in patients with psychogenic nonepileptic seizures. *Epilepsy Behav.* 2011 Aug;21(4):364–6. PMID: 21737353.

12. Brigo F, Nardone R, Ausserer H, Storti M, Tezzon F, Manganotti P, Bongiovanni LG. The

diagnostic value of urinary incontinence in the differential diagnosis of seizures. *Seizure.* 2013 Mar;22(2):85–90. PMID: 23142708.

Chapter 7.3

1. Crompton DE, Berkovic SF. The borderland of epilepsy: Clinical and molecular features of phenomena that mimic epileptic seizures. *Lancet Neurol.* 2009 Apr;8(4):370–81. PMID: 19296920.

2. Thijs RD, Kruit MC, van Buchem MA, Ferrari MD, Launer LJ, van Dijk JG. Syncope in migraine: the population-based CAMERA study. *Neurology.* 2006 Apr 11;66(7):1034–7. PMID: 16606915.

3. Muppidi S, Razavi B, Miglis MG, Jaradeh S. The clinical utility of qualitative electroencephalography during tilt table testing: A retrospective study. *Clin Neurophysiol.* 2018;129(4):783–786. PMID: 29448152.

4. Sheldon R. How to differentiate syncope from seizure. *Cardiol Clin.* 2015;33(3):377–385. PMID: 26115824.

5. Crompton DE, Berkovic SF. The borderland of epilepsy: Clinical and molecular features of phenomena that mimic epileptic seizures. *Lancet Neurol.* 2009 Apr;8(4):370–81. PMID: 19296920.

6. Shmuely S, Bauer PR, van Zwet EW, van Dijk JG, Thijs RD. Differentiating motor phenomena in tilt-induced syncope and convulsive seizures. *Neurology.* 2018;90(15):e1339–e1346. PMID: 29549227.

7. Monté CP, Monté CJ, Boon P, Arends J. Epileptic seizures associated with syncope: Ictal bradycardia and ictal asystole. *Epilepsy Behav.* 2019;90:168–171. PMID: 30576964.

Chapter 7.4

1. McGuire S, Chanchani S, Khurana DS. Paroxysmal dyskinesias. *Semin Pediatr Neurol.* 2018;25:75–81. PMID: 29735119.

2. Wadi L, Medlej Y, Obeid M. A child with hyperekplexia and epileptic myoclonus. *Epileptic Disord.* 2018;20(4):279–282. PMID: 30078784.

3. Raina GB, Cersosimo MG, Folgar SS, et al. Holmes tremor: Clinical description, lesion localization, and treatment in a series of 29 cases. *Neurology.* 2016;86(10):931–938. PMID: 26865524.

4. Thorpy MJ. Classification of sleep disorders. *Neurotherapeutics.* 2012;9(4):687–701. PMID: 22976557.

5. Tinuper P, Bisulli F, Provini F. The parasomnias: Mechanisms and treatment. *Epilepsia.* 2012 Dec;53 Suppl 7:12–9. PMID: 23153205..

6. Alfonsi V, D'Atri A, Scarpelli S, Mangiaruga A, De Gennaro L. Sleep talking: A viable access to mental processes during sleep. *Sleep Med Rev.* 2019;44:12–22. PMID: 30594004.

7. Honda K, Hashimoto M, Yatabe Y, et al. The usefulness of monitoring sleep talking for the diagnosis of dementia with Lewy bodies. *Int Psychogeriatr.* 2013;25(5):851–858. PMID: 23425512.

8. Moore DM, Rizzolo D. Sandifer syndrome. *JAAPA.* 2018;31(4):18–22. PMID: 29517619.

9. Treiman DM. Violence and the epilepsy defense. *Neurol Clin.* 1999;17(2):245–255. PMID: 10196406.

10. Hilger E, Zimprich F, Pataraia E, et al. Psychoses in epilepsy: A comparison of postictal and interictal psychoses. *Epilepsy Behav.* 2016;60:58–62. PMID: 27179193.

11. Leung AKC, Leung AAM, Wong AHC, Hon KL. Breath-holding spells in pediatrics: A narrative review of the current evidence. *Curr Pediatr Rev.* 2019;15(1):22–29. PMID: 30421679.

12. Dreissen YE, Tijssen MA. The startle syndromes: Physiology and treatment. *Epilepsia.* 2012;53 Suppl 7:3–11. PMID: 23153204.

13. Dicpinigaitis PV, Lim L, Farmakidis C. Cough syncope. *Respir Med.* 2014 Feb;108(2):244–51. Epub 2013 Nov 5. PMID: 24238768.

14. Madkour O, Elwan O, Hamdy H, Elwan H, Abbas A, Taher M, Abdel-Kader A. Transient ischemic attacks: Electrophysiological (conventional and topographic EEG) and radiological (CCT) evaluation. *J Neurol Sci.* 1993 Oct;119(1):8–17. PMID: 8246015.

15. Kwon Y, Yang Y, Jang JW, Park YH, Kim J, Park SH, Kim S. Left dominance of EEG abnormalities in patients with transient global amnesia. *Seizure.* 2014 Nov;23(10):825–9. doi: 10.1016/j.seizure.2014.06.014. Epub 2014 Jul 2. PMID: 25037277.

16. Payne LE, Gagnon DJ, Riker RR, Seder DB, Glisic EK, Morris JG, Fraser GL. Cefepime-induced neurotoxicity: A systematic review. *Crit Care.* 2017 Nov 14;21(1):276. PMID: 29137682.

17. Ekici A, Yakut A, Kural N, Bör Ö, Yimenicioğlu S, Çarman KB. Nonconvulsive status epilepticus due to drug induced neurotoxicity in chronically ill children. *Brain Dev.* 2012 Nov;34(10):824–8. PMID: 22445289.

18. Janssen S, Bloem BR, van de Warrenburg BP. The clinical heterogeneity of drug-induced myoclonus: An illustrated review. *J Neurol.* 2017 Aug;264(8):1559–1566. PMID: 27981352.

19. Woodward OB, Naraen S, Naraen A. Opioid-induced myoclonus and hyperalgesia following a short course of low-dose oral morphine. *Br J Pain.* 2017 Feb;11(1):32–35. PMID: 28386402.

20. Azar NJ, Bangalore-Vittal N, Arain A, Abou-Khalil BW. Tiagabine-induced stupor in patients with psychogenic nonepileptic seizures: nonconvulsive status epilepticus or encephalopathy? *Epilepsy Behav.* 2013 May;27(2):330–2. PMID: 23524471.

21. Burkhard PR. Acute and subacute drug-induced movement disorders. *Parkinsonism Relat Disord.* 2014 Jan;20 Suppl 1:S108–12. PMID: 24262159.

Chapter 8.1

1. Serafini A, Gerard E, Genton P, Crespel A, Gelisse P. Treatment of juvenile myoclonic epilepsy in patients of child-bearing potential. *CNS Drugs.* 2019 Mar;33(3):195–208. PMID: 30747367.

2. Agarwal M, Fox SM. Pediatric seizures. *Emerg Med Clin North Am.* 2013;31(3):733–754. PMID: 23915601.

3. Chen J, Xie L, Hu Y, Lan X, Jiang L. Non-convulsive status epilepticus after cessation of convulsive status epilepticus in pediatric intensive care unit patients. *Epilepsy Behav.* 2018;82:68–73. PMID: 29587188.

4. https://charliefoundation.org

5. Reilly C, Agnew R, Neville BG. Depression and anxiety in childhood epilepsy: a review. *Seizure.* 2011;20(8):589–597. PMID: 21741277.

6. Plevin D, Smith N. Assessment and management of depression and anxiety in children and adolescents with epilepsy. *Behav Neurol.* 2019;2019:2571368. Published 2019 May 2. PMID: 31191736.

7. Çelen Yoldaş T, Günbey C, Değerliyurt A, Erol N, Özmert E, Yalnızoğlu D. Behavioral problems of preschool children with new-onset epilepsy and one-year follow-up: A prospective study. *Epilepsy Behav.* 2019;92:171–175. PMID: 30660968.

8. Rajapakse T, Buchhalter J. The borderland of migraine and epilepsy in children. *Headache.* 2016;56(6):1071–1080. PMID: 27103497.

9. Nabbout R, Andrade DM, Bahi-Buisson N, et al. Outcome of childhood-onset epilepsy from adolescence to adulthood: Transition issues. *Epilepsy Behav.* 2017;69:161–169. PMID: 28256379.

10. Martínez-Ferrández C, Martínez-Salcedo E, Casas-Fernández C, Alarcón-Martínez H, Ibáñez-Micó S, Domingo-Jiménez R. Long-term prognosis of childhood absence epilepsy. Epilepsia ausencia infantil. Pronóstico a largo plazo. *Neurologia.* 2019;34(4):224–228. PMID: 28325560.

11. Yuskaitis CJ, Ruzhnikov MRZ, Howell KB, et al. Infantile spasms of unknown cause: Predictors of outcome and genotype-phenotype correlation. *Pediatr Neurol.* 2018;87:48–56. PMID: 30174244.

12. Yacubian EM. Juvenile myoclonic epilepsy: Challenges on its 60th anniversary. *Seizure.* 2017;44:48–52. PMID: 27665373.

13. Duran MH, Guimarães CA, Medeiros LL, Guerreiro MM. Landau-Kleffner syndrome: Long-term follow-up. *Brain Dev.* 2009;31(1):58–63. PMID: 18930363.

14. Asadi-Pooya AA. Lennox-Gastaut syndrome: a comprehensive review. *Neurol Sci.* 2018;39(3):403–414. PMID: 29124439.

Chapter 8.2

1. Krumholz A, Wiebe S, Gronseth GS, et al. Evidence-based guideline: Management of an unprovoked first seizure in adults: Report of the Guideline Development Subcommittee of the American Academy of Neurology and the American Epilepsy Society. *Neurology.* 2015;84(16):1705–1713. PMID: 25901057.

2. Kwan P, Brodie MJ. Effectiveness of first antiepileptic drug. *Epilepsia.* 2001 Oct;42(10):1255–1260. PMID: 11737159.

3. Marson AG, Al-Kharusi AM, Alwaidh M, et al.; SANAD Study group. The SANAD study of effectiveness of carbamazepine, gabapentin, lamotrigine, oxcarbazepine, or topiramate for treatment of partial epilepsy: An unblinded randomised controlled trial. *Lancet.* 2007 Mar 24;369(9566):1000–1015. PMID: 17382827

4. Glauser TA, Cnaan A, Shinnar S, et al.; Childhood Absence Epilepsy Study Group. Ethosuximide, valproic acid, and lamotrigine in childhood absence epilepsy. *N Engl J Med.* 2010 Mar 4;362(9):790–799. PMID: 20200383.

5. Rowan AJ, Ramsay RE, Collins JF, et al.; VA Cooperative Study 428 Group. New onset geriatric epilepsy: A randomized study of gabapentin, lamotrigine, and carbamazepine. *Neurology.* 2005 Jun 14;64(11):1868–1873. PMID: 15955935.

6. Meador KJ, Baker GA, Browning N, et al.; NEAD Study Group. Fetal antiepileptic drug exposure and cognitive outcomes at age 6 years (NEAD study): A prospective observational study. *Lancet Neurol.* 2013 Mar;12(3):244–252. PMID: 23352199.

7. Tomson T, Battino D, Bonizzoni E, et al.; EURAP Study Group. Comparative risk of major congenital malformations with eight different antiepileptic drugs: A prospective cohort study of the EURAP registry. *Lancet Neurol.* 2018 Jun;17(6):530–538. PMID: 29680205.

8. Meador KJ, Pennell PB, May RC, et al.; MONEAD Investigator Group. Fetal loss and malformations in the MONEAD study of pregnant women with epilepsy. *Neurology.* 2020 Apr 7;94(14):e1502–e1511. PMID: 31806691.

9. Arfman IJ, Wammes-van der Heijden EA, Ter Horst PGJ, Lambrechts DA, Wegner I, Touw DJ. Therapeutic drug monitoring of antiepileptic drugs in women with epilepsy before, during, and after pregnancy. *Clin Pharmacokinet.* 2020 Apr;59(4):427–445. PMID: 31912315.

10. Birnbaum AK, Meador KJ, Karanam A, et al.; MONEAD Investigator Group. Antiepileptic drug exposure in infants of breastfeeding mothers with epilepsy. *JAMA Neurol.* 2020 Apr 1;77(4):441–450. PMID: 31886825.

11. Bagnato F, Good J. The use of antiepileptics in migraine prophylaxis. *Headache.* 2016;56(3):603–615. PMID: 26935348.

12. Parikh SK, Silberstein SD. Current status of antiepileptic drugs as preventive migraine therapy. *Curr Treat Options Neurol.* 2019;21(4):16. Published 2019 Mar 18.

13. Honnekeri B, Rane S, Vast R, Khadilkar SV. Between the person and the pill: Factors affecting medication adherence in epilepsy patients. *J Assoc Physicians India.* 2018;66(7):24–26. PMID: 31325256.

14. Glauser T, Ben-Menachem E, Bourgeois B, et al.; ILAE Subcommission on AED Guidelines. Updated ILAE evidence review of antiepileptic drug efficacy and effectiveness as initial monotherapy for epileptic seizures and syndromes. *Epilepsia.* 2013 Mar;54(3):551–563. PMID: 23350722.

15. Beghi E, Gatti G, Tonini C, Ben-Menachem E, et al.; BASE Study Group. Adjunctive therapy versus alternative monotherapy in patients with partial epilepsy failing on a single drug: A multicentre, randomised, pragmatic controlled trial. *Epilepsy Res.* 2003 Nov;57(1):1–13. PMID: 14706729.

16. Kwan P, Brodie MJ. Epilepsy after the first drug fails: Substitution or add-on? *Seizure.* 2000 Oct;9(7):464–468. PMID: 11034869.

17. Semah F, Thomas P, Coulbaut S, Derambure P. Early add-on treatment vs alternative monotherapy in patients with partial epilepsy. *Epileptic Disord.* 2014 Jun;16(2):165–174. PMID: 24776953.

18. Millul A, Iudice A, Adami M, Porzio R, Mattana F, Beghi E; THEOREM Study Group. Alternative monotherapy or add-on therapy in patients with epilepsy whose seizures do not respond to the first monotherapy: An Italian multicenter prospective observational study. *Epilepsy Behav.* 2013 Sep;28(3):494–500. PMID: 23892580.

19. Abou-Khalil B. Selecting rational drug combinations in epilepsy. *CNS Drugs.* 2017 Oct;31(10):835–844. PMID: 28975553.

20. Kwan P, Brodie MJ. Early identification of refractory epilepsy. *N Engl J Med.* 2000 Feb 3;342(5):314–319. PMID: 10660394.

21. Schiller Y, Najjar Y. Quantifying the response to antiepileptic drugs: Effect of past treatment history. *Neurology.* 2008 Jan 1;70(1):54–65. PMID: 18166707.

22. Kwan P, Arzimanoglou A, Berg AT, et al. Definition of drug resistant epilepsy: Consensus proposal by the ad hoc Task Force of the ILAE Commission on Therapeutic Strategies. *Epilepsia.* 2010 Jun;51(6):1069–1077. PMID: 19889013.

Chapter 8.3

1. Treiman DM, Meyers PD, Walton NY, et al. A comparison of four treatments for generalized convulsive status epilepticus. Veterans Affairs Status Epilepticus Cooperative Study Group. *N Engl J Med.* 1998 Sep 17;339(12):792–798. PMID: 9738086.

2. Kapur J, Elm J, Chamberlain JM, et al.; NETT and PECARN Investigators. Randomized trial of three anticonvulsant medications for status epilepticus. *N Engl J Med.* 2019 Nov 28;381(22):2103–2113. PMID: 31774955.

3. Ferlisi M, Shorvon S. The outcome of therapies in refractory and super-refractory convulsive status epilepticus and recommendations for therapy. *Brain.* 2012 Aug;135(Pt 8):2314–28. PMID: 22577217.

4. Eaton JE, Meriweather MT, Abou-Khalil BW, Sonmezturk HH. Avoiding anaesthetics after multiple failed drug-induced comas: An unorthodox approach to management of new-onset refractory status epilepticus (NORSE). *Epileptic Disord.* 2019 Oct 1;21(5):483–491. PMID: 31708492.

5. Sutter R, Marsch S, Fuhr P, Kaplan PW, Rüegg S. Anesthetic drugs in status epilepticus: Risk or rescue? A 6-year cohort study. *Neurology.* 2014 Feb 25;82(8):656–64. PMID: 24319039.

6. Alvarez V, Drislane FW. Is favorable outcome possible after prolonged refractory status epilepticus? *J Clin Neurophysiol.* 2016 Feb;33(1):32–41. PMID: 26840875.

7. Pugin D, Foreman B, De Marchis GM, et al. Is pentobarbital safe and efficacious in the treatment of super-refractory status epilepticus: A cohort study. *Crit Care.* 2014 May 21;18(3):R103. PMID: 24886712.

8. Krishnamurthy KB, Drislane FW. Relapse and survival after barbiturate anesthetic treatment of refractory status epilepticus. *Epilepsia.* 1996 Sep;37(9):863–867. PMID: 8814099..

9. Treiman et al. A comparison of four treatments for generalized convulsive status epilepticus..

10. Alvarez, Drislane. Is favorable outcome possible after prolonged refractory status epilepticus?.

11. Rosati A, De Masi S, Guerrini R. Ketamine for refractory status epilepticus: A systematic review. *CNS Drugs.* 2018;32(11):997–1009. PMID: 30232735.

12. Holtkamp M. Pharmacotherapy for refractory and super-refractory status epilepticus in adults. *Drugs.* 2018;78(3):307–326. PMID: 29368126.

13. Rai S, Drislane FW. Treatment of refractory and super-refractory status epilepticus. *Neurotherapeutics.* 2018;15(3):697–712. PMID: 30704686.

Chapter 8.4

1. Zangiabadi N, Ladino LD, Sina F, Orozco-Hernández JP, Carter A, Téllez-Zenteno JF. Deep brain stimulation and drug-resistant epilepsy: A review of the literature. *Front Neurol.* 2019 Jun 6;10:601. PMID: 31244761.

2. Fisher R, Salanova V, Witt T, et al.; SANTE Study Group. Electrical stimulation of the anterior nucleus of thalamus for treatment of refractory epilepsy. Epilepsia. 2010 May;51(5):899–908. PMID: 20331461..

3. Matias CM, Sharan A, Wu C. Responsive neurostimulation for the treatment of epilepsy. Neurosurg Clin N Am. 2019;30(2):231–242. PMID: 30898274.

4. Skarpaas TL, Jarosiewicz B, Morrell MJ. Brain-responsive neurostimulation for epilepsy (RNS® System). Epilepsy Res. 2019;153:68–70. PMID: 30850259.

5. Chan AY, Rolston JD, Rao VR, Chang EF. Effect of neurostimulation on cognition and mood in refractory epilepsy. Epilepsia Open. 2018;3(1):18–29. Published 2018 Feb 13. PMID: 29588984.

6. Vining EP, Freeman JM, Ballaban-Gil K, et al. A multicenter study of the efficacy of the ketogenic diet. Arch Neurol. 1998 Nov;55(11):1433–1437. PMID: 9823827.

7. Chen W, Kossoff EH. Long-term follow-up of children treated with the modified Atkins diet. J Child Neurol. 2012 Jun;27(6):754–758. PMID: 22532541..

8. Muzykewicz DA, Lyczkowski DA, Memon N, Conant KD, Pfeifer HH, Thiele EA. Efficacy, safety, and tolerability of the low glycemic index treatment in pediatric epilepsy. Epilepsia. 2009 May;50(5):1118–1126. PMID: 19220406.

Chapter 8.5

1. Meador KJ. Epilepsy surgery. Compr Ther. 1989 Mar;15(3):33-8. PMID: 2706925.

2. Meador et al. *J Epilepsy* 1989;2:21–25.
Kwan P, Arzimanoglou A, Berg AT, et al. Definition of drug resistant epilepsy: Consensus proposal by the ad hoc Task Force of the ILAE Commission on Therapeutic Strategies. *Epilepsia.* 2010 Jun;51(6):1069–1077. PMID: 19889013.

3. Callaghan B, Schlesinger M, Rodemer W, Pollard J, Hesdorffer D, Allen Hauser W, French J. Remission and relapse in a drug-resistant epilepsy population followed prospectively. *Epilepsia.* 2011 Mar;52(3):619–626. PMID: 21269287.

4. Banerjee PN, Filippi D, Allen Hauser W. The descriptive epidemiology of epilepsy: A review. *Epilepsy Res.* 2009 Jul;85(1):31–45. PMID: 19369037.

5. Kwan P, Brodie MJ. Early identification of refractory epilepsy. *N Engl J Med.* 2000 Feb 3;342(5):314–319. PMID: 10660394..

6. van Mierlo P, Carrette E, Hallez H, et al. Ictal-onset localization through connectivity analysis of intracranial EEG signals in patients with refractory epilepsy. *Epilepsia.* 2013 Aug;54(8):1409–1418. PMID: 23647147..

7. Wiebe S, Blume WT, Girvin JP, Eliasziw M. Effectiveness and efficiency of surgery for temporal lobe epilepsy study group. A randomized, controlled trial of surgery for temporal-lobe epilepsy. *N Engl J Med.* 2001 Aug 2;345(5):311–318. PMID: 11484687..

8. Engel J Jr, McDermott MP, Wiebe S, et al., Early Randomized Surgical Epilepsy Trial (ERSET) Study Group. Early surgical therapy for drug-resistant temporal lobe epilepsy: A randomized trial. *JAMA.* 2012 Mar 7;307(9):922–930. PMID: 22396514.

9. Engel J Jr, Wiebe S, French J, et al. Practice parameter: Temporal lobe and localized neocortical resections for epilepsy. *Epilepsia.* 2003 Jun;44(6):741–751. PMID: 12790886..

10. Burneo JG, Shariff SZ, Liu K, Leonard S, Saposnik G, Garg AX. Disparities in surgery among patients with intractable epilepsy in a universal health system. *Neurology.* 2016 Jan 5;86(1):72–78. PMID: 26643546.

11. Sperling MR, Barshow S, Nei M, Asadi-Pooya AA. A reappraisal of mortality after epilepsy surgery. *Neurology.* 2016 May 24;86(21):1938–1944. PMID: 27164679..

12. Roberts JI, Hrazdil C, Wiebe S, Sauro K, Vautour M, Wiebe N, Jetté N. Neurologists' knowledge of and attitudes toward epilepsy surgery: A national survey. *Neurology.* 2015 Jan 13;84(2):159–166. PMID: 25503624.

13. Created by HS with arrows; data are from Jerome Engels Jr.'s book, *Seizures and Epilepsy* 2nd edition (New York: Oxford University Press, 2012).

14. Erba G, Messina P, Pupillo E, Beghi E; OPTEFF Group. Acceptance of epilepsy surgery among adults with epilepsy: What do patients think? *Epilepsy Behav.* 2012 Jul;24(3):352–358. PMID: 22658431.

Chapter 8.6

1. Kadima NT, Kobau R, Zack MM, Helmers S. Comorbidity in adults with epilepsy—United States, 2010. CDC. *MMWR.* 2013;62(43):849–853.

2. Fiest KM, Patten SB, Jetté N. Screening for depression and anxiety in epilepsy. *Neurol Clin.* 2016;34(2):351–viii. PMID: 27086983.

3. Nye BL, Thadani VM. Migraine and epilepsy: Review of the literature. *Headache.* 2015;55(3):359–380.

4. Shahien R, Beiruti K. Preventive agents for migraine: Focus on the antiepileptic drugs. *J Cent Nerv Syst Dis.* 2012;4:37–49. Published 2012 Feb 26. PMID: 23650466.

5. Leach JP, Mohanraj R, Borland W. Alcohol and drugs in epilepsy: Pathophysiology, presentation, possibilities, and prevention. *Epilepsia.* 2012;53 Suppl 4:48–57. PMID: 22946721.

6. Shmuely S, van der Lende M, Lamberts RJ, Sander JW, Thijs RD. The heart of epilepsy: Current views and future concepts. *Seizure.* 2017;44:176–183. PMID: 27843098.

7. Tényi D, Gyimesi C, Kupó P, et al. Ictal asystole: A systematic review. *Epilepsia.* 2017;58(3):356–362. PMID: 27988965.

8. Feldman L, Lapin B, Busch RM, Bautista JF. Evaluating subjective cognitive impairment in the adult epilepsy clinic: Effects of depression, number of antiepileptic medications, and seizure frequency. *Epilepsy Behav.* 2018;81:18–24. PMID: 29455082.

9. Sen A, Capelli V, Husain M. Cognition and dementia in older patients with epilepsy. *Brain.* 2018;141(6):1592–1608. PMID: 29506031.

10. Aji BM, Larner AJ. Cognitive assessment in an epilepsy clinic using the AD8 questionnaire. *Epilepsy Behav.* 2018;85:234–236. PMID: 30032813.

11. Latreille V, St Louis EK, Pavlova M. Co-morbid sleep disorders and epilepsy: A narrative review and case examples. *Epilepsy Res.* 2018;145:185–197. PMID: 30048932.

12. Beghi E. Social functions and socioeconomic vulnerability in epilepsy. *Epilepsy Behav.* 2019;100(Pt B):106363. PMID: 31300385.

Chapter 8.8

1. DailyMeddailymed.nlm.nih.gov.

2. Arya R, Giridharan N, Anand V, Garg SK. Clobazam monotherapy for focal or generalized seizures. *Cochrane Database Syst Rev.* 2018;7(7):CD009258. Published 2018 Jul 11. PMID: 29995989.

3. Wiffen PJ, Derry S, Bell RF, et al. Gabapentin for chronic neuropathic pain in adults. *Cochrane Database Syst Rev.* 2017;6(6):CD007938. Published 2017 Jun 9. PMID: 28597471.

4. Strzelczyk A, Zöllner JP, Willems LM, et al. Lacosamide in status epilepticus: Systematic review of current evidence. *Epilepsia.* 2017;58(6):933–950. PMID: 28295226.

5. Davidson KE, Newell J, Alsherbini K, Krushinski J, Jones GM. Safety and efficiency of intravenous push lacosamide administration. *Neurocrit Care.* 2018;29(3):491–495. PMID: 29949010.

6. Abou-Khalil B. Levetiracetam in the treatment of epilepsy. *Neuropsychiatr Dis Treat.* 2008 Jun;4(3):507–523. PMID: 18830435.

7. Kapur J, Elm J, Chamberlain JM, et al. Randomized trial of three anticonvulsant medications for status epilepticus. *N Engl J Med.* 2019;381(22):2103–2113. PMID: 31774955.

8. Reich SG. Essential tremor. *Med Clin North Am.* 2019;103(2):351–356. PMID: 30704686.

9. Panebianco M, Prabhakar H, Marson AG. Rufinamide add-on therapy for refractory epilepsy. *Cochrane Database Syst Rev.* 2018;4(4):CD011772. Published 2018 Apr 25. PMID: 29691835.

10. Gomes D, Pimentel J, Bentes C, et al. Consensus protocol for the treatment of super-refractory status epilepticus. *Acta Med Port.* 2018;31(10):598–605. PMID: 30387431.

11. Trinka E, Höfler J, Leitinger M, Rohracher A, Kalss G, Brigo F. Pharmacologic treatment of status epilepticus. *Expert Opin Pharmacother.* 2016;17(4):513–534. PMID: 26629986.

12. Bagnato F, Good J. The use of antiepileptics in migraine prophylaxis. *Headache.* 2016;56(3):603–615. PMID: 26935348.

Chapter 9.1

1. Niaz FE, Abou-Khalil B, Fakhoury T. The generalized tonic-clonic seizure in partial versus generalized epilepsy: Semiologic differences. *Epilepsia.* 1999 Nov;40(11):1664–1666. PMID: 10565598..

2. Chin PS, Miller JW. Ictal head version in generalized epilepsy. *Neurology.* 2004 Jul 27;63(2):370–372. PMID: 15277642..

3. Gilliam F, Steinhoff BJ, Bittermann HJ, Kuzniecky R, Faught E, Abou-Khalil B. Adult myoclonic epilepsy: A distinct syndrome of idiopathic generalized epilepsy. *Neurology.* 2000 Oct 10;55(7):1030–1033. PMID: 11061264..

4. Cutting S, Lauchheimer A, Barr W, Devinsky O. Adult-onset idiopathic generalized epilepsy: Clinical and behavioral features. *Epilepsia.* 2001 Nov;42(11):1395–1398. PMID: 11879340..

5. Nicolson A, Chadwick DW, Smith DF. A comparison of adult onset and "classical" idiopathic generalised epilepsy. *J Neurol Neurosurg Psychiatry.* 2004 Jan;75(1):72–74. PMID: 14707311.

6. Marini C, King MA, Archer JS, Newton MR, Berkovic SF. Idiopathic generalised epilepsy of adult onset: Clinical syndromes and genetics. *J Neurol Neurosurg Psychiatry.* 2003 Feb;74(2):192–196. PMID: 12531947.

7. Reichsoellner J, Larch J, Unterberger I, et al. Idiopathic generalised epilepsy of late onset: A separate nosological entity? *J Neurol Neurosurg Psychiatry.* 2010 Nov;81(11):1218–1222. PMID: 20802210..

8. Mayville C, Fakhoury T, Abou-Khalil B. Absence seizures with evolution into generalized tonic-clonic activity: Clinical and EEG features. *Epilepsia.* 2000 Apr;41(4):391–394. PMID: 10756402..

9. Beniczky S, Rubboli G, Covanis A, Sperling MR. Absence-to-bilateral-tonic-clonic seizure: A generalized seizure type. *Neurology.* 2020 Oct 6;95(14):e2009–e2015. PMID: 32817392.

10. Fakhoury T, Abou-Khalil B. Generalized absence seizures with 10–15 Hz fast discharges. *Clin Neurophysiol.* 1999 Jun;110(6):1029–1035. PMID: 10402089.

11. Rocamora R, Kurthen M, Lickfett L, Von Oertzen J, Elger CE. Cardiac asystole in epilepsy: Clinical and neurophysiologic features. *Epilepsia.* 2003 Feb;44(2):179–185. PMID: 12558571..

12. Rugg-Gunn FJ, Simister RJ, Squirrell M, Holdright DR, Duncan JS. Cardiac arrhythmias in focal epilepsy: A prospective long-term study. *Lancet.* 2004 Dec 18–31;364(9452):2212–2219. PMID: 15610808.

13. Bestawros M, Darbar D, Arain A, Abou-Khalil B, Plummer D, Dupont WD, Raj SR. Ictal asystole and ictal syncope: Insights into clinical management. *Circ Arrhythm Electrophysiol.* 2015 Feb;8(1):159–164. PMID: 25391254.

14. Shih TT, Hirsch LJ. Tonic-absence seizures: An underrecognized seizure type. *Epilepsia.* 2003 Mar;44(3):461–465. PMID: 12614405.

15. Lavin PJ. Hyperglycemic hemianopia: A reversible complication of non-ketotic hyperglycemia. *Neurology.* 2005 Aug 23;65(4):616–619. PMID: 16116129.

16. Stayman A, Abou-Khalil BW, Lavin P, Azar NJ. Homonymous hemianopia in nonketotic hyperglycemia is an ictal phenomenon. *Neurol Clin Pract.* 2013 Oct;3(5):392–397. PMID: 29473606.

17. Knupp K, Wirrell E. Progressive myoclonic epilepsies: It takes a village to make a diagnosis. *Neurology.* 2014 Feb 4;82(5):378–379. doi: 10.1212/WNL.0000000000000091. Epub 2014 Jan 2. PMID: 24384640..

18. Kälviäinen R, Khyuppenen J, Koskenkorva P, Eriksson K, Vanninen R, Mervaala E. Clinical picture of EPM1-Unverricht-Lundborg disease. *Epilepsia.* 2008 Apr;49(4):549–556. PMID: 18325013..

19. Canafoglia L, Barbella G, Ferlazzo E, et al. An Italian multicentre study of perampanel in progressive myoclonus epilepsies. *Epilepsy Res.* 2019 Oct;156:106191. PMID: 31446282.

20. Crespel A, Gelisse P, Tang NP, Genton P. Perampanel in 12 patients with Unverricht-Lundborg disease. *Epilepsia.* 2017 Apr;58(4):543–547. PMID: 28166365.

21. Bhatt AB, Popescu A, Waterhouse EJ, Abou-Khalil BW. De novo generalized periodic discharges related to anesthetic withdrawal resolve spontaneously. *J Clin Neurophysiol.* 2014 Jun;31(3):194–198. PMID: 24887600.

22. Santamaria J, Chiappa KH. The EEG of drowsiness in normal adults. *J Clin Neurophysiol.* 1987 Oct;4(4):327–382. doi: 10.1097/00004691-198710000-00002. PMID: 3316272.

23. Atalla N, Abou-Khalil B, Fakhoury T. The start-stop-start phenomenon in scalp-sphenoidal ictal recordings. *Electroencephalogr Clin Neurophysiol.* 1996 Jan;98(1):9–13. PMID: 8689999.

24. Haykal MA, El-Feki A, Sonmezturk HH, Abou-Khalil BW. New observations in primary and secondary reading epilepsy: Excellent response to levetiracetam and early spontaneous remission. *Epilepsy Behav.* 2012 Apr;23(4):466–470. PMID: 22386591.

25. Koutroumanidis M, Koepp MJ, Richardson MP, et al. The variants of reading epilepsy. A clinical and video-EEG study of 17 patients with reading-induced seizures. *Brain.* 1998 Aug;121 (Pt 8):1409–1427. PMID: 9712004.

Chapter 9.3

1. Chen-Block S, Abou-Khalil BW, Arain A, et al. Video-EEG results and clinical characteristics in patients with psychogenic nonepileptic spells: The effect of a coexistent epilepsy. *Epilepsy Behav.* 2016 Sep;62:62–5. PMID: 27450307..

2. Eaton JE, Meriweather MT, Abou-Khalil BW, Sonmezturk HH. Avoiding anaesthetics after multiple failed drug-induced comas: An unorthodox approach to management of new-onset refractory status epilepticus (NORSE). *Epileptic Disord.* 2019 Oct 1;21(5):483–91. PMID: 31708492..

INDEX

Tables, figures, and boxes are indicated by an italic *t*, *f*, and *b* following the page number.